"When it comes to breakthrough therapy for eye problems, Dr. Abel is THE source for reliable, up-to-date information."
—Ronald Hoffman, M.D., host of WOR's "Health Talk" and author of *Intelligent Medicine*

"Dr. Robert Abel's *The Eye Care Revolution* is really several books in one, for it sees the eye as a gateway to an overall strategy for health, wholeness, and vitality. He provides a map through the chaos of illness based on the idea of "alliances for healing." We learn to rely upon our own healing capacities, informed common sense, and the guidelines in the book. We form alliances with our physicians, where caring becomes an essential ingredient in healing; and where the skill and technology of western medicine is allied with the wisdom of ancient healing traditions. My wife and I have been fortunate to come under the care of this remarkable physician and man. His book is a personal kindness to everyone."
—Julian Gresser, Chairman of Alliances for Discovery, Santa Barbara, California

"Dr. Robert Abel is one of the most respected eye physicians in America, and his limitless knowledge shines through in this book. Written with the special kind of love that only comes from a doctor who cares, he deftly delineates practical methods for treating the major eye problems. Like a magical prism, he is able to pull in light from all corners of the earth and separate out only the most brilliant parts . . . the parts you (and your eyes) need to get better."
—Alan Keith Tillotson, Ph.D., A.H.G., Director of the Chrysalis Natural Medicine Clinic, and author of *The One Earth Herbal Sourcebook*

"As a long time proponent of preventive medicine, I appreciate Dr. Abel's emphasis on steps we can all take, starting today, that will improve our eye health through proper nutrition and lifestyle. *The Eye Care Revolution* is an excellent resource for both the clinician and the patient."
—Kenneth H. Cooper, Founder and CEO of The Cooper Clinic, Dallas, Texas

THE EYE CARE

REVOLUTION

*Prevent and Reverse
Common Vision Problems*

REVISED AND UPDATED

Robert Abel, Jr., M.D.

KENSINGTON BOOKS
http://www.kensingtonbooks.com

This work is dedicated to my late mother Ruth, in whose eyes I could do no wrong, except that I didn't know much about nutrition.

KENSINGTON BOOKS are published by

Kensington Publishing Corp.
850 Third Avenue
New York, NY 10022

Copyright © 1999, 2004 by Robert Abel, Jr.

All Kensington titles, imprints and distributed lines are available at special quantity discounts for bulk purchases for sales promotion, premiums, fund-raising, educational or institutional use.

Special book excerpts or customized printings can also be created to fit specific needs. For details, write or phone the office of the Kensington Special Sales Manager: Kensington Publishing Corp., 850 Third Avenue, New York, NY 10022. Attn. Special Sales Department. Phone: 1-800-221-2647.

Kensington and the K logo Reg. U.S. Pat. & TM Off.

ISBN 0-7582-0622-4

First Kensington Trade Paperback Printing: July 1999
Revised and Updated Edition: January 2004
10 9 8 7 6 5 4 3

Printed in the United States of America

Contents

Appendices

Acknowledgments

The Eye Care Revolution would not be what it is without the contribution of Neenyah Ostrom, whose wisdom, counsel, and steady hand were always available. My deepest appreciation goes to Lee Heiman for his great support and help in structuring the manuscript, and to Allan Graubard, who provided careful editing and fine-tuning of the finished work. My thanks also go to Tracy Bernstein for her continuing interest in the project.

I am extremely grateful to Dr. Nai-Shing Hu and Alan Tillotson for sharing their expertise in Chinese and Ayurvedic medicine; to Dr. Ralph and Sharon Milner for evaluating portions of the pediatric section; to Dr. Joe Ternes for his insights into eye muscle movements and stress reduction; to Dr. Jay Jemail for sharing her knowledge about learning disabilities; to Glenn Herringshaw for sharing his knowledge of optics; and to Vicki Accardi for her assistance in assembling the charts and graphs for the book. Thanks, too, to Susan Hussey for providing tips about natural cosmetics, Dr. Barbara de Lateur for weight-training and rehabilitation information, and Dr. Anil Patel for sharing his research into natural models for preventing and treating cataracts. I am grateful to my friend and teacher, Dr. Don Willard, for introducing me to the biochemistry of wine. All the trips to New York would not have been possible without my sister Nancy Abel Hoffenberg and her husband Hack Hoffenberg who put me up and put up with me while providing invaluable advice and counsel.

I am grateful to Penny Edwards for her information about selected nutrients. My partners at Delaware Ophthalmology Consultants (DOC) deserve thanks for their support and patience throughout the book-writing process: Andy Barrett, M.D.; Brent Bond, M.D.; Gordon Bussard, M.D.;

Judy Holloway, O.D.; Harry Lebowitz, M.D.; Jeff Mainolfi, O.D.; Jonathan Meyers, M.D.; Ralph Milner, M.D.; and Arunon Sivilinghan, M.D. Special thanks go to Ed Becker, M.D., for his constant encouragement. I'd also like to thank the DOC team—support services, technicians, and all the administrative, clerical, and billing staff—who assisted me during the writing of *The Eye Care Revolution*.

I owe a great debt to the people who taught and inspired me over the years: the late Dr. Chaim Sheba (in Israel); Dr. "Vaidja" Mana (in Nepal); Dr. Sandoc Ruit (in Nepal); Dr. Venkataswami and his sister Dr. Nachiar at the Aravand Eye Hospital (in Madurai, India); the late Dr. Irving Leopold at Mt. Sinai Hospital (in New York City); Dr. Thomas Duane, chief of ophthalmology at Thomas Jefferson University during my medical education; and Dr. Herbert Kaufman, chief of ophthalmology at Louisiana State University during my fellowship. I'd like to thank my patients for giving me the insights to make many of these connections and help them heal their own diseases.

My deepest appreciation goes to my father Robert and stepmother Nancy, whose parental support never wavered, as well as to Valla and Gus Amsterdam.

Finally, I want to thank my children—Lauren, Ari, and Adam—who provided constant energy and support. I have no way to thank my dear wife Mike, whose research and healthful pantry got me involved in learning about healthful foods to nourish our bodies and our eyes.

Foreword

As a heart surgeon who uses hair thickness sutures to repair capellini-sized vessels, I have always treasured my eyes' ability to view the world outside me. In his unique book, *The Eye Care Revolution*, Dr. Robert Abel has shown me that the eyes also provide a window into our bodies which we can use to assess our health and potentially heal illness. Opening our minds to the wonders of the eye's secrets requires an individual talented and respected in both the science of conventional medicine and the art of the healing spirit. Dr. Abel has accomplished this task by fulfilling his own definition of a Zen doctor. He is a healer who becomes aware—using all five senses as well as intellect and intuition—of the entirety of a patient and his or her disease. In his meticulously woven tale of the eye and its ailments, Dr. Abel reveals unique insights into his patients and their illnesses, often highlighted by his "Tips." Common eye problems are discussed together with a comprehensive medical explanation and a survey of complementary options to treatment. He covers overarching health concerns including the role of nutrition and lifestyle by convincingly arguing that the same environmental hazards affecting the eye will hurt the body.

And Dr. Abel goes one step further. He addresses the spiritual aspects of disease which are so frequently overlooked. He recognizes that illness provides an opportunity for personal growth for all involved and he wants to be the catalyst. Dr. Abel sings to his surgery patients when he wheels them to and from the operating room. He calls his patients before and after surgery to guide them in their recovery, addressing issues beyond the basic management of the healing eye. Dr. Abel sees that physicians and patients are partners on the road to health, and I support his vision that caring is part of curing. Healing is a partnership in finding the core cause and exploring all options. We can learn much from Ayurvedic medicine, Chinese medicine and basic nutrition to keep our eyes and hearts strong and healthy; Dr. Abel is charting the course.

Only an internationally recognized physician with Dr. Abel's credentials could lead the maturation of conventional approaches to ophthalmology that we are witnessing. He is respected as a technically gifted surgeon who performs the latest high-tech eye surgery, has patents on artificial corneas and is an acknowledged leader in complementary medicine for the eyes. He connects the eye to the mind and body in order to restore vision, prevent disease, and provide insights into improved health generally.

Pythagoras designed the caduceus, the sword with two entwining snakes, as the symbol for healing. One snake represents reason or science and the other represents intuition or art. Dr. Abel has combined these two aspects in his methods dealing with eye problems. *The Eye Care Revolution* is about taking care of the harmony among mind, body and spirit in order to preserve a lifetime of vision. As the fox advises in Antoine de Saint-Exupéry's masterpiece, *The Little Prince*, "It is only with the heart that one can see rightly. What is essential is invisible to the eye." His unique approach to the causes and treatments of common eye disorders are both enlightening and beneficial. Many treatments that we have used in cardiovascular disease including antioxidants also appear to have a role in healing the eye. He carefully draws analogies with other organ systems as well which provide the reader with heretofore unrecognized insights. The eyes are the portal to the body and may be the first clue to problems in other areas.

I support Dr. Abel's hypothesis that we need to secure the best of high-tech modern medicine as well as the age-old remedies of other medical systems. Dr. Abel provides his patients with options and more importantly integrates them into their own care. He teaches that you are the shepherd of your body, the guardian of your health and that you make a difference. He helps patients observe and become their own medical detectives. When Western medicine doesn't have an answer he searches elsewhere. He is not only able to perform the highest level eye surgery, but to share insights in maintaining vision and reducing the likelihood of recurring disease.

My interest in Dr. Abel's work was piqued by his ability to demonstrate how the eye is directly related to the heart. If the heart fails or a patient requires certain potent cardiac drugs, cataracts and other eye conditions may occur. But they don't have to. The French paradox, which revealed that wine benefits the heart, also showed that wine benefits the eyes.

Grapes, green leafy plants, fish, eggs and sulfur-bearing vegetables such as onions and garlic are helpful to the eyes as well as to the rest of the body. Correcting a bad digestive tract, increasing activity, drinking water and exercising has proven effects on healing. Since the eye is intimately connected to the body, a total approach to health and healing is mandatory.

Dr. Abel provides valuable tips which we can start implementing immediately. He feels that glaucoma is a disease of stress and has found that maintaining a healthy colon, deep breathing, exercise and certain natural substances complement Western medicine in saving vision. Some of his recommendations include treating "pink eye" with iodine, resolving headaches by massaging the neck, using exercises for computer ailments and correcting inadequate eyeglass prescriptions. He has learned that Tai Chi, Chi Kung and Yoga have salutary effects for the eye. He has found that visual imagery is important to direct people toward self-healing, humor is a valuable medicine and love is the ultimate vitamin.

Dr. Abel is drawing a picture for a global perspective of eye care and has shown us that doctors can be more than technicians. He is a healer for the 21st century and a role model for future physicians.

Mehmet Oz, M.D.
Columbia University

Introduction
A Global View of Health Through Your Eyes

This is not simply a book about eyes. In these pages, you and I will explore how the eyes serve as a mirror of general health and reflect symptoms of hidden imbalances. We don't go from well to ill in an instant, nor do we develop glaucoma, ulcers, or heart failure overnight. Ill health usually results from a gradual deterioration. Such deterioration can often be reversed—*if we detect it early enough.* Getting older does not have to bring loss of sight, hearing, and energy. You *do* have options other than a daily diet of synthetic pills, laser treatments, and surgery to preserve your eyes and your vision throughout your lifetime, and I will reveal them to you in *The Eye Care Revolution.*

Safeguarding vision is one of our aging population's primary concerns. In a Louis Harris poll, when people were asked their greatest fear, 26 percent responded "cancer"; 25 percent responded "loss of vision." In a 1998 poll in which middle-aged respondents were allowed multiple choices, Elizabeth Sloan found 85 percent feared losing vision to 81 percent fearing cancer. Vision loss is understandably very frightening, but today there is no need for people to be blinded by cataracts, glaucoma, diabetes, or even macular degeneration.

I have dedicated my professional life to preserving vision. I have practiced ophthalmology for thirty years as a founding partner in a ten-doctor eye care practice in Delaware. I operate on four hundred cataract patients a year, but I treat six times that number without surgery. Even though modern cataract surgery is superb and the majority of my fellow ophthalmologists advise their patients that there is no alternative, I've discovered other ways to treat cataracts. My patients know that *they have choices.*

I discovered these alternatives because I finally realized that, in performing cataract surgeries, I was operating on a symptom. A cataract or any abnormal growth is a response to physical and environmental effects. Like other chronic conditions, eye disease must be addressed in a broader framework that includes diet, lifestyle, and increased health care options.

This book will show you ways to avoid or reverse degenerative eye diseases. But to use these prevention techniques, we must also heal your body and improve your general health. That is why I will discuss subjects like cancer, heart disease, Alzheimer's disease, obesity, and other health problems that may seem inappropriate in a book on eye care. Each of these conditions affects the eyes and, in many cases, the eyes can reveal the presence of these conditions before symptoms become overt. As you'll discover, the eye has many hidden connections to and within the body that can have enormous impact on vision and eye health.

Diseases are symptoms of deeper imbalances. In February 1998, *New York Times* health columnist Jane E. Brody noted the newly recognized association of gum infections with heart disease. I've come to realize that poor circulation and a weak heart can cause macular degeneration and low-tension glaucoma—both serious degenerative eye diseases. Certain drugs prescribed for medical reasons can accelerate cataracts, while medications prescribed to treat eye conditions can worsen asthma. *The Eye Care Revolution* is about treating the whole person, not just the symptom. By looking for deeper causes, I have found I can more effectively prevent and treat common eye diseases.

As an eye specialist, I must concern myself with medical problems in general. Doctors are beginning to view their patients as whole people instead of as collections of symptoms; physicians are increasingly giving patients nutritional advice as well as prescribing supplements for themselves and their families. In my practice, I spend much of my time fielding phone calls, faxes, and e-mails from fellow optometrists and ophthalmologists asking me what supplements I recommend. In response, I always ask, "Is this for you or your family?" The doctor's response is usually, "For myself, actually." When I then inquire whether he or she suggests vitamin supplements to patients, I'm often told that there's not enough scientific information to recommend nutritional management. That many doctors think the science is good enough for *them*, but not good enough to recommend to their patients is indeed something to think about.

I have learned that every system in the body is interrelated, and the eye is the window on the whole. An eye condition may reflect a hidden chronic (or even acute) illness. For example:

- A *woman told me that she was going to have a lobe of her left lung removed. She had a lesion that her doctor suspected might be cancer, and it couldn't be approached in any less invasive way. When I examined her eyes, I saw lesions on her retina that indicated infection with a parasite called histoplasmosis. Found in chicken droppings, histoplasmosis can be inhaled through the lungs and passed to the eyes. I suggested that she tell her doctor. He agreed that histoplasmosis might very well be the cause of her lung lesion, and she was spared this major surgery.*

- A *65-year-old New York executive visited me after being informed that he would need a cataract operation. I realized that his blood pressure and cholesterol lowering medications were affecting his liver—and therefore his vision—and suggested natural alternatives to those drugs. I recommended specific vitamins and predicted that his cataract changes would stop, if not improve (but that is a story for later). I gave the same advice to my father when he showed early cataract changes in 1968. Twenty-four years later, at the age of 90, my dad continues to have 20/20 vision.*

- A *73-year-old woman came to me with double vision. Although she had been given an eyeglasses prescription to correct the condition, it persisted. When she told me she was taking Atenolol, a high-blood-pressure medication, I knew something was wrong. She was the fifth person I'd seen who had developed double or disturbed vision (strabismus) while on Atenolol; the other four had responded positively to discontinuing Atenolol and switching to another medication, and this patient did, too. I suspect that this may be a widespread phenomenon, particularly among older people who are being treated by more than one physician. One physician may not observe the complications (drug-related or not) obvious to a doctor with a different specialty.*

Our arrogant belief in the supremacy of Western medicine is just bad medicine. We tend to forget that modern medicine is a relatively new invention. Chinese civilization, for example, has had an effective, plant-based medical system for four thousand years. Even today, 80 percent of the world uses such a plant-based medical system. In certain cases, synthetic drugs are necessary and we should take advantage of them, but in other situations natural preparations may be safer and equally effective. And that's where complementary medicine comes in. In 1990, for instance, my son Ari, who was visiting from college, was suffering from severe asthma attacks. He agreed to be examined by a Chinese medical doctor in our community, who prescribed a combination of herbs that were so effective that they eliminated the need for three out of four of Ari's asthma medications. (I am very careful about suggesting that patients, especially those with eye disease, try something new like consulting a Chinese medical doctor, and I follow each patient's course closely.)

Another man, who suffered from recurrent redness of the eyes, learned that his condition was associated with irregular eating patterns and, at one point, with a urinary tract infection. Chinese medicine was helpful in this case as well. Chinese traditional doctors know that the digestive organs are related to the eye. Afterward, I sent ten more patients with chronically red eyes (resistant to all but strong, steroid eye drugs), on an individual basis, for treatment with Chinese herbs. Not only did the patients' eyes clear up; their skin conditions, sinusitis, and asthma also disappeared.

As these patients' cases illustrate, high blood pressure, diabetes, and other chronic conditions—as well as the drugs used to treat them—can contribute to eye problems and diseases. The eyes are a partner to the body. They are nourished by blood (heart and circulation), oxygen (lungs), nutrition (digestion and circulation), and removal of toxins (kidney and liver). They are regulated by glands and hormones, are associated with remote parts of the body, and act as an extension of the brain itself. What we eat, drink, and breathe is integrally related to our body chemistry and, therefore, to the condition of our eyes. In *The Eye Care Revolution*, you will learn how all these ingredients—nutrition, supplementation, drugs, breathing, and relaxation—interact to produce eye health (or disease). You'll also gain some knowledge about Chinese medicine, about the Ayurvedic medicine practiced in India and Nepal, and about naturopathic health systems whose insights predate the Roman Empire and still endure today.

Nutrition has a major influence on health. The American diet is generally unbalanced—low in many nutrients, but high in saturated fats and simple sugars. This high level of saturated animal fats and refined carbohydrates (simple sugars) has been implicated in the rise of chronic, noninfectious diseases such as coronary artery disease, diabetes, stroke, cancer, arthritis, gallstones, dental cavities, and digestive disorders. Sugar may also contribute to susceptibility to infectious diseases. I will explain how the foods we eat—and the foods we may neglect eating—affect our eye/body health.

In the Chinese traditional medical text *Bo Wu Gi*, written between 265 and 420 A.D., it was said that the less one eats, the broader the mind and the longer the life span. Hippocrates (who lived even earlier, around 500 B.C.) also knew that diet, exercise, and a balanced lifestyle were necessary for a harmonious body. Modern, scientific studies show that eating wisely extends one's life span. The more we eat, the more energy we must expend in metabolizing our food; the excess is stored as fat even in places such as our waists, arteries, and vital organs. The combination of junk food consumption, lots of TV watching, and very little exercise is leading to obesity, even among our children. In middle age, there is a decrease in glucose clearance, enzyme synthesis, and immune responsiveness. Eating too much decreases our thinking ability and our muscle mass, and hastens aging. Obesity has been associated with many diseases, including gallstones, diabetes, heart disease, hypertension, and degenerative joint disease. We all agree that being considerably overweight is not healthy, and this is a condition we can cure. I'll show you how to balance your diet, eliminate empty calories and packaged foods, and still feel satisfied.

Many of the very same high-calorie foods we eat in such abundance are actually less nutritious than the food we give our pets! When we change our dietary habits and address our real nutritional needs, we take a giant step toward improving our general health and resolving conditions we don't even associate with our diet:

- Patients treated with the essential fatty acid DHA and glucosamine sulfate for their dry eyes experience an improvement in their arthritis.
- Nuts and chocolate, high in the essential amino acid arginine, can trigger attacks of herpes on the lip, eye, and elsewhere. Avoidance of these foods, along with taking a supplement of L-lysine (another amino acid), counteracts this tendency toward herpes outbreaks.
- Bilberry, the northern European blueberry, was said to provide the advantage for English fighter pilots to win the Battle of Britain. The British were outnumbered but, because of the phytonutrient in the berries they ate (called anthocyanidin), they had superior night vision.
- Many packaged foods have artificial, hard fats within them that are not designed to contribute to health; they are strictly engineered to keep the product stable for long periods of time. And just because a food is labeled *low-cholesterol* or *diet* doesn't mean that you shouldn't read the nutrition label carefully. This is even more important now that fat substitutes (such as Olestra) are being introduced in "low-fat" foods that don't explicitly state they contain these artificial substances that have unknown long-term effects. (We already know their short-term effects: diarrhea, bloating, and abdominal pain.)

Specific nutritional supplements have value in treating specific diseases. For instance, folic acid is helpful to people with carotid artery disease and prevents nervous system-related birth defects, which are often fatal. Vitamin E shows benefit in preventing Alzheimer's disease, heart disease, cataracts, and prostate cancer, among other conditions. Large studies are showing the value of these and other supplements and providing the science to explain their effects.

There are also supplements that specifically encourage eye health. It is well known that antioxidants—vitamin C, vitamin E, lutein, and other carotenoids—are of particular importance to eye health, since they inhibit the damaging effects of oxygen and ultraviolet (UV) light on the retina. I will be highlighting these antioxidants in several later chapters. Because zinc, selenium, magnesium, taurine, and bioflavonoids (from fruits and vegetables) play important roles in stabilizing the normal metabolism of retinal tissue, I will also be discussing these nutritional elements, together with medicinal herbs, in Chapter 15.

Total health management requires more than just medication, nutrition, and supplementation. It includes exercise, stretching, consumption of pure water, proper breathing, socialization, alternative health care options, meditation, and relaxation. Using this formula to create fundamental good health is crucial to general eye health, as you will learn in *The Eye Care Revolution*. I'll explain specific eye conditions and diseases and reveal alternatives to treating these conditions with surgery or prescription drugs.

Over the years, I have personally adopted many of the health-supporting practices I share in *The Eye Care Revolution*, such as improving my eating habits, exercising (I practice Tai Chi and yoga, plus work out), and meditating. Stretching in conjunction with exercising increases flexibility and balance; you don't need to succumb to ligament contraction and progressive loss of height with age. I believe these lifestyle changes have made me not only a healthier person but also a better doctor.

Healing energy is not mysterious. I will show you how to increase body energy (known as *chi*, pronounced "chee" in Chinese medicine) and teach you to relax with the help of deep breathing and meditation. I'll suggest nutrients for your eyes that also help your general well-being. As you develop better habits, healing energy will connect many parts of your body.

Many insights can be gained from Chinese and Ayurvedic (Indian) medicine, especially in terms of their concept of the mind and the body as one, an integrated system. For instance, Chinese medical practitioners connect the health of the eyes to the health of the liver. A Chinese traditional physician may treat an eye symptom by addressing the liver disease causing (or contributing to) it.

Western practitioners also understand the connection between the eyes and the liver. The yellowing (jaundice) of the white of the eyes is a well-known indication of serious liver diseases like hepatitis or cirrhosis. It is impossible to make the eye symptom—the jaundice—disappear without curing the underlying liver disease.

In Ayurvedic medicine, the eyes have to neutralize fire, that is, light. Light is thought of as fire because it damages tissues. Western medicine now also understands that light damages tissues. When light focuses on the retina, it causes a breakdown in visual pigments. This reaction creates an electrical response that is sent to the brain and interpreted as vision. Ayurveda describes the eye as a bag filled with water that helps to dissipate the heat of light. The eyes use tears (water again) and eyelids to protect them on the outside, and liquid to protect them on the inside. It's important to drink a lot of water—eight glasses a day—(as we'll discuss in more detail later) to hydrate the body as a whole and contribute to making the fluids that protect the eyes.

I have studied these Eastern concepts and methods in detail, checking information in as many authoritative sources as possible, and I certainly didn't adopt these new ideas and practices immediately. But because of my strong belief in the value of interactive medicine—working with my patients and using concepts and methods from many disciplines around the world—I feel compelled to share what I have learned to be of value with my patients. I do my best to be a medical thinker. I believe that both Western and Eastern medical treatments (sometimes labeled *conventional* and *alternative*) can be used together—as appropriate—to improve the health of the body and of the eyes. I also believe that you and your doctor should be able to work together to evaluate these therapies in the truly interactive health care setting that you should have. After you read this book, I hope you will demand more from all your caregivers and yourself.

As Western physicians, we've already realized that, to learn the most about a patient and at the same time be perceived as a caring provider, we must use all our senses. We must listen to the patient in a caring dialogue that leads to diagnosis. We must look the patient in the eye while communicating. Through our words, eye contact, and touch, we encourage the patient to become involved in the process of conquering ailments. The patient empowered can empower the doctor. There is no greater confidence-builder for the doctor than feeling that the patient is confident and, as a result, is more of a participant in his or her treatment.

An empowered patient can also devise disease-prevention strategies, which should be our first line of defense against illness.

For instance, it's possible to control or eliminate many of the factors that contribute to the development of serious eye diseases (other than heredity, of course). Cataracts, as I will explain in Chapter 6, are caused in part by damage from excessive exposure to sunlight. The free radicals produced by sunlight's ultraviolet rays cause the proteins in the eye's lens to deteriorate, clump together, and harden into a cataract. Wearing sunglasses that protect your eyes against UV light, therefore, is one step you can take to help avoid developing cataracts.

Glaucoma is a disease of the optic nerve. When the optic nerve is damaged in glaucoma (perhaps partially due to increased eye pressure), a certain amount of sight can be lost. We now know that we can control glaucoma by lowering stress (through exercise and stress-management techniques like meditation), supporting the blood vessels that supply the optic nerve with oxygen and other nutrients (through diet and supplementation), and lowering internal eye pressure (first through medication, then by using more natural means which I'll describe in Chapter 7). By taking these steps, we can prevent or minimize vision loss from glaucoma.

Macular degeneration, formerly the blinding scourge of older age, is very much a disease of poor digestion. It can be prevented or stopped from progressing by eating foods rich in substances that specifically support the macula (the center of the retina), such as carotenes like lutein (found in spinach and many vegetables) and lycopene (found in tomatoes). In Chapter 8, I will share with you all I have learned about preventing and stopping (for some) this blinding condition through nutrition and supplementation.

Diabetes can be managed by the patient (under a doctor's supervision) so that potentially blinding diabetic eye disease does not develop. Every diabetic can construct a program (in consultation with a physician and possibly another expert, like a nutritionist) to control blood sugar levels through diet, supplementation, weight loss, and exercise. No diabetic needs to go blind today—there are too many options available to us to prevent diabetes-related vision loss. I'll tell you about specific foods and supplements that you can add to your diet to help prevent (or control) diabetic eye disease in Chapter 9.

Patients heal their own ailments; I only help them to do so. To that end, I use a combination of nutrition, medications, lifestyle modifications, and herbs.

Because I practice interactive medicine, I am commited to discovering what works best for each individual patient while having the fewest side effects. This doesn't mean I don't use conventional drugs. Whenever they are necessary, I prescribe them. I want my patients to be comfortable and empowered to take control of their own health.

I have a different perspective on many aspects of medicine because I have stepped "outside the box" of being a traditional, Western physician. Throughout *The Eye Care Revolution*, you will find Dr. Abel's Tips for dealing with various conditions and treatments. Some of these tips may conflict with current Western medicine, because I am neither an Eastern practitioner nor solely a Western physician, but a doctor in the middle who looks at the whole.

As a traditional ophthalmologist who explores the latest discoveries— from whatever medical tradition they originate—I use what works best for my patient. Many alternative therapies, for example, are less toxic than currently available medical treatments. And they are easily obtainable and safe. When no conventional therapy is available to treat a condition, I investigate all potential treatments for saving a patient's vision and health. Sadly, there are no miracles, and I am deeply disappointed if no therapy is effective. To me, this situation provides even more of an incentive to discern what new therapies might even now be growing in our own backyards.

Sometimes, exploring options (even when other ophthalmologists have given up) can result in a sudden cure.

For example, there was Ken who, at 48 years of age, developed optic nerve inflammation (optic neuritis)—a frustrating condition in which the eye's main nerve swells up and, and, if left unattended, can degenerate, causing vision loss. To make matters worse, Ken has only one usable eye; he was born with cataracts and glaucoma, leaving him blind in his left eye. After examining him, two excellent retina specialists concluded that his condition, an unusual complication of diabetes and poor circulation, was untreatable. He came to me in despair about losing his remaining vision.

I took Ken to see Dr. Nai-shing Hu, a practitioner of Chinese traditional medicine, who evaluated his tongue, pulses, physical appearance, and symptoms. Four weeks after Dr. Hu prescribed a combination of Chinese herbs, Ken was no longer hunched over as he had been for years, his thick scaly skin had softened, the redness in his palms and soles of his feet was gone, and the vision in his eye had returned to 20/20. His acute optic neuritis was under control. Ten years later, Ken no longer takes Chinese herbs, but he does take vitamin supplements: a multivitamin; a B complex vitamin; Vitamins A, C, and E; the minerals magnesium, chromium, and selenium; and he's added soy to his diet to stop potential blood vessel growth that could threaten his vision. Ken maintains tight control over his blood sugar level, and continues to have 20/20 vision in that one eye.

People with macular degeneration are also told all too often that nothing can be done for them. After appearing on television's *700 Club* in April 1997 to discuss nutritional management of macular degeneration, I received many calls from desperate viewers who'd been told that their eye conditions were due to aging and that they would lose some or all of their vision. Not true! As I have found (and as I told these callers), the dry form of macular degeneration can be halted. Occasionally some vision can even be restored with proper nutritional management.

The paradigm is shifting. A major eight-year prospective study published in 2001 conclusively showed that supplementation with antioxidants and zinc can alter the course and vision loss in macular degeneration (this will be described in Chapters 8 and 23). Overnight many ophthalmologists began recommending vitamins to their patients with or at risk for AMD. Furthermore, a 2001 survey showed that 80 percent of eye care specialists now believe that the regular use of lutein can minimize macular degeneration. That is, four out of five doctors feel that yet another vitamin can help AMD patients and recommend it. This was reported by the Jefferson Davis Associates Lutein Eye Health Study, in which 150 ophthalmologists and 150 optometrists were interviewed.

No one knows everything there is to know about healing and medicine. That's why I rely on colleagues who are knowledgeable about Western herbs, Ayurvedic medicine and Chinese medicine. They have spent ten or more years gaining this knowledge—in other words, the same amount of time that it took me to complete my medical education. I could never hope to reach their level of knowledge in these subjects while maintaining my practice as an ophthalmologist. Every health practitioner, whether traditional or alternative, is in the same position; no one can learn everything about every discipline. This is why you yourself must become a medical detective, and refuse to accept "nothing can be done" from any doctor without exploring every other safe option you can identify.

If your doctor is impatient, harried, or distracted, he or she won't be able to give you the proper amount of time required to deal with your problem. Worse yet, he or she won't be able to make the observations that are crucial to your improvement. Both doctors and patients must expand their vision, become better listeners and observers, and act together to solve medical problems. Your doctor should be willing to work with you. A true healer would not impose a bad diagnosis on the patient in a rushed fashion on the basis of inadequate information. The most valuable physicians of tomorrow will work with each of their patients carefully. Many doctors with these characteristics are practicing today, and I'll show you how to identify them.

The Chinese use the same word for both crisis and opportunity. Likewise, you should take a recent medical scare as an opportunity to redefine how you feel, how you live, and who you are. The purpose of *The Eye Care Revolution* is to help you prevent and reverse disease.

You don't need to become sick to transform your life and health or to take a global view of life and health. A revolution is occurring in health care. *The Eye Care Revolution* will show you how to take full advantage of the new thinking in medicine today.

I am just as I appear—a caring medical doctor who believes in interactive health care. Your wellness is important to me.

PART I

AWAKENING

CHAPTER 1

A Doctor Steps Outside the Box

• An older woman came to see me about her glaucoma. Despite treatment by another eye doctor, her vision was deteriorating. She had asthma as well as glaucoma, and I discovered that the medicine she was taking for her asthma was making her glaucoma worse, while the medicine she was taking for her glaucoma was worsening her asthma! She was plunging into increasingly poor health because of a very simple fact: the mechanical model of medicine—in which people go to different specialists to be treated for diseases in different parts of the body—fails to examine the whole individual. Her eye doctor had probably forgotten the long-term impact of the glaucoma eyedrops on this patient's asthma (if he or she even knew she had asthma) and the doctor treating her asthma almost certainly didn't realize that his prescription was worsening her glaucoma. As soon as I recognized that the medications were worsening both of the patient's diseases and managed to talk with her doctors, her medicines were adjusted and her glaucoma and asthma stabilized.

• A 52-year-old man from North Carolina asked me what could be done for his macular degeneration, a condition that can result in blindness. Five years earlier, after noting a decline in his already nearsighted vision, he'd learned that he had early degenerative changes in his retina (the first sign of macular degeneration). At about the same time, he began suffering chest pains—an altogether new symptom. On the advice of friends, he underwent ten chelation therapy treatments for his chest pain. (During chelation, a controversial procedure, a chemical circulates through the bloodstream and *sometimes helps clogged arteries. In other words, chelation, which was designed to remove metals from the body, may reverse hardening of the arteries.) He got immediate relief from his chest pain, and also noticed that, by the end of the chelation treatments, his vision had improved markedly. His health was good for about four years, but then his chest pains returned. This man's new HMO refused to pay for chelation therapy, so he was forced to undergo coronary bypass surgery. The charge for the bypass was $50,000. The cost of chelation treatments would have been $3,000. Fortunately, the bypass surgery was successful; the man's chest pain was relieved, and he was able to return to normal activity. Yet his vision continued to deteriorate. I was able to assure this patient that there were other options, including nutrition, he could pursue to stabilize his vision. After three months of an improved diet and taking specific vitamins, he reported that his vision had stabilized.*

• *Accompanied by her daughter, a 78-year-old woman came to see me because she'd had a sudden hemorrhage in her left eye, causing her to lose most of her vision there. After the examination, I asked her why she thought she'd experienced the bleeding in her eye (which was due to macular degeneration) and how she thought we might best protect the other eye. Just in case the problem was hereditary, I asked her daughter what she was doing to avoid losing her sight. Once I had their full attention, I pointed out that we all have choices; we don't have to remain passive while degenerative diseases overwhelm us. As a Zen doctor, I try to use an acute illness to awaken people to the need for a new life program.*

The Evolution of the Zen Doctor

The term *Zen* refers to a branch of the Buddhist religion—a faith that emphasizes meditation as a path to achieving individual enlightenment and awareness. Zen Buddhists practice a form of meditation that involves concentrating themselves very intently on an idea or problem so as to comprehend it as completely as possible. I use the expression *Zen doctor* to describe those in the healing arts who seek to become aware—using all five senses, as well as intellect and intuition—of every relevant aspect of a patient's illness in order to arrive at the best possible therapy for it. (In using the term *Zen* I am not, in any way, comparing my level of concentration to that of a Buddhist monk or anyone else who can meditate intensely.)

I also pride myself on having learned to think "outside the box"—

beyond the usual, automatic and conventional responses to various medical conditions. I recognize just how interconnected the eyes are to the rest of the body, and I know that I cannot treat eye diseases effectively without paying close attention to those connections. I've learned, for example, that taking certain vitamins can stop or slow certain degenerative eye diseases, like cataracts. These ideas are anathema to many doctors, because they've been trained to practice medicine in a very narrow way.

I understand their reasoning, because I received exactly the same narrow training. For many years, I was a typical ophthalmologist. I saw patients in my office, performed consultations, and did surgery two or three days a week. As the routine wore on me, I looked for ways to break it. I began learning Tai Chi, partly to build strength and balance, but mostly to reduce the stress in my life. My Tai Chi teacher, Alan Tillotson, is also an alternative medicine practitioner. He became an essential participant in the circumstances that changed my life and my medical practice.

I realized one day that my son's asthma had became intractable. Various oral medications and two types of inhalers were not preventing him from having severe, almost nightly, asthma attacks. Convinced that traditional medicine was only adding more drugs to his system and not solving his nightly attacks, I consulted Alan, who referred me to a Chinese medical doctor, Nai-shing Hu, with whom I made an appointment. Dr. Hu was confident that she could help and she prescribed a variety of Chinese herbs. Not only did my son's health improve dramatically; my own life was changed forever.

I witness other people changing their lives in response to health crises nearly every day. Dealing with a serious illness—your own or that of a loved one—provides an opportunity to reexamine your whole life. A major goal of my practice is to help patients dealing with life-altering situations to respond in ways that enhance their future health.

I am a successful, board certified ophthalmologist who's practiced medicine for thirty years. I'm concerned about medical practice in general because of what I've seen over the years. I'm also willing to step "outside the box," expand my horizons, and attempt new approaches—like trying nutritional therapy to stop a cataract's growth before resorting to surgery—when I see that an alternative treatment might be productive and it poses less risk to the patient than conventional therapy does.

Few ophthalmologists either understand this concept or take it seriously. Nevertheless, treating individual patients requires individually tailored methods. No physician can treat every case of the same illness exactly the same way because of differences in age, gender, body type, or the presence of other illnesses.

Nor am I concerned about being considered a traitor to the medical community by way of my beliefs here—I have always said exactly what I think, without necessarily conforming or being politically correct. Unfortunately, my penchant for seeking answers and for rejecting rote responses did not find ready support during my medical school years. At medical school, there were, in fact, few opportunitites for free thinking or expression. I am sure that many of my esteemed professors found my constant questioning of their teachings as tedious as I found them, but I felt compelled to search for broader contexts and more penetrating answers.

Am I alone in finding it strange that modern physicians ignore medical systems that have existed for thousands of years? Why is it that we are so slow to integrate some Eastern concepts and practices into our medicine? Acupuncture is not the only technique to come out of Chinese medicine, but it's probably the only one most physicians could name. Ayurvedic (Indian) medicine also uses many herbs widely recognized for their effectiveness that broad-minded Western doctors are beginning to employ. In my practice, if the end result is therapeutic for patients whom other doctors consider beyond help, I am satisfied. I can state with confidence that certain alternative treatments are effective because I have seen them work.

One of my patients, Cathie, developed a significant cataract in one eye when she was only 36 years old. She was also very nearsighted. She'd consulted another doctor who'd recommended cataract surgery as her only option, and was just waiting for her to schedule it. But Cathie wasn't eager to have the surgery because she knew that her healthy eye (which did not have a cataract) would not adjust well to the difference in image size that would result. She came to me knowing that I had used other remedies to stop cataracts from getting worse and, in some cases, to reverse them. I suggested she try an Ayurvedic herbal formula, both in eyedrop and oral form, and her vision improved significantly. From being able to see only one of the larger letters on the eye chart (20/200 vision), Cathie's vision improved to 20/30. A year after beginning the herbal treatment, her cataract problem returned, and I performed cataract surgery. As a believer in interactive medicine, I always try the least invasive approaches first. Only when they fail to produce the desired results do I move on to the more dramatic treatments favored by Western medicine.

As an ophthalmologist, I treat many older individuals. Older people frequently fall and break bones, which are treated by an orthopedist. The falls themselves may be caused by an unsuspected vision problem, which is the province of the ophthalmologist, but we generally don't see these patients until they come limping into our offices. Several studies in the medical literature indicate that poor vision in one eye—resulting in lack of depth perception—is a major risk factor for hip fractures. To try to prevent hip and other fractures in the older people whose vision I correct, I question them about how much and what kinds of medications they are taking, because overmedication can also cause falls in elderly people.

Sometimes being "outside the box" doesn't even require investigating alternative approaches to treatment, but simply paying close attention to what a patient has to say. For instance, a man called a New York radio talk show that I was being interviewed on and asked me why his eyes were suddenly tearing (weeping) every time he sat down to read the newspaper. The problem had started, he told me, after he got new glasses. He'd returned to his ophthalmologist, who told him that he had early cataracts and might need surgery in six months. After talking with him for a few minutes, it became clear to me that the problem this gentleman was experiencing was due to his new glasses: the optical center was not in the right place for him to be able to read without straining his eyes. He didn't have the tearing before he put on his glasses to read, and he didn't have it with distance vision, when he wasn't wearing the glasses. I advised him to return to the eyeglasses shop, explain his problem, and have his glasses adjusted to correct it.

Throughout my training, I was always taught that vision therapy—using eye exercises to strengthen the eyes and improve vision—was bunk. In Appendix F: Eye Aerobics, you'll learn about scientific techniques that are investigating how eye muscle movement is integrated with language in the brain. As we learn more about the brain's interactions with the eyes, we are also learning that eye movements may even be able to repattern the brain's learning mechanisms.

I perform surgery when it becomes necessary, or when the patient grows frustrated by a lack of progress in resolving his or her symptoms utilizing other methods (nutritional therapy, of course, does not work as quickly as surgery). I enjoy being able to rely on highly technical diagnostic and therapeutic equipment, with which the latest cataract surgical techniques can be performed—no-stitch, no-patch surgery, using eyedrops for anesthesia instead of injections, to minimize discomfort. I want to make my patients as comfortable as possible, whether we're using a surgical intervention or a nutritional one; it's better for them, and for me.

Corneal transplant surgery is another modern medical marvel that I use to restore sight. For anyone with a corneal scar (a condition that will not respond to herbal therapy), the surgery can now be done on an outpatient basis. Patients often say, "Doctor, I'm glad to have you for my surgeon. You're the best." I'm always happy to hear my patients say that.

If I am the best for them though, it's because I try to get the best out of each patient. I help them transform a sometimes frightening experience into a health-affirming one. By making my patients partners in their own care, I may appear to be the "best" doctor many people have ever had.

Vision is of primary importance in our modern society. We have erected stunning skylines, created museums to house fine art, built multicinema theaters, and drenched our minds with TV commercials made by people who recognize the primacy of visual stimuli. Our language is replete with expressions alluding to sight, including: "Look out," "See you later," "I'll see to it," "Outta sight." We begin relationships based on physical appearance and often end up judging books by their covers. We rely on our vision to transport us through the streets and along the information superhighway, as well as to make judgments that govern nearly every other aspect of our lives. I suspect that the profound need to maintain vision drew me into a field in which so much good can be done. Once I learned about alternative methodologies, I realized I could help even those people who had partially lost their sight.

Macular degeneration is a vision-threatening disease in which the central part of the retina is damaged. Many ophthalmologists consider macular degeneration to be an untreatable, progressive, and ultimately blinding condition. Research has shown, however, that certain nutrients can halt the progression of macular degeneration in many cases. I was consulted by an 82-year-old woman with macular degeneration, for example, whose other doctors had told her that, while nothing could be done, she wouldn't become *totally* blind. Unhappy with this bleak assessment of her future, she was delighted when I was encouraging about stabilizing or improving her condition. On my recommendation, she began drinking one glass of red wine nightly (red wine contains numerous antioxidants that counteract retinal damage), in conjunction with specific vitamin and mineral supplementation. (For details on preventing and treating macular degeneration, see Chapter 8.) Three months later, her vision had improved by three lines on the eye chart in one eye, and by two lines in the other. She couldn't have been happier.

Yes, there are simple solutions to some progressive problems. In most cases, there is no need to lose vision. How many times has a person with poor vision or macular degeneration been told that nothing more can be done? I cannot accept this, and you should not either. It *is* occasionally the case, and I am terribly disappointed when it is. I certainly don't give up until I have tried every useful therapy I can find, whether it's part of conventional or of alternative medicine. Of course, most people can improve their sight through low-vision aids or simply by turning up the light to see better, especially if they are older. If you have been told that nothing can be done to improve your vision, you can probably find resources in your community, including organizations that provide low-vision counseling, to help you identify your best options. (See the Resource Guide at the back of the book.)

The eyes are the key to the body. A good ophthalmologist should be able to look into the eyes and understand the patient's state of health. I will explain later how each part of the eye can provide a different type of information about the patient's health and lifestyle. But in general, an eye exam should (1) determine your best vision; (2) note the state of your health; and (3) help identify lifestyle implications for maintaining vision and longevity.

A *friend of my brother-in-law in Puerto Rico was diagnosed with open-angle glaucoma and warned that he would go blind if he didn't obey all his doctor's recommendations. He came to me for a second opinion, and I found that he had elevated internal eye pressure as well as other risk factors for glaucoma, but had sustained no damage to his optic nerve. In other words, he did not have active glaucoma. His smoking and other habits, however, were contributing to a condition that could progress to glaucoma. Although it wasn't what he wanted to hear, I told him that he could take charge of all of these habits, maintain his vision, and improve his overall health. If your doctor, even an eye doctor, doesn't advise you to stop smoking, who will? This patient was also a somewhat nervous individual. Knowing that stress plays an important role in the development of glaucoma, I advised him to investigate various stress-reduction techniques, including exercise, meditation, and visualization.*

Very traditional physicians who are unfamiliar with such new techniques may understandably find themselves uncomfortable advising their patients to try them. They make sense to me because I have tested them. They've helped many of my patients, without introducing any of the risks that prescription drugs can carry with them. Most doctors don't question conventional treatment strategies, and don't think about the larger boundaries to a condition. The best pioneers in medicine, however, have had to be revolutionaries to get their ideas heard.

Ignaz Semmelweis, a nineteenth-century Hungarian obstetrician, for example, was thought to be radical because he insisted that doctors wash their hands before delivering babies. In the 1920s, Alexander Fleming found that fungus made a compound that killed bacteria, but it wasn't until the 1940s that his penicillin was developed as an antibiotic drug. More recently, Harvard professor Kilmer S. McCully, M.D., was ridiculed because he argued that the B vitamin folic acid could reduce hardening of the arteries—which it does by lowering the amount of homocysteine (an amino acid) in the blood. If physicians had the time to examine the concepts and therapies considered alternative medicine today, they would find that many are not so revolutionary after all.

While preparing a lecture on anesthesia, I learned that an Italian practitioner named Valverdi was the first Western doctor known to use compression of nerves to numb an arm or a leg. The Shao-lin monks in China probably taught this technique to the Italian merchants who first visited China via the Silk Road in the Middle Ages. In turn, the merchants brought the information back to Venice with them when they returned home. The Shao-lin monks practiced the defensive art known today as kung fu, in which an attacker is neutralized by a blow to a pressure point. (By the way, this kung fu technique is the basis of Mr. Spock's "Vulcan grip" in *Star Trek*.)

Throughout my medical education and practice, I've tried to share with patients and colleagues the knowledge and insight I've been fortunate enough to gain—sometimes through the most coincidental of events. A dirt-ball fight during which I got smacked in the right eye at age 11, sustaining a corneal abrasion and inflammation, had the serendipitous effect of introducing me to my future mentor in the field of ophthalmology, Dr. Irving Leopold at Mt. Sinai Hospital in New York City. The pain from this injury and my permanently enlarged pupil had the further effect of engaging my interest in eye health, leading me into a career in ophthalmology and teaching me compassion for other people with eye problems.

Even during my rigidly controlled medical education, I pushed the envelope whenever possible. When I had the opportunity in medical school to join a committee developing a new curriculum for medical students, I jumped at it. Our committee proposed a curriculum that enabled medical students to take elective courses for the first time. I went further, however, suggesting that an elective course could be taken at any university hospital, and offering myself as a guinea pig. I established a precise set of goals, enlisted a mentor, and completed all missed assignments and examinations; I even promised I would spend an extra year in medical school if necessary (which it was not). As a result of this bargain, I spent three months (1968) working in Israel with Dr. Chaim Sheba, medical director of Tel-Hashemir Hospital and vice president of Tel Aviv University. This remarkable man (who read fourteen languages and spoke thirteen) transformed the lives of both Arabs and Jews at the major military hospital in

Israel, using his medical acumen and charisma. He made certain to sit on each patient's bed and touch him during the examination, making each feel like the most important patient in the hospital.

Thereafter, I spent time as an adjunct professor of ophthalmology in Guadalajara, Mexico, performing surgical missions and teaching courses in other Mexican towns. Later, I worked in Tunis, Tunisia, with Project Orbis, a program that flies ophthalmologists around the world to teach ophthalmologic techniques to local doctors, and subsequently brought one of their residents to Delaware for a surgical fellowship. I also had the opportunity to perform cataract surgery workshops in Amman, Jordan, with SEE International, an organization that recruits ophthalmologists to perform surgical missions as well as sponsoring international teaching programs.

In 1992, during a sojourn in Brazil, I sought out native healers to ask them about the natural methods they used to treat eye diseases. Most recommended colorful fruits and vegetables that are rich in vitamins, and some taught me about specific native herbs. In northern Brazil, where practitioners are descendants of people brought from Nigeria, eating red ants for better vision is still a common regimen. I had already learned that red ants were prescribed by native doctors in Nigeria and China for the same reason. Only recently have Western chemists realized that the pigment in the skeleton of the red ant is similar to the pigment in the bilberry or grape, which nourishes the rods in the retina to improve night and peripheral vision. From this experience, among others, I learned that remedies passed down through the generations (even when a population is uprooted and moved) can not only prove to be very effective but also have a solid scientific foundation that explains their effectiveness. It's scary that your grandmother might know more than your doctor, but I recommend listening to both.

In 1996, with my son (who was studying to be an ophthalmologist), I spent time in Kathmandu, Nepal, and at the Aravind Eye Hospital in Madurai, India. In Kathmandu, I met Vaidja (which means Doctor) Mana, who, in a family history spanning seven hundred years, is the twenty-first generation to become a physician. He is the keeper of original Sanskrit herbal formulas passed down in his family from antiquity. As one of the most eminent authorities on Ayurvedic medicine in Nepal, he personally picks and processes herbs that he then compounds into specific formulas, using them to treat a variety of illnesses, including asthma, multiple sclerosis, hepatitis, multiple myeloma, breast cancer, and many others. Dr. Mana explained to me how generations of doctors have used herbs to treat chronic disease, including eye diseases, without any of our fancy

Western equipment. With all our sophisticated technology in the United States, we have neglected simpler therapies that have worked for centuries.

In Nepal I also met an outstanding ophthalmologist and humanitarian, Dr. Sandoc Ruit, who has created an eye institute in Nepal (employing many local people), funded primarily through his own surgical practice. This gifted physician also performs medical missionary work in Tibet, where the shortage of adequate medical care is shocking.

In Madurai, India, I met the legendary ophthalmologist, Dr. Venkataswami, and his sister, Dr. Nachiar, at the Aravind Eye Hospital. Together, they have found some answers to the seemingly overwhelming eye care problems of their country. My son and I spent time working at the Madurai eye hospital, where we observed ophthalmologists being trained to manage the tremendous number of cases of blindness caused by cataracts and other conditions in India.

Drawing on my international experiences, I have tried over the years to emulate the great teachers in my field: Dr. Thomas Duane at Jefferson Medical College, Dr. Irving Leopold at Mt. Sinai Hospital, and Dr. Karl Anstreicher, a retired psychiatrist in Wilmington, who created a clinic for my city's underprivileged, staffed by volunteer physicians. Along the way, I've discovered that we continue to be students as well as teachers. On the one hand, we must continue to learn; on the other, we need to share the gifts that we have been given. It's the chain letter of caring. We need to stop, look, listen, evaluate, and integrate. We are privileged, in the United States, to have the highest quality nurses, technicians, optometrists, and ophthalmologists, as well as the most sophisticated technology. Now we need to open ourselves to learning about medical systems and practices that are not as technologically sophisticated, but that have proved themselves to be remarkably effective over the centuries.

In the United States, education is almost as readily available as water. Research projects, advanced clinical skills, and good patient care proliferate in metropolitan areas. But true healers—like Drs. Ruit, Mana, Venkataswami, Sheba, and others—employ touch, compassion, and the wisdom of the ages to augment their modern medical skills. They draw on ancient, indigenous medical systems as well as on modern science and empower the patient to find his or her own solutions.

Our most famous physician in the West, Hippocrates, was a student of the great mathematician Pythagoras, who is thought to have created the symbol that represents the medical profession, the caduceus. The dual, spiralling snakes of the caduceus represent the interweaving of science (or rationality) and art (or intuition) in the field of medicine. In practicing modern medicine, we technologically oriented physicians sometimes forget that, in addition to all our science, there is still an *art* to healing. Other physicians are beginning to join me in rediscovering that forgotten art.

The Eye Care Revolution describes the changes happening in a world in which doctor and patient are beginning to communicate in new ways. Eye illnesses are symptoms that should awaken us to look more closely at ourselves and seek new paths to a healthier life.

PART II

THE BODY AS A WHOLE

CHAPTER 2

The Eye as Mirror

The eye is a mirror of general health. We look outward and see an entire world through our eyes. As an eye doctor, I can look into your eyes and see into *your* world, the physical world of your health. Knowing how profoundly interrelated are the health of the eyes and the health of the body, I also know that it is often impossible to treat eye disease without healing the rest of the body and its underlying disharmony as well. The one is intimately connected to the other. But few people are aware of this connection.

Even some of my colleagues are prone to ignore the relationship between the eye and the brain. For instance, headaches can start in the eye, which is why I will teach you eye exercises to relieve eyestrain. (See Chapter 5.) Headaches can also move down the body and cause pain in other areas, so it's also necessary to look for the eyes' remote connections there. As I do with my patients, I will show you how to identify the root cause of your suffering, not just the symptom that has your immediate attention.

I am not alone in realizing that we must identify root causes of conditions to treat them successfully, as numerous reports in the medical literature now show. The case of a 41-year-old woman who developed a type of progressive night blindness called retinitis pigmentosa was described in a medical journal by her physicians because she was simultaneously suffering from rheumatoid arthritis, a thyroid condition (Graves' disease), and a bowel disorder (Crohn's disease). This woman's physicians suggested that an underlying autoimmune disorder was causing all of these conditions—a conclusion that showed their understanding of the eye-body connection.

Many conditions can be first diagnosed by looking in the eye: liver disease, diabetes, high blood pressure, hardening of the arteries, heart disease, and brain tumors can often be detected in the eyes before they are apparent anywhere else. Conversely, eye problems can sometimes cause symptoms elsewhere.

The body's systems have myriad connections that we are just beginning to unravel. A bacterial infection that begins in one part of the body, for instance, can result in infection in distant parts of the body. It was first suggested in the eighteenth century that mouth infections could contribute to the development of arthritis, and twentieth-century studies are confirming that connection. Untreated gum and mouth infections can also increase the risk of heart disease and stroke.

Hidden Connections Between Your Eyes and Body

When I look in your eyes, I learn about your general health. I can only treat your eyes by addressing problems or diseases that you have in the rest of your body as well. I would prefer, however, to help you prevent disease than try to remedy it once it's developed. And prevention requires understanding how the eyes and the body interact, a field of knowledge that is expanding each and every day.

How Do We Know?

How do we know that the eye and body are connected, and that treating one influences the other?

- We feel our bodies' energy, or aches; for instance, we feel a cold coming on before the symptoms become obvious.
- We observe the history of events in our lives—how symptoms have come and gone and what made them better or worse.
- We listen to other peoples' stories, and the order in which their symptoms developed.
- We learn from doctors who have accumulated evidence of these connections from their own patients' experiences.
- We learn from the scientific literature and the popular press.
- Physicians and researchers follow ongoing studies and plan future research.

As an ophthalmologist, I continue to learn about the eye-body connection, one patient at a time. Even in a major research study involving hundreds of patients, the observing physicians must still make their determinations one patient at a time. Each case of scratchy eyes, elevated eye pressure, and blurry vision can only be evaluated individually. Because I believe in the value of individual case studies as much as in the value of large-scale studies, you will find abundant references in *The Eye Care Revolution* to remedies that are known to have had a positive effect on patients, but that haven't yet been subjected to formal scientific testing.

Ultimately, you are your own scientific laboratory. If you are aware of the order of events, how your body feels, and can compare how your eyes see from day to day, you can perform your own scientific study on whether taking a pill or an herb improves your vision over a specified period of time.

I'd also like to share with you some important information (aspects of which flatly contradict the conventional wisdom) that has been gathered from several studies that have followed thousands of patients over many years. From these extensive studies, we have learned a great deal, not only about general eye health, but also about how to prevent common eye diseases like cataracts. The major long-term studies of eye health I'll be referring to include the following:

- **The East Baltimore Eye Survey** examined 5,308 individuals in East Baltimore. The survey found that, contrary to preconceptions about glaucoma, approximately 40 percent of people with this condition have normal, not elevated, internal eye pressure. It further confirmed that many people with elevated intraocular pressure never develop the optic nerve damage consistent with glaucoma. (The Beaver Dam Eye Study reached the same conclusion.)

- **The Beaver Dam Eye Study** examined eye disease in a community in Wisconsin. Among other findings, the study documented the increased incidence in macular degeneration with age, finding that it occurs in 14.4 percent of people ages 55–64, in 19.4 percent of people ages 65–74, and in 36.8 percent of those 75 and older.

- **The Chesapeake Bay Watermen's Study** followed individuals who had increased lifetime exposure to ultraviolet light and examined the correlation of that exposure with the development of cataracts and macular degeneration. Watermen who were exposed to higher levels of ultraviolet light over long periods of time had higher incidences of cataracts and macular degeneration in later life.

- **The Eye Disease Case-Control Study** is working to determine the specific risk factors for developing age-related macular degeneration. This is an ongoing, multicenter study; its final conclusions have not yet been published.

- The Early Treatment Diabetic Retinopathy Study (ETDRS) has provided important guidelines for treating different types of diabetic retinal disease.
- The Physicians' Health Study will follow 50,000 male physicians over the years, examining many aspects of their health, including cataract formation. The study is also looking at the development of various diseases in relation to nutrition, smoking, and other factors. This study has already established that the risk of developing cataracts increases with smoking, and that some nutritional factors (*such as vitamins*) are protective against cataracts. This and similar large studies are accumulating so much patient information that they will provide important data for years to come. The Physicians' Health Study is still ongoing.
- The Nurses' Study will follow over 120,000 female nurses, examining the same factors as the Physicians' Health Study, including the relationship of cataracts to smoking and diet. It is also an ongoing study.
- The Age-Related Eye Disease Study (AREDS) In this study, 4,600 people have been enrolled in a randomized, double-blind clinical trial sponsored by the National Eye Institute to evaluate the role of beta-carotene, vitamin C, vitamin E, and zinc in the development and progression of macular degeneration and cataracts.

Studies that follow thousands of people over several years have the particular value of allowing us to spot trends and understand disease processes in ways that shorter, smaller studies may not. Other important studies are mentioned in Chapter 23.

The Paradigm Shift

There is an old story about three men who bumped into an elephant in the dark. One grabbed hold of the tail, the second grabbed a leg, and the third encountered the trunk. After they stumbled out of the forest the next day, they each described their encounter. Each of them believed he knew what an elephant was, having only experienced one part. Medicine, in many respects, is also operating in the dark, and it takes all of us together sharing the information to restructure the paradigm of healing.

Tradition is usually the enemy of progress. This is nowhere more true than in a classic medical education, which is generally resistant to change and to new therapies, some of which are actually new and others of which are newly adopted but older than Western medicine itself. Remember: we doctors are trained to treat disease by prescribing drugs and operating. We are sometimes at a loss when disease is subtle or does not respond to a medication. This is one of the reasons why it can take years for medicine to accept changes institutionally. Our medical system has attained supremacy by conquering, temporarily, microbes using a biomedical model that examines, then treats, the body piecemeal. We physicians now must recognize that we've been treating symptoms, not root causes, and begin to change the way we deal with preserving health and treating illness.

Eighty percent of the world uses plants as pharmaceuticals; our herbal and pharmaceutical therapies originally came from plants, too. Closed systems, like our current medical system, fail to promote creativity, flexibility, or evolution. We tend to approach knowledge one study at a time, yet for a full understanding of how a biological system works, we cannot follow the action of one chemical compound in the body without investigating how it interacts with others. Likewise, we cannot fully study a drug that works on the eyes without understanding its effects elsewhere in the body.

Today's scientists are beginning to shift their attention, their understanding and the paradigms that guide their thinking, from the part to the whole. When physicians say "no" to heart surgery as a first choice for treating heart disease, for example, they are then able to embrace new methods for unclogging arteries. Pioneering physicians like Dean Ornish have showed us that diet, exercise, and meditation can reverse heart disease to varying degrees. Bernie Siegel, M.D., has shown us that love is part of therapy. Larry Dossey, M.D., has described the power of meditation, and Andrew Weil, M.D., has reminded us that the body will heal if we give it a chance and don't interfere too much.

As you read this book, you'll begin to understand something essential: that what we call disease is merely a symptom of a deeper imbalance in the body as a whole. With this ancient knowledge newly in your grasp, you will learn to work *with* your doctor instead of having him or her work *on* you. You will learn to become a physician-extender for your own healthcare. You will find out about adding herbs to your medicine. You may even learn to substitute herbs for prescription drugs in some cases, under your doctor's supervision. You will learn how to make changes in lifestyle and attitude, increase your fitness, and institute preventive measures. The mind is powerful; it can help to prevent or to perpetuate disease.

Twenty Healthful Tips for Your Eyes and Body

The former UCLA basketball coach John Wooden's motto was, "Learn every day as if you will live forever; live every day as if you will die tomorrow." It is in that spirit that I offer you these twenty tips to enhance the health of your eyes and body.

Making changes in our lives is a three-step process: First, you must form an *intention* to make changes; second, you must set specific *goals* to achieve; and third, you must *seek advice* on the best way to implement the changes needed to achieve your goals.

Every goal may not be attainable; it's unlikely, for instance, that any amount of physical and mental striving will restore an ailing, 70-year-old man to the physical state he was in when he was 20. If you set *achievable goals*, however, with the main objective of improving your physical and mental well-being, you'll find that arthritic pain can be minimized; headache frequency and severity can be reduced; vision can be improved; weight can be controlled; and energy levels can be dramatically increased. But don't feel you must create all this change by yourself: Enlist the help and support of your family and medical providers, find support groups of people interested in changing their lives in similar ways, and refer to this book and others for new perspectives on subjects like exercise, weight control, stress reduction, and alternative methods of dealing with physical and emotional illness.

Even people with limited mobility or those who are confined to a wheelchair can improve their fitness. At the Johns Hopkins School of Medicine, for instance, a weight-resistance exercise program was designed specifically for the disabled. The program achieved incredible results for the participants, including better brain function, improved physical performance, and a more positive outlook on life. Similar programs might be available in your area. If you are physically challenged, check with your physician or physical therapist to see if he or she knows of one.

Tip 1: Observe Nature

- Just as you are aware of the changes of seasons, be aware of the changes and renewal in yourself. Most cells in our bodies die and are replaced at a rapid rate. Our retinal photoreceptor cells, in fact, are destroyed and remade with every glimmer of light.
- Recognize that your diet varies according to the time of year, and is dictated by your body type.
- Try to find the harmony and balance of nature in your work, play,

intellectual pursuits, family responsibilities, and every aspect of your life.

• Use water, pets, and flowers to rejuvenate your spirits and empty your mind temporarily of the day's obligations. Learn to balance your life, and make time for recreation, relaxation, and friendship.

Tip 2: Manage Your Diet

• Keep in mind that most traditional diets are plant-based. Our modern diseases (like cavities, obesity, cancer, and diabetes) did not arise until we began eating refined sugar and white flour, large amounts of saturated fats, and artificial substances (like today's "fake fats," artificial sweeteners, and hydrogenated products).

• Remember that a balanced diet does not mean eating equal amounts of all the different types of foods. Over the past century, nutritionists have developed various food pyramids, emphasizing the importance of certain foods over others that should be consumed in small quantities. As our knowledge about nutrition has grown, the food pyramids have been revised by nutritionists to emphasize the importance of vegetables, fruits, and grains over the other food groups. I feel that water should be the base of every food pyramid. We need to drink much more water (eight to ten 8-ounce glasses daily) than we currently do.

Tip 3: Stock Up on Supplements

• Think of dietary supplements as an insurance policy to ensure that some of the nutrients you need aren't falling between the cracks.

• Build up your antioxidant bank account. In most illnesses, there is an overabundance of free radicals—the "bad guys" that attack our cells—and too few antioxidants—the "good guys," that combat free-radical damage. One way you can help guard against illness every day is to concentrate on building up your antioxidant bank account through diet and supplementation.

• Make sure you have adequate amounts of the water-soluble vitamins, vitamin C and the B vitamins. People who are on diuretics, who exercise vigorously, who live in hot climates, or who urinate frequently because of diabetes or some other condition need to be especially careful not to become deficient in the water-soluble vitamins.

• Take a good daily multivitamin. Taking your multivitamin every day should be as automatic as brushing your teeth.

• Boost your levels of the fat-soluble vitamins: vitamins A, E, D, and K. It's helpful to take these vitamins *with* a meal, since the fat in the meal will help your body absorb the vitamins more effectively.

• Remember that minerals are also essential to good health: calcium, magnesium, and zinc are three major minerals we need. Magnesium is particularly important, because magnesium deficiency is implicated in macular degeneration, glaucoma, asthma and other lung diseases, leg cramps, migraine headaches, diabetes, and heart disease. Every cell needs both magnesium and potassium. The minerals chromium, selenium, boron, and copper are also required by our bodies.

• Be aware that the essential fatty acids—the "good fats"—are nutrients in which many Americans are deficient. Essential fats aid digestion, protect the lining of blood vessels, line nerve and retinal cells, contribute to building immunity, and generally act as lubricants all over the body (in the skin, joints, and the bowel). Fifty percent of the fat in the brain is the essential fatty acid DHA. The essential fatty acids also help to protect against dry eyes, glaucoma, loss of bone mass, and arthritis. "Bad fats," like the saturated fats in meat or the transfats in margarine, tend to edge out the "good fats," preventing us from being able to use them properly. Because the typical American diet has such a high percentage of saturated fats, it's generally helpful to take essential fatty acids as a supplement, rather than relying entirely on food sources.

• Take advantage of the "super foods" that contain more than one type of nutrient or phytochemical. Soy is an example of a super food, since it contains not only plant estrogens but also strong anticancer substances like genistein and daidzein.

Tip 4: Drink Your Way to Health

• Be sure you drink six to eight glasses of water (8–10 ounces each) every day. Most of our body is made up of water, and dehydration is a major contributor to many chronic conditions, such as dry eyes, arthritis, and kidney disease.

• Try to consume only filtered or highly rated bottled water. Tap and groundwater can become contaminated with many substances, including pesticides, agricultural runoff, and microbes that can make us seriously ill. Having a water filter at your kitchen sink, or in your entire house, will remove some of these substances and ensure that the water you drink for your health truly enhances it.

Tip 5: Breathe Deeply

• Never forget that breathing deeply contributes to health in many ways. It is a great stress-reducer, for instance, and controlling your breathing is the first step to learning mind/body control techniques like meditation. I look at it this way: you're going to be breathing anyway, so why not do it properly? Deep breathing has other advantages, including increased lung volume, improved diaphragm strength, increased oxygenation of your body, and an enhanced feeling of well-being.

• Perform these two exercises to make a habit of deep breathing: (1) take ten deep breaths, morning and evening, before you brush your teeth; and (2) take one long, sustained deep breath every time you look at your watch. I promise you'll feel better for it.

Tip 6: Improve Your Digestion

• Be aware of your bowel patterns; a sudden change can indicate a serious condition, such as bowel cancer. Other, minor intestinal problems, like developing bloating or gas, can be signs that you are not absorbing your food well, and so are not getting the maximum nutrition from what you're eating or from the supplements you are taking. Poor digestion can contribute to the development of macular degeneration, arthritis, acne, anxiety/stress, colitis, and hemorrhoids. A lifetime of fast foods, hurried meals, and poor digestion will slowly decrease your immunity and health, resulting in conditions like macular degeneration and glaucoma (and serious illnesses in other parts of the body) later in life.

• Drink water between meals. This helps speed food through the digestive tract and aids in maintaining regularity.

• Be conscious of your fiber-to-meat ratio, particularly if you are suffering from constipation, bloating, or indigestion. All these conditions could signal a need for more fiber. Eating bran or oatmeal in the morning can decrease your cholesterol and help eliminate toxins from your bowel.

• Avoid antacids. Many people who have recurrent digestive problems don't realize that they lack sufficient stomach acid to digest their food properly. Taking antacids on a regular basis can contribute to this problem instead of solving it.

• Be aware that a wide variety of foods and supplements can aid in digestion. They include: lactobacillus ("friendly bacteria"), digestive enzymes, Omega-3 fatty acids, papaya, and ginger, among others.

Tip 7: Protect Your Liver

- Understand that when the liver weakens, disease appears. All food is processed in the liver and dispersed throughout the body. Enzymes, which are required to digest food properly, are synthesized in the liver. Both glutathione (an antioxidant that protects against cataracts) and glycogen (the form in which sugar is stored for later usage) are made and stored in the liver. The liver stores fat and the fat-soluble vitamins. It also detoxifies and regulates the entire body. Observations of native peoples show that when they lived solely on organic foods, they did not develop cancer and other degenerative diseases. Refined foods, extra fat, salt, sugar, and environmental contaminants accumulate in the liver.

- Remember that the liver is the sentinel organ that helps to maintain normal metabolism, immunity, and your sense of energy. Renowned cancer specialist Max Gerson, M.D., felt that a healthy liver would not allow cancer cells to take hold. It is impossible to test the liver by examining a single function. Therefore, peripheral signs such as digestive problems, sinusitis, skin disease, and generalized feeling of fatigue, may be your first warning that your liver and body are requesting some dietary realignment to rid the body of accumulated toxins.

- Know your medications—many of them are metabolized in the liver. Know how long you need to be on those medications and whether there are natural alternatives.

- Improve your energy level. When you exercise, be sure to move your waist, which will massage your liver. Feed your body nutritious foods and plenty of water. Treating liver disorders is the basis for treating the eye in Chinese traditional medicine. The future may even prove that some unusual conditions, like retinal degeneration and Alzheimer's disease, begin with a weakening of the liver.

Tip 8: Enhance Your Immunity

- Be aware that you, like most Americans, may be chronically immune-compromised. How can you expect to fight colds without your tonsils and adenoids, tissues that collect microbes and keep them from invading the rest of your body? Start building up your immune system with what you eat. Even if your tonsils and adenoids have been removed, you still have three basic ways to protect yourself against viruses and bacteria: (1) reducing your consumption of refined sugar and flour, transfats, caffeine, alcohol, nicotine, and processed foods; (2) adding vitamin C and other antioxidants, essential fatty acids, and herbs like echinacea to your diet; and (3) getting adequate sleep, and reducing your stress level through relaxation.

• Remember that not only the nose and throat, but also the eyes can be entry points for infectious agents. Although it is rare, viruses have been known to enter people through the eyes—one fatal case of the Hong Kong "bird flu" in 1997, for instance, was transmitted through the eyes. Such events should remind us that our eyes can allow microbes to enter our bodies.

• Understand that, with age, your immunity tends to decline. Using nutrition and supplements, however, immunity can be bolstered, so that in older age you can avoid infections and degenerative diseases like cancer.

Tip 9: Control the Aging Process

• Keep your mind and body active to help you not only feel younger, but *be* biologically younger than your chronological years. Some of the elements that go into staying physically fit and psychically young include: keeping your spine supple and strong; encouraging your colon health; protecting your liver; eating a nutritious diet; keeping your joints flexible through gentle, stress-resistant exercises (which are excellent for older people); and drinking adequate water for lubrication.

• Remember that older age does not have to mean loss of memory. There are naturally derived supplements that can improve memory, including herbs like *Ginkgo biloba* or gota kola; minerals like magnesium; vitamin E; supplements like coenzyme Q10 (CoQ10, which helps electrons flow into specialized cell components), DHA, alpha-lipoic acid, and L-carnitine (which transports fatty acids into the cells' mitochondria). Be careful with hormones like DHEA and melatonin, whose long-term effects have not been fully evaluated in controlled clinical trials. Be sure to see a practitioner who is an expert on these hormones and knows how to evaluate their safe use.

Tip 10: Prevent and Control Allergies

• Understand that an allergy is actually a sign that your immune system is working overtime trying to rid your body of the irritant causing the reaction. Allergic reactions can lead to sinusitis and middle ear infections. Asthma, a condition rooted in the same type of immune response as allergy, can be either chronic or life-threatening. Hidden food allergies can also result in numerous types of chronic misery, from diarrhea to fatigue, to unexplained rashes, even to gall bladder disease. Science is now beginning to explore the possibility that food allergies may contribute to many diseases, so don't take your food allergies lightly.

• Take action to fight your allergies by identifying their causes including your medications, which might even include your eyedrops. For example, one of my patients had been dizzy for six months. She had consulted a new internist, who asked every question except "What eyedrops do you take?" I suspected that this patient's glaucoma eyedrops were making her dizzy. And indeed, after she stopped using them, her symptoms disappeared.

• Utilize an elimination diet, during which you eliminate suspect foods like dairy, wheat, and shellfish.

• Make whatever changes are needed to improve your digestion.

• Take natural antihistamines like vitamin C and quercetin (found in red onions and garlic, or available as a supplement). Quercetin is being used effectively against allergic conditions like hay fever.

Tip 11: Recognize the Link Between Dry Eyes and Arthritis

• Realize that dry eyes and arthritis can be helped by the same remedies, a fact which suggests that a problem with membranes is common to both.

• Become wary of the nightshade plants, which grow in the dark as well as in the light: tomatoes, white potatoes, green peppers, eggplant, peas, and cucumbers. Eliminate these foods from your diet individually, so you can determine if one or more of them is worsening either your dry eyes or your arthritis.

• Take a combination of glucosamine and chondroitin sulfate, available separately or together in supplements. It has been shown to improve symptoms of arthritis dramatically.

• Supplement your diet with essential fatty acids or eat foods that are rich in them.

• Consume Knox gelatin, which studies have shown can keep you from having to undergo hip replacement surgery. Knox gelatin is made from cartilage, the same substance in our joints that is destroyed by arthritis.

• Try a topical treatment for arthritis as simple as cayenne pepper (or Tabasco sauce) mixed into Vaseline and applied to the sore joint. A more expensive version of this topical treatment is Capsicum, a lotion or cream made with extract of hot peppers as its active ingredient.

Although this does not address the cause of the problem, it can reduce pain and swelling in joints.

• Take steps to avoid developing osteoporosis (bone loss). Regular exercise is a must. If you are a woman you may also want to consider estrogen replacement therapy (if appropriate), a "designer estrogen" like Raloxifene, or alternatives to estrogen replacement therapy like natural progesterone, which my colleague John Lee, M.D., has found helpful in preventing osteoporosis. (Naturally, you should consult your physician about using any hormone replacement therapy, whether natural or manmade.) Finally, be sure to eat calcium-rich foods including dark, leafy green vegetables. That's where cows get their calcium. A warning: one million people annually fracture a hip or vertebra due to osteoporosis.

Tip 12: Take Steps to Prevent Cataracts, Cancer, and Coronary Artery Disease

• Read up on the very positive news coming our way these days about the preventive and therapeutic value of foods and supplements. Studies herald the effectiveness of nutrition in preventing cataracts, heart disease, cancer, and a host of other conditions—why not take advantage of what we already know? Increase your antioxidant levels by stocking up on vitamins A, E, C, folic acid, and selenium (a mineral important in cancer prevention). Since much of the soil our foods grow in is now more or less depleted of minerals (especially selenium), it's essential that we use supplements to make up for what's deficient.

• Don't forget about the role of environmental factors in causing cancer. Pesticides and other toxic chemicals have been linked to higher rates of cancers in certain populations. Be sure you wash vegetables and fruits carefully to remove pesticide residues. Soil contaminants, as well as microbes from chicken and pig farms, are polluting the rivers that provide the drinking water for some of us.

• Become aware of potentially damaging substances in your personal environment. As glands concentrate the chemicals we take in, they somewhat reflect our environment. Environmental estrogens—found in plastics and chemical substances—are thought to be linked to higher rates of hormone-sensitive cancers like breast, uterine, thyroid, and prostate cancer.

• Be sure you understand that hormone replacement therapy for women past menopause is a subject of much debate. On the one hand, estrogen replacement is linked to increased breast and uterine cancer, gall bladder disease, and phlebitis (blood clots). On the other, estrogen replacement has been shown to lower cholesterol, increase bone density, halve the risk of developing Alzheimer's disease, increase longevity, and contribute to the health of the eyes. Taking hormone replacement therapy is a personal decision that each woman should make with her physician and family. Natural hormone therapies may be the best available options.

• Try to reduce stress. Stress is a major contributor to the development of cataracts, heart disease, and cancer because it uses up the circulating and cellular antioxidants that protect against these conditions.

Tip 13: Sidestep Your Stress Triggers

• Learn to identify what triggers stress in your body and your mind. If you think about it, you'll realize that certain events or conversations will always cause you to tense up and perhaps then to develop a headache, a muscle knot, or a bad mood. By identifying the cause and dealing with it, you can often reduce a mountain to a molehill. If something a work associate, husband, wife, or child is doing is really upsetting to you, for instance, try discussing it calmly with that person. You'll be surprised how often something as simple as a conversation will help resolve a stress-inducing problem.

• Understand that stress can build up in your muscles, and that you can develop habitual sore spots, or trigger points in your body.

• Try to reduce your stress by stretching and exercising, deep breathing (even just taking ten deep breaths), and meditating. Or try massage, a relaxing way to increase circulation, lower blood pressure, improve flexibility, adjust your spinal alignment, and decrease toxins. You can also try taking magnesium to reduce tension headaches and herbal preparations to help induce relaxation and add balance to your life.

• Consider working with a therapist if none of these stress-reducing methods works for you.

Tip 14: Exercise Regularly

• Make sure to make exercise a regular part of your lifestyle. A study that compared two groups of nonsmoking men found that those who exercised daily (by walking a mile) lived longer than those who did not exercise at all. Exercise is good for the body and the mind, and contributes appreciably to physical and mental health and longevity.

• Develop a routine. Exercise at the same time every day, if possible, so that it becomes a habit, even a pleasure.

• Stretch first, to loosen and relax your muscles and joints. Many good books are available if you don't know how to start. Make sure you have a physical exam before beginning an exercise program, if you have been inactive for many years.

• Choose a form of exercise you can do easily and enjoy: walk, jog, bicycle, play tennis or your favorite sport, do yoga or Tai Chi. Walk up and down the staircase in your home if that's the only exercise easily available to you.

Tip 15: Encourage Energy to Flow Through the Spine

• Know that you don't have to get shorter because ligaments contract as you get older, nor do you have to undergo back surgery, which has been found to be a profoundly depressing experience. Having a backache or back surgery produces a very bad mood, whereas having a flexible back allows you to work and play normally.

• Remember that having a strong and flexible back results in good posture, which allows energy flow throughout the body. In Eastern thought, the flow of energy through the spine is the force behind creativity itself.

Tip 16: Have a Positive Attitude Toward Life

• Don't underestimate the power of the mind, or how intimately body and mind are connected. Your mind can heal, or it can weaken. You can choose which way to direct your mind. The medical literature contains many examples of people dying from self-fulfilling prophecies—that is, from having made up their minds that their conditions were hopeless and thus closing off the possibility of getting well again. The medical literature is also full of examples of people who used the power of their minds to help cure their illnesses. Remember, the mind is connected to the body not only through nutrition, but also through thought in ways that science is only now beginning to understand.

• Be aware that depression is a normal response to certain situations, and that it often cures itself. If it continues, though, don't hesitate to get help, whether from family, friends, community, or a therapist. Prolonged depression can be dangerous: eating disorders, self-destructive habits like drinking and smoking, and isolation from harmonious influences in your environment are all symptomatic of a harmful bout of depression.

Tip 17: Control Your Environment as Much as Possible

• Avoid smoke and air pollution, both of which are major contributors to the development of eye diseases like cataracts.

• Limit your exposure to industrial and agricultural toxins, including the fumes from new carpeting. Choose organic foods and install a water filter. Avoid using cleansing fluids like ammonia and bleach; numerous brands of natural cleansers are now available. Be careful with personal-care products, and use organic shampoo and soap whenever possible, because it's gentler on the skin, scalp and eyes.

• Protect yourself and your family against toxins in foods. Be mindful of the pesticides on fruits and vegetables, the hormones and antibiotics in meat, and bacterial contamination of meat, fish, eggs, poultry, vegetables, and even fresh fruit juices. None of us can control our environment completely, but the health of our body and our eyes requires that we screen harmful substances from our environment as much as we can.

Tip 18: Seek Interactive Care

• Find a doctor who listens to and works with you. I learn from my patients. They have a disease, and they carry its history within their bodies and minds. A good doctor will help a patient relate that history in the most informative way, so that the best treatment can begin. Of course, if your doctor doesn't know what treatment is best for you, he or she should seek out other experts' opinions as well as asking for your help. A delightful neighbor told me she was suffering from sharp pains in her sinus for four weeks before she went to her eye doctor. He sent her to an ear, nose, and throat specialist, who did an X ray and told her two things: she didn't have sinus disease, and he didn't know what she had. Unfortunately, he didn't do anything else. Four weeks later she saw a neurologist, who diagnosed a painful neurological condition called "tic douloureux" (French for "painful spasm"), which has specific Western and Eastern treatments. So if you have a doctor who doesn't know, doesn't help you find an answer, and doesn't refer you to another doctor, move on. Select compassionate, well-trained doctors who observe and listen.

• Be willing to get actively involved in your own care: read, write letters, ask questions, and make lists. Come in with your questions written down. Ask for more than a three-word diagnosis in Latin. Ask for the second-most probable cause. What are the treatment options? What's the best case/worst case? What can you do to aid in your recovery? Ask the doctor and the pharmacist about side effects of any prescribed drugs. As you think about your problem after leaving the doctor's office and come up with new clues or new questions, share them with the doctor or his or her staff.

• Look for a physician who treats you as a whole person, not as a collection of symptoms. Is he or she listening to you? Does he or she ask about other problems you might be having? Has he or she asked if you are on any medications? Has he or she asked you to go home and think about when your problem began and any internal or external clues? Our goal is not to have you take medications with possible side effects or undergo a surgical procedure only to have the problem return. None of us can predict the outcome of any treatment 100 percent of the time, because people and their conditions are different. Select physicians who look at you as an individual and not as a list of symptoms.

• Find a doctor who understands the power of prevention.

Tip 19: Seek Alternatives

• Search for options in your health care, as well as in your personal environment. Add nutrition, exercise, and even herbal advisers to your health care regime. Check out alternative solutions to problems, particularly if the traditional medical options are not to your liking, or have not been successful.

• Be aware that a paradigm shift is occurring in modern medicine away from the Cartesian model (which separates the mind from the body) and toward the Eastern model, which recognizes the interaction between mind and body. Ancient medical systems did not have advanced diagnostic testing and therefore had to rely on the arts of observation, listening, and the use of clinical judgment. Keep in mind that the intertwined snakes of the caduceus, the symbol of the medical profession, signify science and intuition. Both are required for the most effective practice of medicine.

• Keep your doctor informed of any alternative solutions you are pursuing. For example, your doctor needs to know what supplements and herbs you're taking, just as you need to judge how he or she can help you achieve optimum health.

Tip 20: Take Personal Inventory

• Examine your own body each day—perhaps in the shower or bath. You can gauge your health and nutritional state by judging how quickly cuts and abrasions heal. You can take note of any significant changes in the appearance of warts or moles. You can check your body for any suspicious lumps or bumps. You can judge the strength of your nails and hair.

- Keep a dietary diary. If you feel especially good, or not your usual self, when you get up in the morning, check your diary to see what you ate in the past twenty-four hours that could account for the way you feel.
- Revisit your goals periodically.
- Don't expect improvement over the short term. Don't continue to take any supplement if you don't notice definite improvement. Adopt the Chinese method of measuring progress in terms of 100 days. If you take a vitamin or supplement for 100 days and the condition you're taking it for hasn't improved, reevaluate your approach.
- Work with a nutritionist if you need help developing a nutrition plan.

Twenty-first century healers will try natural methods before putting potentially toxic substances into your body. They will attempt to treat the root of a disease, not just its symptom. They will treat the whole person, not just the disease. And they will practice prevention rather than waiting until a disease develops to address an underlying imbalance.

Remember, you can be chronologically old, biologically mature, and mentally youthful. In *The Eye Care Revolution*, I will teach you methods of pursuing your goals, as well as ways to implement my tips and suggestions to achieve the best eye and body health possible by determining what works best for *you*.

CHAPTER 3

Uncovering Hidden Imbalances: Becoming a Medical Detective

Before I explain how to manage eye diseases—either by employing traditional methods or by becoming your own medical detective to ferret out root causes—I will teach you how to look deeper into yourself and your life in general. Having a disease does not only mean taking a pill or blindly following doctor's orders. For many people, prescription drugs and even surgical (or other invasive) procedures may be necessary, but they—and their unwanted side effects, like pain or nausea—can often be avoided. Remember, the most effective and least disruptive therapy is your goal.

Help your doctor discover the underlying cause of your condition, so that he or she can treat you more accurately. By examining your past medical and personal history, you will begin to think like a medical detective and an active partner in your health care, rather than like a passive victim. Do some digging into your own health history. No one knows it better than you. You may well find the roots of your current problem in information that only you have.

Here's an example of what I mean. At the completion of your eye exam, you may be told that you have a condition or disease that needs treatment or correction. You will probably be given some quick advice, perhaps a prescription, and instructed to return after a specified period of time. Well, if that's all that happens, that's not quite enough. What's missing is a search for the underlying causes of your condition, and if your eye doctor doesn't initiate this search, you may want to begin it on your own.

Why and how you did you develop this problem with your eyes? What aspects of your lifestyle or environment might have contributed to its development? Few eye diseases occur overnight, so when, to the best of your recollection, did your problem begin? What were you doing? Had you just returned from visiting another country? What had you been eating? Review your diet and environment. What other messages did your body give you before the symptom or disease appeared?

In my practice, I ask my patients these questions—not to place blame for developing an eye problem on *them*, but to help them understand the root causes of their condition and then become proactive in resolving it. There are no guarantees in life. If you *do* become ill, consider it a signal that you should redouble your efforts to improve your overall health.

The more understanding we gain about how our bodies function and how they respond to various stimuli—including food, drink, sleep, stress, and many other facets of modern life—the more control we can exert over our health and our lives. Unfortunately, we will not always be successful—I would not be a responsible physician if I told you I knew the secret to maintaining perfect health—but we *can* learn to influence our health positively. While acknowledging that fluctuation in the health of our bodies is a natural part of life, I also believe that there are many ways we can improve our basic health, and my goal in *The Eye Care Revolution* is to share them with you.

Now let's return to the eye doctor's office. You've just completed a questionnaire, answered additional questions posed by a technician, physician's assistant, or the doctor, and undergone an extensive eye exam. A well-trained eye doctor has given you a diagnosis. In responding to that diagnosis you will benefit by considering it not just as an end in itself, but as a symptom of an underlying imbalance.

Remember as well that your symptom does not always originate where you feel it most. Symptoms are like the leaves of a tree; the root is elsewhere. Nerves connect and exchange information all over the body. It's possible that earlier symptoms you didn't particularly notice were closer to the actual source of the problem, but that the problem only came to your attention later as a remote, referred pain like a headache caused by a basic strain. Clues to the origin of pain and disease do exist, however, and I'll help you become a medical detective—your own—to track them down and address the problem at its source.

Table 1 gives examples of how to do this—how to "think backwards." Starting with the most obvious symptoms, you can identify the underlying body system (heart, bowel, lung), involved and then determine a deeper cause (infection, allergy, disease).

Here's an example of the kind of "thinking backwards" we do in daily life. Suppose you notice seagulls circling a shopping mall sixty miles inland. Why are there gulls this far inland? you ask yourself. Well, the immediate

Table 1. Outer/Middle/Inner Manifestations of Disease

Symptom	Possible Intermediary Mechanism	Example of a Possible Deeper Cause
Headache	Tight neck or back muscles	Unequal leg length
Migraine headache	Blood vessel spasm	Stress, light, or hormones
Twitching eyelids	Low magnesium	Hypertension or being overweight
Seborrhea (oily skin)	Gallbladder and liver imbalance	Dietary fats
Sinusitis	Food allergy	Poor digestion
Double vision	Strabismus (crossed eyes)	Hereditary farsightedness or drug side effect
Poor vision	Retinal vein occlusion	Circulatory problem or high blood pressure
Corneal ulcer (Mooren's disease)	Enzymes that break down collagen	Hepatitis C
Cataract	Iritis, or steroid use, or poor nutrition	Previous trauma Leaky gut
Blurred vision	Optic nerve swelling	Brain tumor
Age-related macular degeneration	Poor circulation to retina	Poor circulation to the whole body
Chronic simple glaucoma	Blocked aqueous fluid flow out of eye	Chronic lung disease
Low-pressure glaucoma	Poor circulation to eye	Low blood pressure, especially at night

These are just a few examples of underlying conditions or imbalances that can cause seemingly remote symptoms. It is by no means a complete compendium, and none of the entries may apply to you. This information is presented simply to illustrate the point.

answer is that there's food in the mall's dumpsters. But beyond that—by thinking backwards—you realize that they wouldn't be coming inland unless there weren't enough food for them along the shore. If you continue thinking backwards, you might ask yourself what could be happening along the shore—construction work? some pollutant killing off the birds' usual prey? just too many gulls competing for a limited food supply?—that's forcing them to go farther afield.

Now let's look at sinus infection and headaches over the eye. At first glance, the headache might be related to tension, pain in the eye, or an infection in the sinuses. Your doctor can perform tests to help identify the underlying condition or cause for the headache. Treating only that area, however, may not eradicate the problem, if it has a deeper cause.

Illustrating this scenario is the case of one of my patients, who had long suffered from a recurrent sinus infection. Her previous doctor had been in the habit of prescribing antibiotics every time the disease and its sinus headache returned. But there began to be fewer and fewer comfortable days between recurrences. Since she was unhappy about taking antibiotics all the time, she sought a second opinion and came to see me. I felt it was important to consider another possibility—that a food allergy was affecting her digestion and, therefore, her whole body. We worked together on an elimination diet and found that dairy products were triggering her sinus headaches. The dairy foods were stimulating a mucin response as an allergic reaction, and the sinus—essentially a closed space with a very narrow duct—became clogged by the mucous material produced in response to her consumption of dairy products. The bowel, although it cramped, was capable of expelling the mucus, but the sinus was not. When she drank milk, mucus resulted, and the infections took root in the warm, moist place.

Eye problems reflect problems elsewhere in the body. The earlier you detect a previously unsuspected cause (e.g., your itchy eyes may be due to the neighbor's cat), the faster you will make the connection. These examples may ring true for you or someone you know, or they may appear far-fetched. Nevertheless, searching for the root cause of surface symptoms is an important exercise in uncovering hidden imbalances within you.

PART III

HOW WE SEE

CHAPTER 4

Light and the Eye

• I asked an older man with early cataracts what he did for pleasure: did he read, watch TV, walk, or do a lot of driving? He told me that he drove a lot, but really didn't watch television or read anymore. I realized that he had discontinued these activities because, like so many other people, he thought they would make his declining vision worse. I told him that this was not true, and that he should use his eyes—because, if anything, using the eyes strengthens them. He had fallen prey to one of the myths about eyes that I most want to dispel: that overusing your eyes will harm them. In fact, if you do not use your eyes, you may lose the visual acuity you have.

• A 51-year-old horticulturalist came to see me with moderate cataracts and declining vision in both eyes. I asked him what he thought the cause of his cataracts might be. His only answer was that his father, who had also worked outdoors, had developed cataracts at an early age. As I questioned him, he recognized that he'd rarely worn sunglasses. Only then did he understand the connection between his and his father's occupations and their early cataracts. Light, especially its ultraviolet component, is the major cause of cataract formation worldwide.

Light is the great love the eyes can't live with and can't live without. While it allows us to see, too much of the wrong kinds of light can severely damage our eyes (and skin) over time.

Determining the *refraction* of light by the eye—how the eyes bend and focus light to produce vision—is the foundation of the routine eye exam.

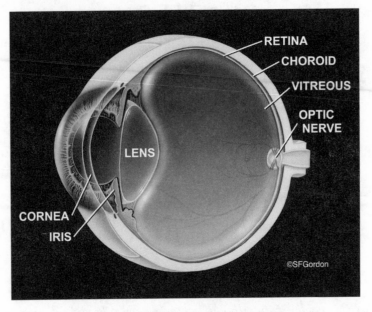

RETINA
CHOROID
VITREOUS
OPTIC
NERVE
LENS
CORNEA
IRIS
©SFGordon

Figure 1. Anatomy of the Normal Eye

It's important, therefore, to understand a little bit about the eyes and how they use light to create vision.

The eyes are designed to provide minimal interference to light's progression through them to the retina. In fact, only two structures interrupt the passage of light inside the open eye—the *cornea* and the *lens*, both of which filter and focus light. (See Figure 1.)

The eyeball has three layers: Its tough outer coat is made of the connective tissue collagen. In the front of the eye, that collagen layer forms the *cornea*, which is clear. The collagen covering the rest of the eyeball is white—the "white of the eye"—and is called the *sclera*. The collagen layer completely encircles the outside of the eye and continues all the way back to the brain as the outer coating of the optic nerve.

The middle layer of the eye is the vascular or nutrition-bearing layer. Its frontmost portion is the *iris*, the colored portion of the eye. The pupil is the opening in the iris and, in a healthy eye, is usually dark. Behind the iris is a muscular structure called the *ciliary body* where some of the eye's fluid is formed.

The innermost, third layer of the eye is the *retina*, which lines the posterior two-thirds of the eye. The retina is a complicated structure, and its deep layers contain the *photoreceptor cells*—the rods and cones that turn light into sight. It is nourished by the layer beneath it, called the *choroid*. The retina is composed of a network of nerve fibers which coalesce to form the *optic nerve*. The optic nerve resembles a giant cable transmitting information from the back of the eye to the brain.

The eye is filled with fluid; its only internal structure is the *lens*, which focuses light. The lens is transparent, having no blood vessels or nerves. It is suspended inside the eye by fine filaments from the ciliary body, the circular muscle inside the eye that allows the lens to change shape and focus light.

Besides the ciliary body, the eye's only other internal muscles are within the colored *iris*, where they constrict and dilate the *pupil* to allow more or less light to enter.

There are two types of fluid in the eye. The *aqueous humor* is the clear fluid in the front of the eye, filling the outer chamber that lies between the iris and the cornea. (See Figure 1.) The aqueous humor is secreted from the ciliary body, percolates around the lens, flushes the cornea and the iris, and exits through the *angle* of the eye that can become blocked in glaucoma.

The other fluid in the eye, the *vitreous humor*, is gelatinous in texture. The vitreous humor fills all of the inside of the eye behind the lens. It develops before birth to support the retina and allow blood vessels to nourish the lens during fetal life. Occasionally, bits of cells remain in the vitreous humor after birth and may float around when the vitreous becomes more liquefied in later life. These nuisances are called *floaters*, and occur in most people after the age of 50. Nearly everyone has a few floaters sometime in their lives, and they are usually nothing to be concerned about.

Outside the eye, but inside the skull's orbit, are the six external muscles that regulate the position of the eyes so they move together. The eyeball itself fills only one-quarter of the bony orbit. Besides the six external eye muscles, the orbit contains connective tissue, blood vessels, and lots of fat to cushion the eye from blows. The lids, lashes, and overhanging brow protect against harmful external elements, including the ultraviolet light in natural sunlight.

We live by light, we thrive by light, and we suffer from too much or too little light. We need light to reach the retina to produce sight, just as we need it to reach our skin to produce vitamin D, an essential hormone.

We also need light to regulate the production of *melatonin*, which is made by the brain's *pineal gland*. Light strikes cells in the retina, which communicate directly through the optic nerve to the midbrain, then to the pineal gland. Light suppresses the pineal gland's production of melatonin, and darkness stimulates it, creating the daily tempo known as the circadian rhythm.

The good news is that light allows sight and can create a psychological sense of well-being. The bad news is that too much light, especially ultraviolet (UV) light, can damage the eyes.

What Is Light?

Light is one of the most enigmatic forces in the universe, having both particle- and wave-like properties. Light is measured in wavelengths, which are usually expressed as nanometers (nm). Human beings can see only a portion of the whole electromagnetic spectrum of light emitted by the sun; ultraviolet (UV) and infrared (IR) are both imperceptible to the human eye. What we *can* see falls between 400 and 700 nm and is called the *visual spectrum.*

UV light is invisible to us because it falls below the visual spectrum. Some researchers divide UV into UVA (320–400 nm), UVB (280–320 nm), and UVC (100–280 nm). Near UV light (which is broader than UVA, at 300–400 nm) is found in sunlight close to the purple and blue range of the visual spectrum. *Near-UV light* is used in slow-tanning booths, and has been implicated as a cause of cataracts and corneal disease.

Far-UV light (100–300 nm) is found in sunlight, arc-welding light, and sunlamps. Prolonged exposure to light reflected off sand, snow, and water may produce *snow blindness.* In this condition, the profound concentration of UV rays in the reflected light washes the purple colors out of the retina, leaving a pink afterimage. Prolonged exposure to UV light can also cause corneal burns, abnormal growth of tissue in the eye (pterygia), sunburn, and herpes virus outbreaks.

Nature did not intend for humans to be exposed to so much UV light. The ozone layer in the atmosphere absorbs far-UV light, but the ozone layer has been damaged by air pollution and can no longer absorb as much UV light as it once did. The hole in the ozone layer over the southern hemisphere, which allows more of this damaging UV light to reach Earth, has caused cataracts in animals and in infants in Patagonia, where people wear sunglasses to protect their eyes more than half the year.

Glass, plastic, and windshields filter most UV light, which is why people in cars do not get suntans. Even the eye itself filters out some of the harmful UV light contained in sunlight. As light hits the outer layer of the eye—the clear cornea—some of the UV wavelengths are absorbed by the cornea and filtered out.

The near-UV light that penetrates the cornea is mostly absorbed by the lens. This absorption also occurs at a cost, because if the damaging oxidative effects of the UV light aren't neutralized by antioxidants in the

Table 2. Electromagnetic Spectrum and Light Toxicity to the Eye

Name	Wavelength	Examples (sources)	Physical Findings	How to Prevent
Gamma rays	< 0.3nm	Solar system; radiation devices (affects nucleus of atom)	Skin cancer; catraracts; dry eyes	Avoidance; lead shield
X rays	0.3–100nm	Radiation machine	Same as above	Avoidance
Ultraviolet	100–400nm	Sun, snow, arc-welding, sunlamps, Excimer lasers	Corneal burns; pterygia; sunburn; snow blindness; cataracts	Sunglasses or other protective eyewear; hats; skin lotions
Visible	390–750nm	Sunlight; indoor lights; binocular; indirect operating microscope; electric furnace; eclipse; lasers	Retinal fatigue; solar retinal burns	Oblique light; not looking directly at the sun
Infrared Near IR	750–2000nm	Sunlight; molten steel; glassblowing	Cataracts; corneal burns	Protective glasses
Infrared Far IR	2000–30000nm	Sunlight	Cataract	Protective eyewear
Microwave	30000nm–30cm	Radar; microwave ovens; industrial electric heaters	Cataract	Ordinary care (close door; don't stand around the source, etc.)
Radiowave	30cm–several kilometers	TV; radio	No known hazard	No known hazard

Conversion: 1 nm = 10 Angstroms = 10^{-9} meters.
Short wavelength radiation such as gamma, X ray, and ultraviolet (UV) are the most damaging but are absorbed in the ozone layer in the atmosphere. The UV spectrum ranges from 100 to 400 nanometers (nm). UVA wavelength range is 320–400 nm, but it's more accurate to call this *near UV*. UVB wavelength range is 280–320 nm, and UVC is below 280 nm.

lens, the UV light alters the lens's crystalline proteins so they are no longer transparent. As we age, the clarity of the lens naturally decreases from lifetime exposure to UV light. At the same time, the body's free-radical-fighting capacity also decreases. The increasing cloudiness of the lens is what we call a *cataract*. Unlike the effects of drugs and even smoking, which eventually dissipate, the effects of UV light on the lens are cumulative over time. (Fortunately, there are ways to stop or reverse the damage caused by excessive exposure to UV light. I'll explain them later in this chapter.)

As we age, the natural increasing cloudiness of the lens blocks out the UV light. By allowing far less light to enter the eye, it protects the retina. From birth to age 80, the lens slowly turns yellow and then brown, reducing its transparency dramatically. The increased opacification of the lens in an older person can allow as little as 10 percent of available light to enter the eye. Consequently, older people require much more illumination to see; an 80-year-old can require three times as much light to see as clearly as a 20-year-old. The retina compensates for the decreased amount of light entering the eye by becoming more sensitive. This is why elderly people are slower than younger people to recover their vision when surprised by the headlights of an oncoming car, and after cataract surgery.

Cloudiness of the lens can also create a cloudiness in mood; as people see less, they become more depressed. This is important in terms of evaluating the need for cataract surgery in an older person. Replacing a cataract-clouded lens—which may have been letting in less than 40 percent of available light—with a clear, replacement lens that is transparent is a pleasant surprise to many elderly people. I generally warn my cataract surgery patients that it may take them as long as four weeks to become used to the brightness. I also do not prescribe new glasses for several weeks following cataract surgery.

Blue-violet light (the lower wavelengths of the spectrum) appears to cause the greatest damage to the retina. People with light-colored eyes, large pupils, and/or poor pigmentation of the retina are at increased risk of developing macular degeneration because their retinas are less protected against UV light. Using various antioxidants and sunglasses in combination is helpful in warding off the toxic effects of UV light.

The Eye Exam

While there is much you can do to protect and care for your eyes, you should also have an eye examination at least once a year to ensure your eyes' continuing health, as well as to identify disease in your eyes or in other parts of your body. Don't forget that the eyes are the window through which we can often see illnesses in remote parts of the body.

Three types of professionals generally care for your eyes: opticians, optometrists, and ophthalmologists. The optician is the person who measures you for your glasses and fits them to your face. He or she has usually had special training and passed a state board exam permitting the grinding of lenses and the fitting of glasses.

An optometrist is a college graduate who has had four additional years of optometry school, and learned the art of refraction (correcting vision). He or she knows how to fit contact lenses and diagnose eye conditions and has developed an overview of therapy for ocular disease. In many states, optometrists are licensed to treat as well as diagnose eye conditions. They are not physicians, but they are specialists in eye care. Specialty optometry includes vision therapy; contact lenses; comanagement of ophthalmologic diseases; and therapy.

An ophthalmologist is a specialist who has finished an undergraduate college education and four years of medical school, completed a one- or two-year internship, and spent three or four years in residency training in ophthalmology. Becoming an opthalmologist takes at least twelve years, including college. Some ophthalmologists and optometrists have done additional training in specialty areas. Ophthalmology specialties include the retina; the cornea; external diseases; glaucoma; strabismus (crossed eyes) and pediatric ophthalmology; neuroophthalmology; and ophthalmic plastics.

When you go for an eye examination, vision is usually tested in each eye individually, with or without correction (i.e., glasses). Vision can then be tested with your current glasses correction to determine which is better. Occasionally, the ophthalmic technician or assistant (or the doctor) will put a plastic occluder/cardboard with one or more pinholes in it in front of the eye. This eliminates all the astigmatic waves of light, and is a "cheating device" to minimize the need for glasses and determine what the best vision might be. Later in the eye examination any underlying pathological condition is identified. This brings to mind the misinformation that wearing multiple pinholes (glasses that are opaque, except for pinholes that allow a small amount of light to enter) will improve your vision and correct your eyes; it will not. It simply gives a hint about your best-corrected vision (with glasses). Near vision, with and without correction, is usually tested, especially in those over the age of 40.

The eye examination has seven major components that we'll discuss in detail. They include:

- Visual acuity examination
- Refraction
- Visual field examination
- External examination
- Slit lamp examination

- Tonometry
- Ophthalmoscopic examination

Visual Acuity

The Snellen Eye Chart (you know, the one with the big *E*) is the most commonly used method of measuring visual acuity—that is, how well you can see at what distance. It does not describe all the parameters of vision, including peripheral vision, contrast, and other subtle characteristics. Some people have excellent vision in a dark room, for instance, and others don't. Some people's vision decreases with glare. Some people have good vision for five to ten minutes but fatigue because they are not wearing the right eyeglasses correction. The Snellen Eye Chart does not measure any of these subtleties.

Patients also display different psychological attitudes as they look at the eye chart. Some people find it challenging, while others are afraid of making mistakes. I try to reassure my patients that an eye test is not something you "pass" or "fail"; it's just a measurement. And, if you don't like the measurement you have, there is much we can do to improve it.

Twenty-twenty (20/20) vision simply means that a person can see at twenty feet what it's normal to be able to see at twenty feet. Vision of 20/60 means that a person can see at twenty feet what it's normal to see at sixty feet; in other words, their vision requires an image three times the normal size for them to be able to see it clearly. Vision measured at 20/400 (being able to see only the big *E* on the eye chart) means that a person sees at twenty feet what should be seen clearly at four hundred feet. The definition of legal blindness is 20/200—which implies the best corrected vision, not the person's vision without glasses.

Remember that your vision may actually vary with your mood and even with different times of the day and with the darkness of a room. The doctor may be happy that you see 20/25, but this may not really describe what you're seeing in the real world. You are your own best advocate.

Refraction

Myopia, better known as *nearsightedness,* is defined as seeing better at close range than at a distance. This is because the eye is longer than normal (23 mm is normal), or because the cornea is more curved than normal, which causes light coming from distant images to focus in front of the retina instead of on it. Only by bringing the object closer does the image fall farther back onto the retina and come into focus.

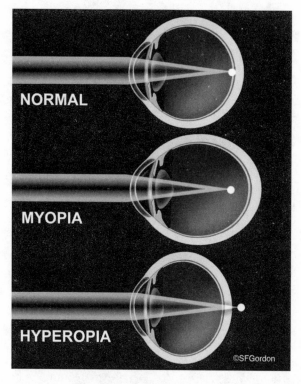

Figure 2. Reflective Errors

Hyperopia, known as *farsightedness,* is defined as seeing better at a distance than close up. This is especially true of younger people who still have *accommodation,* or focus, reserve. A farsighted individual has a short eye or a flat cornea, and doesn't refract, or bend, light enough so that the image is actually behind the retina. This blurred image can be focused on the retina by viewing an object far away or by constricting the ciliary muscle in the eye behind the iris, changing the shape of the lens and accommodating, or focusing, the eye. When the farsighted person gets older, his or her ability to accommodate dwindles, making unaided distance and near vision more difficult. (See Figure 2.)

Astigmatism is another type of refractive error corrected by glasses or contact lenses. The anatomy of the eye is different in every person. The eye's cornea, unlike the dome of a church, does not have the same curve in all directions, and an uneven curve is usually responsible for astigmatism. If light comes to a point because corneal curves are all nearly equal, there is no astigmatism. But if light is broken up such that, in the letter *T*, the horizontal top focuses differently from the vertical body of the letter, then there is astigmatism. Most people have a small amount of astigmatism, but it has no effect on their vision because the tear film neutralizes it.

Refraction—determining how well a patient sees and correcting to "best vision" with glasses or contact lenses—is the cornerstone of the ophthalmic examination. Over the years, the technology used to measure vision has become immensely more sophisticated. Still, getting a good refraction to achieve your best vision depends on the ability of your ophthalmologist or optometrist. There are three ways to refract: The objective method is used by your doctor when he or she shines light into your eye and neutralizes the refraction with hand-held or phoropter lenses (the big device that's put in front of your face when you look at the chart). The subjective method is the one in which you make the decisions of "Better, one or two?" after your present prescription or machine-generated refraction is put in front of you. The latest device, the Marco Epic system, combines methods one and two; it enables you to observe your current and previous prescription with both eyes at the same time. This expensive equipment has helped to standardize refraction but is not available in all doctor's offices.

As Mel Rubin, M.D., and Ben Midler, M.D., indicate in *How to Refract Without Making a Spectacle of Yourself*, there are also certain rules for correcting vision. If the eyes of a farsighted person are overcorrected, for instance, they will relax and lose whatever residual accommodation (focusing power) they had. If the glasses are too strong or the axis of astigmatism is corrected improperly, the glasses won't feel right. The doctor or optician may tell you to try them for a couple of weeks, but if the shoe doesn't fit, don't wear it. You should know right away if your glasses don't have the right prescription in them. If they don't, you may experience excessive tearing (weeping), dizziness, poor depth perception, tiredness, eyestrain, and/or headaches. Did you know that many prescriptions for eyeglasses are filled incorrectly?!

If a person has headaches and other problems from straining to see, then he or she needs his or her glasses corrected. Because this is not always obvious to the eye doctor, a dilated refraction (with short-acting eyedrops that dilate the pupil) is an important part of any exam: it will reveal the actual refraction of the eye. Without dilation, the nearsighted or farsighted patient can simply accommodate (actively focus on the eye chart) and not reveal the correct prescription needed. The art of refraction requires both the doctor's and the patient's participation. We still rely primarily on the patient's feedback to determine which lens is better.

Most people think that you get glasses if you cannot read 20/20 on the eye chart, but that is not necessarily the case. Glasses are not a medication—one dose does not fit all. The need for glasses varies, based on your occupation, your personal and lifestyle needs, and the amount of correction your eyes require.

While most people's vision does not change through the years, this is not true for everyone. Are you secretly farsighted? Have you become more nearsighted? Do you function well despite a new astigmatism? Answers to these questions come from your doctor asking you how old your prescription is, and not relying on the strength of an old prescription, or even on your history of wearing glasses. Again, a *dilated* eye exam will help determine the exact amount of correction a person's vision needs, because with dilated pupils, you cannot change focus through sheer effort.

Some doctors today believe their patients should change their eyeglasses prescription every six months. This may or may not be appropriate. Your eyes are different from every other set of eyes on the planet, so make sure your eye doctor is treating you as an individual. Most eye care physicians don't try to push the sale of glasses. (They are usually betrayed by their own avarice if they do.) If you are suspicious that your eye doctor is suggesting you change your glasses prescription more often than is actually necessary, seek a second opinion.

Children also have vision problems, with one child in four experiencing delayed progress or behavioral difficulties in school as a result. Squinting, rubbing the eyes, closing an eye, having an eye turn, tilting the head, placing the head too close to reading material, having a short attention span, avoiding reading or other close work, even having headaches and dizziness can be signs of a vision problem in a child. (For more on this subject see Chapter 12.)

Color blindness is also more prevalent than you might expect, with one out of eight Caucasian men and boys suffering some form of the condition. In contrast, only one out of thirty women and girls is colorblind. The condition occurs more frequently in boys because the ability to differentiate among all the colors is coded on the X chromosome. Since boys receive only one X chromosome (from their mothers), they are automatically color-blind if the gene for seeing color is defective. Girls, however, have two X chromosomes; therefore, both mother and father's X chromosomes have to contain the genetic defect for a girl to be colorblind. If the condition is mild, people may not recognize it. Other abnormalities of color vision include:

- Hereditary color blindness
- Optic nerve disease, past or present
- Progressive glaucoma
- Progressive macular degeneration or other retinal disease

Visual Field Examination

The *visual field examination* is often done at a separate time from the rest of the eye exam. It measures the responsiveness of the peripheral retina which does not have as many nerve fibers carrying information as does the center of the retina. The photoreceptors in the peripheral retina are *rods*, which are more scattered and thus less sensitive than the *cones* in the center of the retina. As a result, you see only larger and brighter images on the periphery. Visual field examination used to be done by moving a small white ball against a dark background in and out of the patient's line of vision. This technique has been replaced by electronic equipment that can print a computerized version of the visual field that can be compared from exam to exam. The equipment measures the patient's attention span, as well as the consistency, accuracy, and pattern of the patient's responses.

External Examination

In the *external exam,* the doctor scrutinizes the pupils, the lids, the lid margin, the lashes, the tear film layer, the opening of the tear ducts, and ocular motility.

Slit Lamp Examination

A *slit lamp* is the large piece of equipment you look into during the eye exam, placing your chin on a plastic chin rest and resting your forehead against the top of the machine. The slit lamp allows a 10-x magnification of the front portion of the eye to more accurately identify and treat common ocular conditions. Slit lamp examination and ophthalmoscopy are the two most important parts of an eye exam for the asymptomatic patient, as well as for the patient who is not seeing well.

Tonometry

Tonometry measures internal eye (intraocular) pressure, assesses risk for glaucoma, and should be part of a standard eye exam. Normal eye pressure is 10–21 mm of mercury. Erroneously high readings can occur when an individual is under tension, has a tight collar (a condition sometimes referred to as "executive glaucoma"), or high blood pressure. Measurements of eye pressure can also vary depending on the medications the patient takes or even on the time of day. Some people may have abnormally low readings after surgery because of low blood pressure or just because the cornea is more relaxed.

Ophthalmoscopic Examination

The doctor uses an *ophthalmoscope* to look into the eye. The health of the liquid inside the eye (the vitreous humor), the retina, and the optic nerve are assessed during ophthalmoscopic examination. The eyes are often dilated for this part of the exam, so that more of the inside of the eye can be seen. Examination with an ophthalmoscope can reveal hemorrhage (bleeding); vascular disorders (like an artery blockage that is starving the retina); growth of new blood vessels (which can indicate a tumor or overgrowth due to lack of oxygen); and many types of retinal disease. Detecting these serious conditions is only one of the reasons you should have a complete eye exam every year.

The retina, in the back of the eye, is best seen with the pupil *dilated* (that is, opened as far as possible with special eyedrops) so that the doctor can assess the appearance of the optic nerve, the *macula* (center of the retina), the blood vessels as they come through the optic nerve, and the peripheral retina. Although it's not possible to see the *rods and cones* (the photoreceptor cells), it is possible to find holes or tears in the retina.

A variety of techniques is used to look at the retina as well. These include: direct (with a hand-held ophthalmoscope) examination, indirect (when the light's on the doctor's cap and a lens is in his hand) examination, and lenses placed before the eye while you're seated at the slit lamp. Each of these techniques supplies different information.

Ask your eye doctor if he or she is performing a complete eye examination, including dilation of the pupil, so that you know whether to bring someone else along to drive you home afterwards.

Glasses

I find that, no matter what their age, nine out of ten patients who think their vision is going bad can have it improved by new glasses. Don't believe the myth that if you've abused your eyes by reading in low light, sitting close to the television, wearing an outdated prescription, not wearing glasses when you think you should have, or even working at a computer for long hours, you have ruined your eyes. You need to care for your eyes by getting them checked regularly and obtaining answers to your questions from a competent professional, as well as by paying attention to your total body health. You need to know what your best eyeglasses correction is before determining whether any deterioration in your vision has occurred and what its cause may be. Don't jump to the conclusion that your vision will diminish just because your mother had bad eyes, or your paternal uncle went blind—your vision does not have to deteriorate inexorably with age.

Remarkable improvements in glasses design have been made over the years. Lenses are now made from a variety of different materials (see Table 3), and many specialty lenses have been developed for fashion, function, or both. Today, lenses can be made for single vision, either distance or near. They can be *bifocal*, which means having two distinct areas, one in the top half of the lens for distance and the other in the bottom half for reading. Or they can be *progressive*, which means a gradual shift from the distance correction at the top of the lens to the close-up correction at the bottom, without a visible line dividing the two.

In choosing what type of lenses to have in your glasses, remember that they sit in frames that contribute to the weight of the glasses. Frames are made of plastic or metal (stainless steel, titanium, or nickel-based) and come in different styles, sizes, and colors. Frames must fit comfortably on the bridge of the nose, around the ears, and on the face. A good fit will create excellent vision without boundaries.

Presbyopia is the term for losing accommodation (focus power) in middle age. People begin to complain that the light is too dim, the print is too small, and their arms are too short for them to be able to read the printed page in front of them. This condition is not a disease, but a fact of life for which the optical industry has provided many options.

If you see well at distance, you don't need a bifocal and can wear half-lenses. People who are nearsighted and develop presbyopia can have bifocal lenses with a line, or can wear contact lenses with a different prescription for each eye—one for distance vision, one for close-range vision.

Progressive lenses provide another option for people entering the bifocal period of their lives—people ages 40–50 who not only need a prescription for distance vision but for close-up vision as well. Progressive lenses are designed so that the eye convergence moves along the same downward line as the increased power for reading. These progressive lenses have improved to the point that there is no line, as there is in bifocals, which is their major advantage. Their disadvantage is a smaller area for reading; however, there are over 100 lens designs in North America. These lenses require very careful measurement of the pupil for both distance and near. You have to demonstrate where you like to hold your reading material so that there won't be surprises. Despite these considerations, it's better for

Table 3. Glasses

Material	Advantages	Disadvantages
Glass	Most scratch-resistant; comes in many colors; absorbs infrared light; causes the least amount of distortion in vision.	Heavier than plastic or polycarbonate, and can shatter; must be treated with heat or chemicals to be more impact-resistant. Can be dangerous in sports.
Polarized (glass or plastic or polycarbonate)	Reduces glare from surfaces like water, sand, or snow; ideal for driving or outdoor activities.	Polarized glass is thicker and heavier than glass (or plastic) alone.
Polycarbonate plastic	Very impact-resistant; relatively light and thin; has built-in UV protection; safer for sports, but still lightweight enough for comfort.	Second-most expensive (after high-index plastic); soft; doesn't take dark tints well; gives slight distortion in higher powers.
Allyl resin plastic	Lightest material.	Inferior to glass in blockage of ultraviolet light; less scratch-resistance; thicker than other plastics.
High-index plastic	Blocks 100 percent of ultraviolet light; thinnest and lightest plastic. Reduces edge thickness (for nearsighted people).	Most expensive lens material; highly susceptible to scratches; may distort peripheral vision; can shatter.

people who refuse to wear bifocals to have progressive lenses than to neglect to correct their farsightedness. Progressive lenses are more expensive because of their design, and the cost takes into consideration that a certain percentage of lenses will need to be remade for free.

Aspheric lenses are ideal for moderately and extremely farsighted (hyperoptic) individuals. Aspheric lenses are also great for nearsighted people. Their special advantage is that, however serious the correction needed, the lenses remain relatively thin (a far cry from the Coke-bottle look of old).

Sports safety glasses are made of polycarbonate and are specially designed to provide maximum protection for athletes. (Polycarbonate plastic is the material used to manufacture compact discs and Plexiglas.)

Sunglasses

Everyone should have ultraviolet-blocking sunglasses to protect their eyes outdoors in sunlight. Polarized lenses are good, but they may not filter all the ultraviolet. Specifically, they do not filter damaging light in the infrared and blue ranges.

Sunglasses should block most UV light; an optometrist can check your sunglasses to see how efficient they are. Their tint should be uniform throughout (not gradient from top to bottom). You should make sure there's no distortion in the lenses by looking at a straight line (like the top of a door) through each lens while moving your head from side to side.

There are other lens options that don't protect the eyes from UV light as well but provide comfort in outdoor settings. Photochromic lenses change from light to dark, allowing the wearer to have dual functions with the same pair of glasses. The outdoor darkening is not 100 percent, and as the lens ages (after two or three years), it doesn't lighten completely. Chromophores (the molecules that block UV light) are also now placed in contact lenses as well as in intraocular lenses that are inserted after cataract surgery.

Antireflective coating can be placed on any lens (front or back surface) at the time you order your glasses or even afterwards. This is especially good for light-sensitive individuals to have on their indoor glasses, especially if they work under fluorescent illumination.

Even good sunglasses can allow UV light to enter from the side. For this reason, people with light-colored eyes or ocular disease should be especially careful and should consider wearing sun goggles that wrap around the entire eye area. People with a family history of macular degeneration and cataracts also need to be especially careful.

Who Should Wear Sunglasses?

You're an excellent candidate for sunglasses if you have even one of the following:

- Photophobia (light sensitivity)
- Light-colored irises (usually found in combination with fair skin)
- An outdoor occupation and/or recreational activities involving snow, sand, water, or high altitudes
- Ocular infection or iritis
- Cataracts
- Recently performed cataract surgery
- Macular degeneration

- Retinitis pigmentosa
- Family history of eye disease
- Prescriptions for photosensitizing drugs (ask your physician or pharmacist about your prescriptions)
- Tropical travel plans
- Common sense! If you're in very bright sunlight (during the summer, or at midday all year around), always wear sunglasses. You should even wear sunglasses on a bright, cloudy day, because UV light penetrates the cloud cover.

Contact Lenses

Contact lenses are much safer now than they were a couple of decades ago, but they are still not without risk. If misused, contaminated, or badly fitted to the surface of your eye, contact lenses can cause a number of sight-threatening conditions, including: corneal infection, infectious keratitis, and an altered eye surface. The newer forms of contact lenses, however, allow more exchange of air and fluids, and are made with UV blockers.

Contact lenses are prescribed primarily for nearsighted people, but also for farsighted individuals and those who are astigmatic. A complete eye exam is necessary before contact lenses are prescribed in order to:

- Determine the prescription (including measuring the corneal curvature) correctly
- Be certain there is no corneal or external eye disease
- Ensure that the eyes have adequate tear film
- Rule out any internal eye disease

You and your doctor (or fitting technician) should discuss your choices and reach a decision together on the type of contact lenses best for you. You should discuss the different types of lenses—those requiring daily sterilization versus the disposable kind—along with their cost and subsequent maintenance. Be sure to consider potential complications as well as the need for periodic eye examinations. (See Table 4.)

Soft contact lenses are available in many colors. Because the pigment in the lens blocks some oxygen transmission, these lenses must be removed daily. Never sleep in them. There are also cosmetic contact lenses that are very valuable in normalizing the appearance of disfigured eyes, such as a blind eye, an abnormal pupil, or a scarred cornea. Custom-made, hand-painted, hard and soft contact lenses are available to mask these disfiguring conditions.

Table 4. Contact Lenses

Type of Contact Lens	Advantages	Disadvantages
Rigid gas permeable (semi-hard)	Easy to care for; good for correcting astigmatism; cause few allergic reactions or infections.	Can slip off the center of vision more easily than soft lenses; require very accurate measurement; most people need to adjust to them by building up daily wearing time.
Soft lenses, daily wear	Stay in place better than hard lenses; can be disposable; may wear infrequently without adjustment time needed.	Vision may not be as sharp, depending on correction; may be uncomfortable for dry-eyed patients.
Astigmatic soft lenses	Allow people with astigmatism to wear soft lenses instead of hard ones.	These are tight lenses, and often do not move on the eye; for high levels of astigmatism, I recommend a rigid, semipermeable contact lens.
Soft lenses, extended wear	Less handling because of nonremoval, so less potential for contamination from hands.	Periodic cleaning or disposal is necessary; risk of complications, including infection, is higher; artificial tears or wetting solutions are required for comfort.

Optometrists have worked with bifocal contact lenses for years and have been frustrated by the fact that maybe one or two in ten is successful, a dreadful rate of success. Now there are new soft bifocal contact lenses that have more than a 50 percent success rate. This may not sound like a high batting average, but it is excellent considering the adjustment to placing something foreign in your eye and learning a new method of focusing at the same time. Given excellent fitting by your contact lens technician, optometrist, or ophthalmologist, you can successfully avoid glasses indoors. However, I would urge you to have sunglasses for your outdoor and recreational activities. If you have trouble wearing contact lenses, please wear glasses if that's what your eye care specialist recommends. Don't compromise the health of your eyes.

Some contact lenses are used for therapeutic purposes after cataract or refractive surgery. They can serve as bandages to protect and comfort the eye and can also deliver antibiotics directly to the surface of the eye, which avoids having to use injections around the eye. Therapeutic lenses are also used in certain corneal conditions, like abrasions and incisions— any condition in which the cornea needs to heal under the therapeutic contact lens without the eyelid constantly scraping over the corneal injury.

Complications from soft contact lenses include persistent redness, tearing, a conjunctival reaction under the lid called GPC, and potential infection. A serious complication can require the discontinuation of soft lenses; options for a person in this situation include wearing glasses, trying semi-rigid contact lenses, or having refractive (vision-correcting) surgery. Any of these options is preferable to chronically medicating the eye, which can prove toxic over the long term and have adverse consequences for vision. The use of soothing or numbing eyedrops of any kind is contraindicated if you are having a contact lens complication because they may mask important signs of eye irritation and potentially allow ulceration.

Ordering contact lenses by mail is very popular because it enables people to avoid costly eye exams. Unfortunately, one person in ten eventually develops a problem as a result of ordering contact lenses through the mail without seeing an eye doctor. The reasons range from changes in the configuration of the eye to conjunctival reactions to the contact lenses, which, if unattended, can cause not only discomfort but corneal ulceration. While it's efficient to do many kinds of shopping by mail order, under no circumstances would I recommend that anyone order contact lenses through the mail. Have your contact lenses fitted by an expert.

If your eyes show any sign of redness or infection, remove your contact lenses immediately and consult your doctor. Don't wear your lenses longer than medically recommended, and don't share or swap contact lenses (even nonprescription colored lenses) with other people. These are artificial devices which can become contaminated. It's always unwise to be cheap or careless when it comes to your eyes.

Your occupation and lifestyle may dictate what type of glasses or contact lenses is best for you. If it is appropriate for you, refractive surgery may increase the number of choices you have for correcting vision.

Refractive Surgery

People who are not happy with glasses and who cannot wear contact lenses but want to see better naturally now have an increased number of choices in refractive surgical procedures. Each individual must weigh the risks, benefits, and costs here, making sure they are satisfied, after a conversation with their ophthalmologist, that this is the right path for them to take. Remember that glasses and contact lenses have a cost over the years, too.

Before having any type of refractive surgery, a comprehensive eye exam is a must. The cornea, which surgery will change the curve of, needs to be evaluated carefully, as does the general health of the eye (see Chapter 5). In fact, contact-wearing pateints must not wear their soft lenses for three days or their hard lenses for three weeks prior to their eye exam in order to obtain an accurate measurement of the corneal curve. For proper healing after surgery, it's also essential that they avoid prescription soft contact lenses for weeks.

Using surgery to improve vision is not a new idea or even a new technique. As long ago as 1898, a German physician published a report describing using a controlled cut on the cornea to correct astigmatism. It probably had been known for a long period of time that any incision in the cornea reversed astigmatism. In 1953, Professor Hiroshito Sato in Japan started using this technique to flatten the cornea. It was effective, but eventually some corneas got hazy because he made the incisions from the inside as well as from the outside. His and other investigators' research formed the basis for *radial keratotomy* (RK), in which four to sixteen incisions are made in the cornea to flatten it, thereby correcting nearsightedness. As RK became more sophisticated, the optical zone, depth, and the number of the incisions was varied. A study called the "Prospective Evaluation of Radial Keratotomy" (PERK) evaluated the results over ten years and found that many patients who were between three and six diopters of nearsightedness experienced good results, although there was always a small incidence of overcorrections that were sometimes not obvious for several years.

RK has been performed since 1978 in the United States. Four to eight incisions are made in the cornea (based on long-standing formulas) to reduce nearsightedness; arcing incisions can be used to reduce astigmatism. After one year, the results are excellent for 90 percent of patients. Long term, there can be a weakening of the cornea and, with severe injury, a corneal tear can open. A number of people—perhaps as many as 25 percent—become farsighted over time. This procedure is cost-effective but should be performed with the goal of undercorrecting the vision, especially in those who are more than 40 years old, because there is a tendency for the procedure to increase its effectiveness over time. In other words, the amount of correction increases over the years after you have the procedure.

Photorefractive keratoplasty (PRK) has been done for many years in Europe and was approved by the Food and Drug Administration in the

United States in 1996. By 1998, over one million patients had been treated worldwide, and 25,000 had undergone successful procedures in the United States. The advantage is clear: the cornea is not weakened with deep incisions. Instead, an excimer laser is used to shave off cellular levels on the cornea. Long-term results show that from two to six diopters of nearsightedness can be easily corrected by this method. The laser can eliminate astigmatism at the same time. The excimer laser mixes two different laser crystals to create a wavelength in the UV range; this wavelength is absorbed by the cornea. The center of the cornea is shaved in rings, with deeper rings toward the center and shallower rings toward the periphery. This flattens the center of the cornea, thus reducing the nearsightedness. Lasering in the periphery of the cornea can be used to steepen the cornea to help reduce farsighted patients' need for glasses or contact lenses, but it is not quite as accurate.

One side effect of PRK is short-term discomfort. Another, less common, side effect is a visual haze that takes some time to decrease. Topical steroids (eyedrops) are required for four to six weeks after PRK.

Laser-assisted keratoplasty (LASIK) successfully treats up to 12 diopters of myopia. Instead of shaving the surface of the cornea (as is done in PRK), the corneal surface is cut; a flap (or cap) is reflected backwards; laser energy is applied beneath the base; and then the corneal cap is replaced. (The procedure is affectionately called "flap and zap.") The patient experiences very little pain, because the surface of the cornea remains mostly intact (unlike the patient's experience with PRK, in which the surface of the cornea is shaved). LASIK appears to be a better procedure for most nearsighted people and now is used for farsightedness as well. The complications of LASIK consist of transient glare and dry eyes. You must make sure you have a surgeon who is highly skilled and has performed many procedures. Ask what your surgeon's success rate is. Very occasionally, incisions don't heal properly and scar tissue (which interferes with sight) develops underneath the cap. Nonetheless, the risk-versus-benefit ratio is excellent. Because the corneal cap is replaced immediately, 95 percent of patients can see very well the day of surgery. LASIK has replaced other refractive procedures because of less discomfort and greater predictability.

Astigmatic keratotomy (and *photo astigmatic refractive keratoplasty*, or PARK) applies the principle of radial keratotomy in a transverse direction (instead of in a radial direction). Imagine taking the pleat of one's pants and making a cut across it, thereby reducing all the tension in that line. Astigmatic keratotomies can be effective in patients with high astigmatism after a cornea transplant (allowing six months after suture removal so the wound is stable).

Implantation of an *intrastromal corneal ring* (ICR) corrects vision using a completely different approach. The ICR is a sterile plastic ring that is surgically inserted into the cornea. The ring (which, after much research, has evolved into two arcs and is no longer an actual ring) encircles the peripheral cornea and flattens it to correct nearsightedness (just as shaving or cutting the cornea does). The advantage of the ICR is that it doesn't interfere with the center of vision, can be implanted quickly and inexpensively, and is completely reversible.

I began performing radial keratotomy, or RK, in 1980, so I have a broad perspective on the various techniques. If proper measurements (including corneal topography) are made, an RK can provide excellent short-term patient satisfaction. In fact, the satisfaction level is even higher than one would expect. While it is always possible with any of these techniques to lose a line of best-corrected vision after the surgery, most people are willing to take that very slight chance. As with any surgery, there are risks, but the procedure works exceptionally well for people who have small amounts of astigmatism, small refractive errors, stable refractions, and don't want to spend too much money.

The laser procedures are highly technical, expensive, and sometimes fraught with infrequent but unusual complications that may require repeat procedures. PRK is well standardized, less expensive, and causes more initial discomfort. LASIK is more expensive, has become the most popular procedure, and produces the least discomfort of these techniques. Most patients opt to do both eyes at once to shorten the time in which they may not see well (usually one to three days), which is certainly convenient and cost-effective in terms of losing work hours. Myopic patients may want to be less slightly myopic in their nondominant eye so that they can continue to read without glasses throughout middle age, for instance, and the ICR does not allow for that option. It is also important to remember that other conditions often occur in conjunction with myopia, including open-angle glaucoma, retinal tears, or retinal detachment. These potential problems do not disappear, even after the refractive error is normalized.

Intraocular Contact Lenses

The latest refractive prodecure about to become available places contact lenses inside the eyes of people who are very nearsighted. Both the material and technique appear to have been perfected, and may be available in the very near future. A foldable contact lens (made by Staar Surgical Co.) is placed behind the pupil (which is dilated while the surgical procedure is performed), but does not touch the lens of the eye.

A device that was granted an FDA investigational-device exemption (meaning that it can be used experimentally but is not yet available on the market) is the *Artisan Myopia Lens*, which is surgically implanted in the eye to correct very nearsighted vision. Invented by Dutch researcher Jan Worst, M.D., the Artisan Myopia Lens is inserted in front of the iris and held in place by being clipped onto the edge of the iris. Because the surgery is a relatively long one (between fifteen and twenty-five minutes), it is usually performed under general anesthesia. According to Maurice John, M.D., director of the John-Kenyon Eye Center in Jeffersonville, Indiana, and one of two U.S. surgeons allowed to implant the lenses, patients have a "magnificent quality of vision and they are extremely happy after surgery," as he told *Ophthalmology Times* in March 1998. Dr. John predicted that, after it gains full FDA approval, the Artisan Myopia Lens will replace LASIK as the procedure of choice for extremely near-sighted people. In my opinion, the Staar lens is a better choice.

I urge you to seek a well-trained specialist, preferably one with cornea training, and obtain all information about the choices available to you. Ask about the experience of the laser center's support staff and your surgeon's success rate. You will also want to know if he or she will be on call after performing the procedure to care for you if any problems arise. And be sure that your cornea is healthy before you undergo any of these procedures. Refractive procedures can change your life, so you must help assure that they change your life for the better.

Low Vision

It's important to know that even people with very poor vision, either from high refractive errors or scarring of their retina or cornea (as a result of diabetes, macular degeneration, corneal degeneration, or other diseases), may have options to see better. *Low vision* refers to the seeing ability of people who, even after correction, have less than "normal" vision (20/20 to 20/40). This reduced vision cannot be improved with conventional eyeglasses or surgery and interferes with daily life physically, psychologi-cally, and socially. Over twelve million Americans are considered to be visually impaired; only about 10 percent of that number are totally blind. Therefore, the vision of many people can be improved.

The tools that we use to increase vision in people who are classified as having low vision include: spectacle magnification; telescopes; increased light; enhanced contrast; training and adaptation for daily life; electronic magnifiers; and counseling.

For severely visually handicapped people, there is an optical device that can be placed over a book; the individual reader can choose the amount of magnification he or she needs. Obviously, if the magnification is very high, only a few letters at a time can be seen. This often frustrates people and leads to depression. Nevertheless, it allows people who were not able to read at all to have an option to read, however slowly. There are many options for low vision patients; doctors should be on the lookout for people who might benefit from them. We can help these patients with a selection of low vision aids and encouragement.

I have found that at least half of the people categorized as "legally blind" can be helped to enjoy a fuller life with low vision aids and counseling. Such patients are often regarded by ophthalmologists as a failure of their work, but people with low vision need to be able to participate in their family life and society. If you have a loved one who suffers from low vision, call your State Academies of Ophthalmology or Optometry to obtain help and referrals. (See Resource Guide.)

Future Options

Will we actually be able to make the blind see one day? Development of an artificial retina is under way at Johns Hopkins University and North Carolina State University, where researchers have invented a computer microchip that would act as a retina for people with damaged retinas. A tissue thin, delicate biochip is implanted in the retina, where it receives electrical impulses and forwards them to the brain, producing some sight in previously blind individuals. If perfected, the biochip could return at least some level of sight to the nearly one million Americans who have significant macular degeneration or retinitis pigmentosa. This fascinating therapeutic area is still very much in the experimental stage.

Mark Hallet, M.D., clinical director at the National Institute of Neurological Disorders and Stroke, has used PET brain scans to show that, when blind people run their fingers over Braille, the flow of blood to the visual cortex is increased, as if they were actually "seeing" the Braille. This research demonstrates how versatile the brain is in adapting to challenging circumstances. Researchers at the Technion Institute, in Israel, have demonstrated that, by employing visual imagery along with other vision aids, they can enhance vision in normal subjects. They are working now with people who have eye disorders.

British researchers are evaluating a camera worn as a hat that has an electrical connection to the occipital cortex in the back of the brain, allowing vision in people who are blind. These investigators are working on refining the image produced by this technology and reducing the long-term risk of infection.

I urge anyone who has friends or family members who are blind to make the most of life but continue to look for options to increase vision. Seek the help of special therapists who are familiar with the specific physical and emotional problems of people who are blind or have severely impaired vision. Ask your ophthalmologist for referrals.

CHAPTER 5

General Eye Health

A 24-year-old woman came to me complaining that her eyes were tiring very easily; she was worried that her eyesight was weakening. She had not previously been nearsighted, nor were either of her parents, but she now required a mild nearsighted prescription to achieve 20/20 vision. During her eye exam, I noticed that both eyes were slightly bloodshot. After talking to her about her symptoms and her life in general, I discovered that she works many hours every day at a computer. I diagnosed this young woman with a condition we call computer fatigue syndrome. *Researchers have found that focusing your eyes on one location and using your near vision for sustained periods of time—as this young woman was doing working at her computer for hours on end—may change vision, even causing some people to become nearsighted. Most eye doctors know that staring at anything without blinking frequently enough causes the eyes to redden and tire. Studies have shown that, when people are working at a computer, they don't blink nearly frequently enough to keep their eyes from drying out. I advised the young woman to begin taking frequent breaks from her computer (every fifteen to twenty minutes) and to focus her eyes at distance, instead of constantly using them for near vision. Making even very simple changes like taking frequent breaks while doing close work can reduce eyestrain and stop your vision from changing.*

Our eyes, like the rest of our bodies, want to heal themselves, and we can help them do so. By ensuring that our diet contains the proper nutrients, by protecting our eyes from ultraviolet light, chemicals, smoke, and air pollution, and by obtaining proper medical care, we can preserve our eyes—and the vision that's so precious to us—throughout our lifetimes.

We need to protect our eyes both from within and from without. Consuming adequate amounts of vitamins and nutrients will help support and strengthen them from within. Protective sunglasses and gentle care will help shield them from external damage. The eye and its surrounding areas, of course, are quite fragile. The skin under the eyes is particularly delicate, and shouldn't be rubbed. Makeup and eye creams, for instance, should be applied with gentle pats. Inadvertant tugging at the tissue under the eye can result in saggy eyelids as well as bags and wrinkles under your eyes later in life. Rubbing your eyes (when they're tired or itch) can induce swelling (inflammation) and breakage of small capillaries on the surface of the eyes, which can make your eyes feel *and* see worse than they did before you rubbed them. Rubbing the eye can also make tears thicker and intensify the burning sensation that often accompanies itching.

A black eye may look amusing in a movie, but it's no laughing matter for your vision. In fact, a black eye can result in permanently damaged vision, so it's wise to protect your eyes during exercise or outdoor activities like running, biking, or skating. Be alert, too, to the hazards that exercise equipment (at the gym or in your home) can pose to your eyes. Exercise bands—lengths of elastic between two handles that are used to strengthen leg, arm, and abdominal muscles—can cause severe damage to your face or eyes if the elastic recoils unexpectedly (if one handle is dropped, for example, or a foot or hand slips off the elastic). I suggest wearing polycarbonate plastic safety glasses, when appropriate, during exercise, sports, and outdoor activities.

How we use our eyes is directly related to their health and the vision problems we develop (or avoid). It's long been suspected, for instance, that there is a connection between constant close work and developing myopia, or nearsightedness. Researchers at the Primate Research Center at Washington State University tested this suspicion in monkeys whose eyes are very similar to humans'. They restricted the monkeys' vision to fifteen inches—that is, the monkeys weren't allowed to look into the distance. These monkeys subsequently developed nearsightedness, a condition that has not been observed in the wild. This may remind you of the saying, "Use it or lose it." The monkeys who were not allowed to use their eyes to look farther than fifteen inches into the distance lost their ability to see at a distance. If you don't use both your near and far vision, your eyes may weaken, as in the case of our simian friends.

People who spend most of their time outdoors—and presumably looking into the distance—experience very little nearsightedness. The vision tests performed on native Alaskans in the 1930s and again in the late 1960s bear this out quite well. In the 1930s, native Alaskans had no nearsight-

edness. But over the intervening forty years, their lives underwent momen-
tous changes; from living primarily outdoors, they began to live primarily
indoors. By the 1970s, 30 percent of Eskimo children—who lived much
more of their lives inside than their elders—had become nearsighted.

Various types of eye exercises, some as simple as taking a break to look
into the distance, may prevent or even cure mild cases of nearsightedness.
While some of my patients are children, most are not, and children
comprise the usual age group that develops nearsightedness. Adults—
especially those who work on computers, attorneys, accountants, and others who do a lot of close work—occasionally experience occupationally
related changes in refractive error. In response, I provide such people with
information and eye exercises. I, too, am keen to understand just how
well eye exercises, in fact, prevent or cure nearsightedness. Nevertheless,
staring far away to sharpen vision (by relaxing focus) has long been prescribed. In Nepal, herbal doctors advise people with eye problems to stare
at the moon. One-hundred-fifty years ago, our forefathers and -mothers
looked out at the horizon to forecast the daily weather—today, we turn
on the TV and sit close to it.

Although disagreements may persist over just how well looking into
the distance helps vision, one thing is obvious: the more close work we
do, the greater the strain we place on our eyes. Eyestrain, headaches, neck
and backaches, and other aches can result from close work. Until we learn
how best to prevent the stress and strain of modern life from tying our
muscles—particularly our eye muscles—into knots, we will continue to
suffer.

Coping with Eyestrain

What does "eyestrain" really mean? The achy sensation in the eyes
that people are describing when they say they've "strained" their eyes can
be caused by one of several conditions: (1) the inability of one or both
eyes to focus well; (2) the inability of both eyes to track together; or (3)
excessive continuous close work without a break. Only a good eye exam
can determine whether both eyes are centered in the same place or, for
example, if one of the six eye muscles is pulling on the eye a little differently
from others and causing the two eyes to be misaligned. Rarely, a more
serious problem can lead to eyestrain-like symptoms or headache. Headaches around the eyes can also produce symptoms similar to those of
eyestrain. Working under fluorescent lights can cause eyestrain as well as
other problems, including migraine attacks.

The symptoms of eyestrain include: redness, tearing, itching, swelling, burning, blurred vision, headaches, sensitivity to glare, difficulty adjusting to light, worsening of nearsightedness, and decreased concentration. Any of these symptoms can also be related to more serious diseases; each needs to be considered in the context in which it occurs.

Using your eyes intently for hours in an enclosed space without resting contributes not only to eyestrain but also to other health problems. When a person stares at one spot for a long period of time, the brain is focused on balancing everything—keeping the head, neck, and other parts of the body from moving. These days, people stare most intently at the computer screen. This is particularly hard on the eyes, because they're not looking at the entire screen, but only at microimages on it. In contrast, when you watch TV, you're following a panorama on the screen, which doesn't require the brain to be so fixated or the body to be so restricted.

Working at a computer for long periods at a time without a break can result in a condition called "computer fatigue syndrome," which encompasses a host of symptoms: eyestrain; heaviness of the eyelids (eye fatigue); blurred vision; flickering sensations in vision; and headaches. At the same time, neck and back pain can also develop.

It's important for anyone suffering from this ailment of modern life to take frequent breaks, focus on an object across the room, and remember to blink often. A 1997 study in the *American Journal of Ophthalmology* found that computer use is linked to decreased blinking and, therefore, to the development of dry eye symptoms, which can exacerbate eyestrain (see Chapter 11, to learn more about dry eyes and their treatment).

My recommendations for decreasing the eyestrain (and body strain you develop while working at your computer) include the following:

- Set up your computer correctly. The viewing distance from the screen to the eyes should be seventeen to twenty-six inches. The correct viewing angle is 10 to 20 degrees from midscreen to the top of the screen.
- Place reference material next to the screen, with the screen and reference material at the same distance from your eyes.
- Adjust screen brightness and contrast properly.
- Make sure overall room illumination is no more than three times brighter than the screen.
- Use a desk lamp, if possible, instead of an overhead light.
- Control glare from overhead lights and uncurtained windows. Use an anti-glare screen, set up a partition, or move your terminal to an area where glare is less of a problem.
- Rest your feet firmly on the floor. The upper thighs should not touch the supporting surface of the desk or computer table.

- Keep your wrists relatively straight while typing to avoid developing carpal tunnel syndrome (repetitive stress injury).
- Have your eyes examined annually—more often, if necessary. The National Institute of Occupational Safety and Health strongly recommends professional eye care for people who work long hours at computer terminals. Computer use and undiagnosed (or misdiagnosed) vision problems are a bad combination. Farsightedness, nearsightedness, astigmatism, eye-focusing disorders, and poor eye coordination may all worsen from using a computer inappropriately. In fact, studies have shown that people develop a delayed relaxation of the pupil and of accommodation (focus) after six or more consecutive hours of computer work. These eye-fatiguing symptoms may be accumulating daily.

In most cases, simple eyestrain should be treated with a strong prescription of common sense. If you are developing headaches (even migraines) from working too long at your computer without taking a break, schedule regular breaks; set an alarm to remind yourself to take them, if necessary. If the lighting in your work area is bothering you, talk with your supervisor about modifying it. If you haven't seen the eye doctor in a couple of years, schedule an appointment to find out if you need glasses (or a new prescription), or an antireflective coating applied to your current glasses. Unlike some eye conditions that are unavoidable, most cases of eyestrain can be prevented or eased by taking control of other aspects of life and work. Don't continue to suffer from an ailment that it is within your power to heal.

Headaches

Headaches can start in the eye. They can also move down the body and cause pain in other areas, so we must look for the eye's remote connections to them. For instance, a stress headache can make you clench your teeth, causing pain in the jaw joint (the temporomandibular joint, or TMJ), the neck, or the teeth themselves.

Headaches can also be caused by a physical imbalance, like one leg being shorter than the other, or always holding your briefcase in your right hand, both of which cause the body's muscles to be stretched unequally. A headache can also result from having a leg or arm in a cast, from a pulled back muscle, or from wearing high-heeled shoes for long periods of time, which tightens all the muscles in the body.

There are numerous different types of headaches, including: actual muscle pulls, tension headaches, migraine headaches, rebound headaches, cluster headaches, sinus headaches, TMJ-related headaches, and still others. Headaches are so common that they've become synonymous with life's routine problems.

Tension headache is caused by the contraction of muscles around the eyes, face, head, neck, and even the shoulders. Some tension headaches may be caused by an imbalance in some of the naturally occurring neurotransmitters or brain chemicals. Most tension headaches, however, are caused either by physical or by psychological stress (or a combination of both). In stress headaches, muscles constrict (usually in the eyes, face, neck, and back), causing referred pain in the head and/or eyes.

A study from the Johns Hopkins School of Public Health that surveyed 13,000 people by telephone found the following:

1. Women are 15 percent more likely than men to get tension headaches.

2. The age group most prone to headaches is 30–39-year-olds.

3. Some 38 percent of the people interviewed reported having a headache in the previous year.

4. People who developed headaches reported more lost work days and days of decreased effectiveness than people who reported never having headaches.

Cluster headaches, also known as histamine cephalgia, cause an excruciating stabbing pain on one side of the head around the eye or nose and may recur several times within a couple of days. While cluster headaches may occur as variants of migraine headaches, they may also be due to histamine release and therefore be related to allergic sinusitis. The supply of nerves to the head and face is so abundant that we can't always determine the cause of pain because it may be referred pain.

Sinusitis, or an inflammation of the lining of one of the eight sinus cavities, can cause a deep, dull, chronic ache around the eyes, nose, and be referred around the head as well.

TMJ pain, which may be caused by an imbalance in the teeth or jaws, results from a mechanical problem or muscle contraction around the joint where the lower jaw joins the face (on the side of the cheekbone in front of the ear). The nerve distribution in this area of the face is so abundant that one cannot always pinpoint where the pain first originated.

Rebound headache is classically due to the overuse of pain medication and even caffeine or sedatives to treat headache pain. When these substances' effects wear off, the headache rebounds, causing even greater discomfort. Rebound headaches tend to produce mild to moderate dull pain in the head, as well as somewhat diffuse pain over the forehead or back of the head.

Migraine headaches are particularly severe, even debilitating and do recur. I think of migraine headaches as miniseizures of the visual system. Research has shown that, during the aura phase of the migraine headache (when the migraine sufferer may see flickering lights or experience a premonition or "funny feeling") blood flow to the part of the brain governing vision (the occipital cortex) is reduced.

People who have severe migraine auras may experience "positive spontaneous visual phenomena" (PSVP), which result from an interruption of visual information to the brain and which can occur simultaneously with reduced blood flow to the brain. PSVP can be actual visual hallucinations (seeing people who aren't present, for instance), unstructured flashes of light, and structured flashes of light (which usually take geometric shapes). In the worst cases, PSVP can even produce a type of agitated delirium. As well as being associated with migraines, PSVP is associated with cataracts, retinal detachment, brain tumors, stroke, dementia, epilepsy, psychiatric disorders, and drugs. If you suddenly experience the symptoms of PSVP and have not previously suffered from migraine headaches, call your doctor immediately, so he or she can rule out the small chance that you have one of these other, more serious conditions.

At the beginning of a migraine headache, after the blood vessels constrict they dilate excessively, causing the extreme pain associated with migraines. Ergotomine, a product of fungus, is an old migraine treatment that constricts arterial blood supply to the brain, thereby reducing headache pain.

While often caused by stress, migraines can also be initiated by light pulsing at just the right rate. It's been my experience that these "ocular migraines" can be caused by light entering the eye at an angle and stimulating the peripheral retina (unless it's a strobe light, in which case it stimulates the entire retina). The peripheral retina then discharges electrical impulses perceived as flashes of light—as a type of aura. The retina's frequency of electrical discharge grows and then slowly fades over ten to forty-five minutes, leaving younger people with a migraine headache, which is sometimes accompanied by nausea and vomiting. Older people do not experience the same kind of headache. Instead, they tend to develop a "migraine equivalent," in which any postflashing headache or nausea is minimal or unrecognized.

Strobe lights or other visual effects may cause migraines or even seizures. In Japan, a 1997 TV cartoon broadcast featuring a strobe effect caused seven hundred child viewers to have seizures. Even fluorescent lights can cycle at a rate that makes vision very uncomfortable. If you work in an environment with fluorescent light that gives you migraine headaches, you might want to ask your employer to change from fluorescent to phosphorescent lights, which are less likely to have this effect.

People of all ages can develop migraines. In children, migraines often occur without flashing lights but with a funny feeling that precedes the headache. Childhood migraines can be associated with difficulties in relationships; in other words, the child is keeping emotions inside instead of expressing them. Interestingly, older people may see flashing lights for up to ten minutes, which often look like lightning or sparkling dots, but never develop a headache. Perhaps their blood vessels cannot dilate as widely.

No one knows for sure what causes migraines, but studies have suggested that a lack of the neurotransmitter serotonin in the brain is common among people who have migraine headaches.

In susceptible individuals, migraines can be triggered by many different foods and beverages. Every person has different triggers; if you have migraines, a number of these foods may be triggers for you (or none of them may be). Some of the most commonly reported migraine triggers include:

- *Sweets:* Refined sugars, chocolate
- *Fruits and nuts:* Carob, figs, raisins, peanuts, peanut butter, sunflower seeds, sesame seeds, pumpkin seeds, bananas, avocados, and tomatoes
- *Breads and cereals:* Yeast, yeast breads, cheese breads, sourdough bread, doughnuts, granola breads, and cereals
- *Meat and dairy:* Preserved meat, eggs, milk, butter, most cheeses, sour cream, and yogurt
- *Beverages:* Caffeine-containing drinks (coffee, tea, and colas) and alcohol, especially red wine that contains sulfites
- *Chemicals:* MSG (found often in Chinese foods or canned foods), oral contraceptives, estrogen replacement therapy, foods containing nitrites (like hot dogs and cold cuts), spices, and fried foods

While I was examining a patient, I noticed that his wife, Mary, had begun grimacing in pain. When I asked her what was wrong, she said that she was having one of her frequent migraines. In her case the migraine would begin with an aura and then, after about twenty minutes, develop into a severe headache with facial pains. She added that very few remedies relieved her pain. I asked if her neck and back were okay, and she replied that she'd had lumbar (lower back) disk surgery ten years ago. After I spent five minutes massaging her neck and back muscles vigorously, she was amazed at the relief she felt. She suddenly recalled that, six months after her back surgery she'd experienced pain from tightness in her back and neck and had found relief from a chiropractor who massaged her back and neck as I had.

I'm always surprised by patients who know the solutions to their own problems, but fail to use them. It's almost as if they'd rather be given a pill, because that's more acceptable in our society.

Conventional Migraine Therapy

Cafergot, a drug derived from fungi, has been the classic medication used to treat migraines for some time. Now in pill form (each pill containing 1 mg of ergotamine and 100 mg of caffeine), the usual dosage of Cafergot is two pills to start with, followed by an additional pill every half hour (not to exceed six pills in any twenty-four-hour period).

Other oral medications specific for migraine include: Migrinal (dihydroergotamine) and Zomig. Less specific oral medications include: Sansert; Midrin; Fioricet; Esgic-Plus; Phrenalin; and Inderal. You should determine which is most effective for you if you suffer from serious and/or frequent migraines.

An injection of Imitrex can stop a migraine quickly, but may need to be repeated. Imitrex is also available in tablet form. Pain management, with nonsteroidal over-the-counter drugs and prescription drugs like Fioricet or Darvon (or even prescription narcotics, in severe cases), is important. Being alone in a quiet, dark room can sometimes help.

Changing the hormonal cycle, like planning pregnancy or using natural estrogens and progesterones (soy), can sometimes interrupt the migraine rhythm. To prevent migraine recurrence, special combinations of drugs are sometimes prescribed. Ask your doctor about these.

Migraine headache drug development is a very active field of study because of the large percentage of the population that suffers from this debilitating condition, and new drugs to prevent and treat migraines enter the market regularly. As people age, migraine headaches generally become less significant and the attacks get shorter; the flashing lights that accompany the headaches also tend to be less prominent. If you suffer from frequent or severe migraines, you should be under the care of a physician. You should make every effort to identify the factors that trigger the symptoms because avoidance may be far more useful than treatment.

Alternative Migraine Therapy

The following alternative migraine therapies are well worth trying:

- *Magnesium* helps to counter spasms of blood vessels and muscle cramps. It is prescribed by doctors to treat heart and blood vessel diseases. Since vasospasm in the occipital lobe of the brain is associated with migraine, I recommend 500–1000 mg magnesium a day to avert migraine headaches by preventing vasospasm. It is certainly a simple and inexpensive solution that should be tried first, before resorting to prescription drugs.
- 5-hydroxytryptophan is a natural substance available in health food stores and is my first choice after magnesium to treat migraines naturally. Rizatriptan is a potent 5-hydroxytryptophan-type drug that has been found to be effective at 5 and 10 mg levels for acute migraines. To really knock out migraines, try both in combination.
- Herbs such as cayenne pepper, the bioflavonoid quercetin, and vitamin C can help prevent migraine recurrence.
- Try the Western herbs feverfew or stinging nettle. The active compound of feverfew (parthenolide) has been isolated but in a study in which the active compound was compared to the herb, migraine sufferers preferred the herbal remedy available at the health food store right now. This study should serve as a reminder that natural compounds like those found in the whole herb may be more effective because they contain many phytonutrients that may work together in ways we don't yet understand.
- By relieving tension, meditation and other stress-reduction methods can also be very beneficial in preventing migraine headaches.

To treat migraines naturally, I recommend combining the three M's: magnesium, medical detective work, and meditation. The fourth M, medication, should be kept in abeyance to use as a last resort.

If you have increasingly frequent and severe headaches, you should consult your doctor, even though most headaches are caused by stress or by using the eyes improperly (like staring at your computer screen for too long). While it's rare, headaches of increasing severity can signal dangerous conditions, including stroke or brain tumor.

There are other potentially serious disorders that can masquerade as headaches. Headaches caused by these disorders tend to be progressive, constant, and unaffected by light, food, head position, or work. Some of the conditions that can masquerade as common headaches are: high blood pressure; meningitis (which can produce a headache associated with a fever and stiff neck); intracranial aneurysm; blood vessel inflammations in the brain; and brain tumors (which increase the pressure inside the brain). These conditions often cause muscle weakness, double vision, blurred vision, mood changes, and even seizures—so you can see they are far more serious than any other kind of headache.

Improving Night Vision

In my ophthalmology residency, I learned that, with every decade of life, we lose 10 percent of our ability to adapt to the dark. In other words, failing night vision invariably accompanies the aging process. Yes, almost all the older people I talked with told me their night vision was not as good as it had been in their youth. Through my own research, however, I realized that difficulty in seeing at night does have a cause other than aging, and it is this: lack of proper nutrients for the eyes. In other words, declining night vision is a problem that you have the power to help resolve.

Bilberry, a bioflavonoid found in members of the grape family (including English blueberries), has a well-known positive effect on night vision; it helps the eye accommodate to changing light conditions more efficiently. Bilberry contains compounds that: (1) provide purple pigment to your retina (the rods) for night vision; (2) improve circulation in the blood vessels of the eye; and (3) work with vitamin C to strengthen collagen in the eye. Bilberry also prevents inflammation in the eye and has been found to have virtually no toxicity.

Bilberry can be obtained by eating purple grapes, cranberries, or blueberries. The purple pigments in bilberry-related species, the anthocyanosides, help strengthen the purple area of vision that controls adaptation from light to dark and the eyes' response to glare. Bilberry is widely available in supplement form, and is contained in many of the vision-supportive multivitamins. Nondiabetics can eat fresh or frozen blueberries or take the supplement. Diabetics, to avoid the extra sugar, should take the supplement instead of eating the berries. (See Chapter 15 for more information about the supplement.)

Vitamin A can also help improve night vision. Vitamin A is found in spinach and other dark leafy greens, carrots, sweet potatoes, apricots, and cantaloupes. Beta-carotene, the precursor to vitamin A, is found in similar foods. You can take vitamin A or beta-carotene as a supplement.

The Chinese have long known that, to heal the upper parts of the body (like the eyes), the upper part of the plant (like the fruit) should be used. Foods that are yellow (containing the carotene lutein) and orange (containing beta-carotene) help improve your day vision; the blue and purple foods (bilberry and red wine, as we will discuss in Chapter 14) are good for your night vision.

Having an antireflective coating put on your glasses can help reduce glare at night and sharpen your night vision. Any optometrist's office or optical shop should be able to add an antireflective coating to your glasses for a modest charge.

Inflammation of the Eyes

Any inflammation inside the eye is called *uveitis*. The uvea is the vascular, or middle coat, of the eyes. (The eyes' outer coat is composed of the cornea and sclera, and their inner coat is the retina. In the middle are the blood vessels that nourish the eye, pigments, and connective tissues.) When any structure in the uvea becomes inflamed (the iris, the ciliary body, or the choroid), the condition is called uveitis. Fortunately, inflammation usually occurs in the front of the eye, a less serious condition called *iritis*.

In uveitis, the patient may see "floaters" or complain of blurred vision as well as light sensitivity and redness (usually in only one eye). The eye doctor can see that the redness is usually just outside the cornea, and detects cells floating in the anterior chamber. These are either white cells (inflammatory cells) that have leaked out of blood vessels or pigment from the iris.

The most frequent cause of uveitis is trauma. Uveitis is usually self-limiting, although it should be treated to make the patient comfortable and to avoid future problems.

The next-most frequent cause of uveitis is unknown—that is, the cause is indeterminable. If you develop uveitis, however, don't despair of not finding a cause. As your own medical detective, you can start unravelling the clues. If uveitis is a recurrent problem, for instance, there are environmental or internal events you may be able to detect. Ask your doctor to help you, and make certain that he or she does.

The third-most common cause of uveitis falls into a group called *collagen vascular diseases*, which are known to affect connective tissues throughout the body. (These diseases include rheumatoid arthritis, systemic lupus, and polyarteritis.) Sarcoidosis, a disease of unknown cause that affects many organs (principally the lungs) and may involve the eyes, can cause uveitis. Uveitis can also occur as a complication of AIDS. Many people with uveitis and a multisystem disease like sarcoidosis have dry eyes as well.

Conventional Therapy for Inflammation of the Eyes

The conventional treatment of uveitis involves the prompt and intensive use of topical steroids. Throughout *The Eye Care Revolution*, I will remind you that the use of steroid eyedrops is a double-edged sword. This is especially true with uveitis, because the condition can lead to cataract, secondary glaucoma, and even retinal damage. Long-term use of steroids can also lead to glaucoma and cataract, so treating uveitis with steroids increases those risks.

In this case, however, I believe that steroids must be used initially to quiet the inflammation while we are trying to determine a cause. There is often so much redness, light sensitivity, and pain that we need to dilate the patient's pupil and relax the ciliary body with long-acting dilating drugs (such as Homatropine 5 percent twice a day, or Atropine 1 percent twice a day). The effect of these drops may last up to four days, so the patient must be alerted that he or she will experience a little more glare, may not be able to read well, and will have dilated pupils for that length of time.

Occasionally, the inflammation is so severe that a steroid injection beneath the conjunctiva is necessary. If iritis occurs in both eyes, or if the uveitis is in the back of the eye (posterior uveitis), systemic cortisone (pills) may be necessary for a short period of time because vision is threatened. Fortunately, cyclosporin eyedrops, which are generally used to stop corneal transplant rejection, can also be used to treat inflammation without the side effects of steroids. Because cyclosporin eyedrops produce a stinging sensation and are expensive, I use them as a second-line therapy. Nonsteroidal anti-inflammatory drugs (NSAIDs) are not as strong as steroids, and do not have much of a role to play in treating uveitis; some of my colleagues use them for chronic cases of uveitis to reduce the total amount of steroid drugs given over time.

Uveitis is short-lived in people who have suffered trauma, but it may recur when it is due to other causes. People with severe systemic diseases like those already discussed may require long-term treatment.

Alternative Therapy for Inflammation of the Eyes

When people require long-term treatment for uveitis, I worry about both the disease and the long-term use of steroids to treat it. In the past, like other eye doctors, I accepted the development of cataracts and glauocoma as sacrifices that had to be made to retain the vision of people with this condition. In the past five years, however, I have referred patients to Nai-shing Hu, O.M.D., my Chinese medical colleague in Wilmington, who has been able to reduce these patients' steroid use by treating them with herbal medications. Two of eight patients are off topical steroids altogether, and after six months, have been able to discontinue the Chinese herbs as well. These are individuals who've had inflammation of the eye for at least ten years. The other six were able to reduce the amount of medication they needed. I cannot promise that such an herbal therapy will be useful in every case, but I will tell you how to find a Chinese medical practitioner or other herbalist. (See the Resource Guide.)

Allergic Conjunctivitis and Red Eyes

Allergic, or *atopic*, conjunctivitis takes many forms (see Table 5). It may be acute; it may be subtle. It may be seasonal (one type is *vernal*, which means "spring"). It may even be associated with a skin allergy because the eyelid and conjunctiva (which lines the white of the eye and the underside of the lid) are skin-related tissues. Its symptoms include itching, swelling, burning, light sensitivity, or *photophobia*; tearing with watery discharge; and crusting and scaling of the eyelid skin, or *dermatitis*. Swelling and itching are the hallmarks of eye allergies. There are many causes of allergic conjunctivitis, including pollen, foods, eyedrops, chemicals, cosmetics, shampoo, or pets.

When we encounter an *allergen*—any substance we're allergic to—immune cells called mast cells release *histamine* into the surrounding tissues. This is why drugs that combat allergies are called *antihistamines*. The presence of histamine causes swelling and dilation of the blood vessels in tissue, which lead to all the symptoms of allergy—swelling, itching, and redness. Systemic allergic conditions like asthma, sinusitis, or chronic bronchitis only worsen allergic eyes.

Since the allergic response is created by histamine, the goal of treatment is to block its release before symptoms occur. This can be accomplished by several mechanisms, including the use of antihistamines to block the action of histamine after it's been released (these can be eyedrops or pills); drugs that block the mast cells' release of histamine; or even steroids like prednisone or cortisone. All these drugs have drawbacks, however. The best way to deal with an allergy is to identify the offending substance and try to rid yourself of it.

Many eye allergies are seasonal. Hay fever conjunctivitis is a very common type of seasonal allergic reaction caused by histamine release. It is usually related to increased pollen counts; its symptoms include itching, swelling, and sensitivity to light. It may stay with you for as long as three

Table 5. Allergic Eye Conditions

Condition	Description	Conventional Treatments
Seasonal allergies (rhinoconjunctivitis, mild atopic conjunctivitis)	Affect 15 percent of population; causes runny eyes and nose.	Antihistamines; vasoconstrictors; mast-cell stabilizers; NSAIDs; cortisone (for a limited time).
Atopic dermatitis-related eye findings	More severe than seasonal allergies, because symptoms are present all the time; affects 3 percent of all children; can include staph blepharitis, lash loss, and other effects of bacterial skin infection.	Steroids are really the only effective conventional treatment; avoidance of milk products.
Vernal (spring) allergies	Most severe, even disabling, in young people; worse in spring and summer.	Steroids; cyclosporine; surgery.
Contact lens-induced conjunctivitis	May have mechanical cause or be related to preservatives in contact lens solutions.	Switch to semirigid gas-permeable lenses or disposable lenses; change solutions.
Contact allergies	Caused by soaps, shampoos, eye makeup, hair sprays, skin lotions, or iatrogenic (prescription eyedrop).	Discard offending product; use steroid treatment if necessary (for a limited time).
Chemical toxicity	May have any one of a number of sources, including air vents and eyedrop preservatives.	Determine and remove offending chemicals; treat irritation as required.
Dry eyes and pollution	Both increase susceptibility to irritation.	Hydrate with artificial tears; plug eyelid opening into the nose (punctal occlusion).
Staph blepharitis	Lid bacteria release enzymes that cause tiny peripheral corneal ulcers and itchy eyes.	Improve hygiene; topical erythromycin (antibiotic) eye ointment.
Uveitis (intraocular)	Remote causes, including sinus, tooth, bowel, and joint involvement.	Requires medical workup.

seasons of the year, but it should diminish or disappear during the winter months (depending upon where you live and how long you've lived there). Table 5 lists some of the common types of allergic conditions that can affect the eye. While a skin allergy that affects the eye *(atopic dermatitis)* can be related to pollen, it can have other causes, too, including foods. Therefore, this type of red-eye condition may occur in every season, and may be more severe than seasonal allergies. That's why Tables 6 and 7 note that the conventional treatment may be with steroids (an eyedrop and sometimes systemic steroids), despite the danger of side effects.

Vernal (i.e., spring) allergies often occur in teenagers. They frequently

Table 6. Treatment of Allergic Conjunctivitis

Drugs Available Over the Counter (Listed from Weakest to Strongest)		
Description	*Commercial Name of Drug*	*Format*
Artificial Tears		Eyedrops
Mild Vasoconstrictors	AK-Nefrin	Eyedrops
	Allerest	Eyedrops
	Clear Eyes	Eyedrops
	Collyrium	Eyedrops
	Degest2	Eyedrops
	Efricel	Eyedrops
	EyeCool	Eyedrops
	Isopto Frin	Eyedrops
	Murine Plus	Eyedrops
	Naphcon	Eyedrops
	Naphazoline	Eyedrops
	Ocuclear	Eyedrops
	Oxymetazoline (0.025%)	Eyedrops
	Prefrin (tetrahydrozoline 0.5%)	Eyedrops
	Relief	Eyedrops
	Tear-Efrin	Eyedrops
	Tetracon	Eyedrops
	Vasoclear	Eyedrops
	Vasocon	Eyedrops
	Velva-Kleen	Eyedrops
	Visine	Eyedrops
Decongestant astringents	Clear Eyes ACR	Eyedrops
	Preferin-2	Eyedrops
	Vasoclear A	Eyedrops
	Visine A.C.	Eyedrops
	Zincfrin	Eyedrops

Table 6. Treatment of Allergic Conjunctivitis (cont.)

Drugs Available by Prescription Only (Listed from Weakest to Strongest)		
Description	Commercial Name of Drug	Format
Vasoconstrictor/antihistamine combinations	AK-Con	Eyedrops
	Albalon A	Eyedrops
	Naphcon-A	Eyedrops
	Opcon-A	Eyedrops
	Prefrin-A	Eyedrops
	Vasocon-A	Eyedrops
Topical antihistamines	Emedine	Eyedrops
	Livistin	Eyedrops
Mast cell stabilizers	Alomide	Eyedrops
	Opticrom	Eyedrops
	Optivar	Eyedrops
	Patanol	
	Zaditor	
Nonsteroid anti-inflammatory agents. These drugs block one arm of the inflammatory pathway.	Acular	Eyedrops
	Ocufin	Eyedrops
	Profenal	Eyedrops
	Voltaren	Eyedrops
Corticosteroids (mild to moderate). These drugs block both arms of the inflammatory pathway and suppress inflammation.	Alrex	Eyedrops
	Flarex	Eyedrops
	FML	Eyedrops and Ointment
	FML Forte	Eyedrops
	HMS	Eyedrops
	Inflamase Mild	Eyedrops
	Pred Mild	Eyedrops
	Vexol	Eyedrops
Corticosteroids (strong). These drugs suppress inflammation but have potential complications	Ak-Pred	Eyedrops
	Decadron	Eyedrops and Ointment
	Inflamase Forte	Eyedrops
	Lotemax	Eyedrops
	Maxidex	Eyedrops and Ointment
	Pred Forte	Eyedrops

Patients should find the weakest possible strength for over-the-counter formulas that work for them. Prescription formulas are unique to each individual according to his or her symptoms. Discuss the choice of prescription drugs with your ophthalmologist.

Table 7. Antibiotic/Steroid Combinations

Description	Commercial Name of Drug	Active Ingredients	Format
Mild antibiotic/steroid combinations used to treat conjunctivitis	Cortisporin	Hydrocortisone, Neomycin, Polymyxin B	Eyedrops
	FML-S	Fluoromethelone, Sulfacetamide 10%	Eyedrops
Mild antibiotic/steroid combinations Used to treat allergic blepharitis and low-grade infections involving a strong conjunctival reaction	Blephamide	Prednisolone 0.25%, Sulfacetamide 10%	Eyedrops and Ointment
	Isoptocetapred	Prednisolone 0.25%, Sulfacetamide 10%	Eyedrops and Ointment
	Metimyd	Prednisolone 0.5%, Sulfacetamide 10%	Eyedrops and Ointment
	Polypred	Prednisolone 0.25%, Neomycin, Polymyxin B	Eyedrops
	Vasocidin	Prednisolone 0.25%, Sulfacetamide 10%	Eyedrops and Ointment
Strong antibiotic/steroid combinations Used to treat severe intraocular and corneal disease	Maxitrol	Dexamethasone 0.1%, Neomycin	Eyedrops and Ointment 0.05%
	Neodecadron	Dexamethasone 0.1%, Neomycin	Eyedrops and Ointment 0.05%
	Neodecair	Dexamethasone 0.1%, Neomycin	Eyedrops
	Pred-G	Prednisolone 1.0%, Gentamicin 0.3%	Eyedrops
	Storz ND	Dexamethasone 0.1%, Neomycin	Eyedrops
	Tobradex	Dexamethasone 0.1%, Tobramycin 0.1%	Eyedrops and Ointment 0.05%

cause large bumps on the conjunctiva of the lid and on the whites of the eyes. This condition can be very difficult to treat because of its severity.

It is ill-advised for allergy sufferers to wear contact lenses during the allergy season. Furthermore, a condition known as *giant papillary conjunctival hypertrophy* (GPC) can develop during allergy season in people who wear soft contact lenses. GPC is caused by the edge of the lens chafing the conjunctiva underneath the upper lid, giving rise to bumps known as papules that look like an allergy. For a long time, it was thought that this was an allergic condition, but it is now felt to be more of a mechanical one, since discontinuing soft lens wear makes the condition disappear. Treatment is simple: switch to the smaller, semirigid gas-permeable lenses.

If you wear contacts and are experiencing an eye allergy, you could be having a bad reaction to the combination of your contact lenses and topical medication (or its preservatives). Additionally, pollens can stick to contact lenses, worsening the situation. Remember that contact lenses are foreign bodies in your eyes, and you may have to restrict wearing them during allergy season. My recommendation is to wear the semirigid gas-permeable lenses if you have allergies, because they don't pick up as much pollen as soft lenses. I also recommend trying a mast-cell stabilizer (Alomide, Patanol, or Chromolin) for basic therapy, with two or three days of topical steroids, to quiet the eye so the other drops can work properly. One of my partners, Andy Barrett, M.D., calls steroids used this way "pulse steroids," because they're given in a short burst that doesn't allow development of dependence or side effects. If you cannot wear any contact lens because of your allergies, your options are to return to wearing glasses or to have refractive surgery. (See Chapter 4.)

Other environmental compounds we often neglect to think of as provoking an allergy can also suddenly cause red eyes. Soaps, cosmetics, shampoos, and eyedrops may cause this kind of contact allergy. Other chemicals, dirty air vents, dust, molds, food preservatives, and pesticides may elicit similar allergic reactions, as well as possessing their own chemical toxicities.

Other allergic reactions that eye doctors may see include uveitis (inflammation inside the eye, as discussed above) and cornea-transplant reaction. These conditions have symptoms similar to those of the allergies described here, but usually also cause a decrease in vision and marked eye redness. The allergic response is different in these two case, because it is a reaction to a foreign protein (the transplanted cornea a patient receives contains foreign protein). People can develop cornea-transplant reactions after receiving transfusions, flu shots, or other vaccinations (see Chapter 10).

If you have eye symptoms of pain, redness, tearing, and itching, it's important to be sure you don't have severe sinusitis (an inflammation of the sinus cavities that can occur with allergies). Sinusitis can cause swelling and pain in the brow, forehead, cheeks, teeth, and behind the eye. If you experience these or other symptoms that worsen rapidly, or any vision loss (including partial vision loss), call your doctor immediately.

Conventional Therapy for Allergic Conjunctivitis

Many people either do nothing to treat allergic conjunctivitis, or use an over-the-counter antihistamine or vasoconstrictor. If they obtain relief from their symptoms, as three-quarters of people do, they generally continue to use the same over-the-counter drug. What most people don't know is that, over a period of months, the eyes can develop a "rebound redness" after the effects of these drugs wear off. In other words, the

redness can come back. Nevertheless, topical vasoconstrictor and antihistamine drugs can play important roles in managing seasonal allergies.

Over-the-counter lubricant eyedrops, such as artificial tears, can reduce
some of the itching and redness associated with allergic conjunctivitis.
There are three types of artificial tears: preserved, transiently preserved,
and nonpreserved:

- *Preserved tears* are slightly toxic. Frequent administration can
cause problems in people with disturbed corneal surfaces. Patients with
severe dry eyes, a recent corneal transplant, or recent refractive surgery
should use one of the other two types of tears.
- *Transiently preserved tears* have preservatives that degrade upon
contact with either light or the patient's eye. They can be minimally
irritating, but are more cost-effective and convenient than nonpreserved
tears. Transiently preserved tears include Refresh Tears and Gen Teal.
- *Nonpreserved tears* are packaged for single-dose administration (to
avoid bacterial contamination and to decrease all toxicity), and so are
more expensive. There is also a nonpreserved version of Refresh Tears.

I recommend trying transiently preserved tears first because they are
less toxic than the regular artificial tears and less expensive than the
nonpreserved artificial tears packaged in individual doses.

Vasoconstrictor eyedrops (such as Murine, Visine, Naphcon, Vasocon,
Albalon) constrict blood vessels and so whiten the eyes (i.e., remove the
redness) but, with long-term use, the redness returns. It doesn't make
much sense to me for people to use these eyedrops alone, because they
relieve swelling but not itching. There are better choices of eyedrops that
relieve both itching and swelling. (See Table 5.) If you have an over-the-
counter eyedrop, read the label to see what's in it, and ask your doctor
or pharmacist if this type of eyedrop is helpful for your condition.

Antihistamine eyedrops act by decreasing the histamine response that
caused the redness and swelling in the first place. Examples of antihistamine eyedrops are Naphcon-A, Vasocon-A, Albalon-A, Livistin, and the
new Emedine. These antihistamines are appreciated by both patients and
general practitioners because they are effective in decreasing redness,
swelling, and itching in about ten minutes. Likewise, combining a decon-
gestant (a vasoconstrictor) and an antihistamine further helps control
allergies in the short term by causing constriction of blood vessels in
addition to decreasing histamine production.

Mast-cell stabilizers are the most popular type of drug with ophthalmologists because they stop the mast cells from releasing histamine in the first

place. Mast-cell stabilizing eyedrops include Chromolin (Opticrom and Crolon) and the stronger and more rapidly acting Alomide. A newer drug on the market is Patanol, which can both block histamine release and mop up the symptoms because it has an antihistamine effect. Some ophthalmologists still prefer to recommend a separate antihistamine drop, such as Livistin or Emedine, along with Alomide. This alleviates the swelling after it has occurred, which mast cell suppressors do not.

Nonsteroidal anti-inflammatory drugs (NSAIDs) can also play a role in reducing allergy symptoms. These include Acular, Ocufen, Profenol, and Voltaren. The NSAIDs block half the anti-inflammatory response that steroids do, without steroids' serious side effects (including possible cataract formation). None has been approved for use with contact lenses.

Steroid eyedrops are the cornerstone of treatment for all symptoms of eye inflammation (redness, irritation, and itching), including allergies. I must sometimes treat my patients with steroid eyedrops for a short period of time, but I advocate prevention and other methods of treatment for the long term. Steroid eyedrops suppress not only inflammatory cells and swelling, but also scar formation and wound healing. The operative word here is *suppress*; steroids do not cure. To cure the condition, we have to look deeper. It is unwise for people who wear contact lenses and have red eyes to renew their prescriptions for topical steroids because they will generally do just about anything to continue wearing their contact lenses, including overusing the drops. Because of their many negative side effects, I advise using steroids on a "pulse" basis (that is, taking just a short course of steroid eyedrops over a very few days) until the other eyedrops being used can accumulate in the patient's system and have an effect on the ocular allergy. (The side effects of topical steroids are discussed in Chapter 6.)

Nasal steroid inhalers are useful in blocking allergic reactions, and allergists rely on them heavily. However, the eye side effects of all types of steroids—including inhalers—include cataracts and elevated intraocular pressure (a risk factor for glaucoma). Therefore, I use them for as short a period of time as possible (hopefully, no more than one week).

Systemic corticosteroids (like Medrol and Prednisone, in pill form) are used to treat asthma and anaphylactic shock. Because these conditions can be life-threatening, we have no choice but to use these very powerful drugs, despite their dangerous side effects. Steroid pills can also be used to treat severe allergic conjunctivitis and poison ivy. I can't repeat too many times, however, that prolonged use of any form of steroid drugs carries a risk that cataracts or glaucoma will develop. I suggest trying other means of controlling the allergy first, and then, if steroids are absolutely required, limit their use. The steroid pills used most often are: Prednisone,

Medrol, Decadron, and Aristocort. I, like most ophthalmologists, prefer to prescribe Prednisone only when an oral steroid is absolutely necessary. Prednisone is preferred because its oral dose is more easily fine-tuned.

My colleagues suggest treating allergic conjunctivitis with *systemic antihistamines and decongestants.* However, unless the allergic reaction is very severe or there is sinus involvement, I don't believe in treating the eye with something that circulates throughout the entire body and may have side effects. If the patient has sinus symptoms and a runny nose, then antihistamines are useful. Additionally, treating symptoms by preventing histamine release (with systemic antihistamine pills) often causes drowsiness. Thankfully, manufacturers have now formulated nondrowsy antihistamines like Hismanal, Zyrtec, and Allegra.

Epinephrine (adrenaline), which can be administered only by injection, is used to treat asthma and a life-threatening allergic reaction called anaphylaxis, which can occur when you've previously been exposed to an allergen. For example, my partner Harry's wife was stung by bees and had such a violent allergic reaction that she nearly developed anaphylaxis. She now carries a pen containing injectable epinephrine, called Epipen, to restart her heart in case she is exposed to bee venom again.

Cyclosporin, a powerful anti-inflammatory drug, was originally developed to prevent rejection of transplanted organs (heart, liver, kidney, and lung). In pill form, Cyclosporin is also used to prevent cornea transplant rejections. A study published in 1997 showed that Cyclosporin A was totally effective in three out of four patients treated (at a dose of 3–5 mg per kilogram weight daily for twenty-two to forty-eight months) for cornea transplant rejection response. The fourth patient had partial resolution of symptoms. This drug must be monitored carefully, because one patient developed kidney failure that disappeared only when the drug dosage was reduced. Topical Cyclosporin may be helpful for very serious allergic conjunctivitis that has not responded to other therapies. It has now been developed in eyedrop form as an alternative to steroid eyedrops.

And finally, just a reminder: It's wise not to use any eyedrops, which constitute a very concentrated form of a drug, during pregnancy without your doctor's knowledge and permission.

Many of my patients prefer conventional therapies to deal with the misery of allergic reactions and, if that's what makes them feel better, that's what I give them. There are alternative therapies for treating allergic conditions, however, that other patients are eager to explore.

Deeper Investigation and Natural Therapy for Allergic Conjunctivitis

Diet and supplementation play important roles in preventing and treating allergic conjunctivitis. Food allergies to flavorings, colorings, and preservatives (like sulfites, which are used to keep lettuce crisp) may be factors in allergic conjunctivitis. A severe allergy to carmine, a natural red dye used in cosmetics, food, beverages, and medicine, has been reported to cause not only eye itching but occasional anaphylactic reactions. Carefully read the labels on the foods, beverages, medicines, and cosmetics you buy carefully. Some of my patients have discovered that adopting a vegetarian diet (the fat of meat can contain toxins and heavy metals) and eliminating certain allergens can be quite helpful. Middle ear infections, eczema, sinus disease (as I noted above), and many allergic eye conditions are related to food allergies or reactions to chemicals used in processing foods. Dairy and wheat products are the two items that most frequently cause these conditions to flare up.

It's important to recognize that food allergies are extremely subtle and present in a number of remote ways, including puffy eyelids, sinusitis, and headaches. James Breneman, M.D., found a 100-percent success rate in curing gallbladder attacks by eliminating allergenic foods from his patients' diets. Alan Gaby, M.D. and Jonathan Wright, M.D., have instituted the same type of protocol and found that it works.

I prescribe conventional therapies (of which there are many) if they are necessary to treat allergic conjunctivitis in the short term. I prefer to use alternative methods, such as diet and supplementation, for long-term treatment whenever possible.

I've discovered that the adrenal glands are very important in maintaining eye and body health. Providing support for the adrenal glands while relieving stress (an important complement) is an excellent path to follow. Supplementation here includes taking a B vitamin complex (B_6 and B_{12}, especially) and vitamin C (start with 1 gram [1000 mg] a day and slowly work up to 3 grams a day). If increased amounts of vitamin C give you diarrhea, cut back until you find a dosage you are able to tolerate. Combining these vitamins with bioflavonoids is useful in suppressing allergic conjunctivitis. Quercetin, which comes from red onions and garlic, is available in supplement form as well: take 1000 mg a day. Quercitin is a powerful anti-inflammatory—perhaps even more so than bilberry. If you take quercitin, combine it with vitamin C and cayenne pepper.

My other recommendations for naturally combating allergies are:

- Drink filtered or bottled spring water.
- Supplement with essential fatty acids, 500 mg twice a day with a meal and a fat-soluble vitamin.
- Supplement with antioxidants, including vitamin C, Quercitin, and/or bilberry, as discussed above.
- Consume five to ten servings of vegetables and fruits per day.
- Avoid packaged foods, which contain unnecessary (and sometimes hidden) chemicals and transfats that may contribute to your allergies.
- Take an alpha lipoic acid supplement, 100 mg daily. Try it for a month, and then, if it hasn't eased your allergies, stop taking it.
- Use olive leaf extract.
- Take a combination of Chinese herbs. After therapy with Chinese herbs, ten of my patients ended their dependence on topical steroids for their eyes. Amazingly, their asthma and skin conditions also cleared up without the need for antihistamines, systemic steroids, or inhalers.

Floaters and Flashes

Floaters—the little dots that seem to drift around in the fluid of the eye (the vitreous humor)—are common in people over the age of 50 who have experienced some trauma to the eye. Any significant blow to the eye region during a car accident or ball game, for example, can cause floaters to form. A lifetime of other natural wear and tear—such as heavy lifting, coughing, vomiting, straining at the stool, or actually rubbing the eyes—may also lead to changes in the vitreous humor, even if, at the time, such actions don't seem to have serious impact on the eyes.

The vitreous humor has a fibrous portion lining the eyeball; the inner portion of the vitreous is more liquefied. During fetal life, there are blood vessels and cells in the vitreous, and some of them may remain after birth. Occasionally, the entire artery nourishing the back of the lens (the hyaloid artery) remains inside the vitreous after birth. Such leftover blood vessels and cells cause the mild shadows in the vision that we call floaters. (See Figure 3.)

Floaters can be annoying or distressing. Nearsighted people almost always have a certain number of floaters because of the shape of their eyes. In older people, the vitreous transforms from a gel to a more liquid form (a natural change that everyone experiences), and any cells left in the eye become freer to move about, and so are more visible. The number of floaters, therefore, can increase with age.

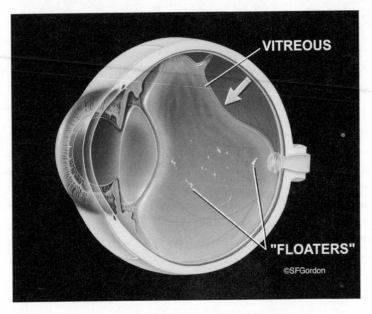

Figure 3. Floaters and Vitreous Detachment

Flashes can appear as lightning, or as vertical or crescent-shaped lines of light. They primarily appear when you are in a dark room (or outdoors in darkness).

Although floaters and flashes are usually harmless, they may be frightening. You should be aware, however, that they can indicate the presence of a serious condition that requires immediate treatment, including posterior vitreous detachment in which the flashes are continuous and the number of floaters increases dramatically. Call your eye doctor immediately to be certain.

Posterior Vitreous Detachment (PVD)

Posterior vitreous detachment (PVD) is usually a benign event that you don't have to worry about. After PVD occurs, you can expect to see a sudden emergence of one or more floaters—usually C-shaped or circular squiggles best noticed in bright illumination, while looking at the horizon, or reading a glossy magazine. Both floaters and flashes can continue to proliferate for ten days after PVD occurs. This passes quickly. The floaters tend to stabilize and disappear within a month or so. If they don't disappear, they may be a sign of a more serious condition.

If the floaters increase, or the flashing is continuous, immediate examination is necessary. Flashes are similar to the "stars" or shimmering light people see when they stimulate their eyes by rubbing, and they are usually simply a normal sign of electrical stimulation of the retina. But when these lights are present without manipulation of the eye, it's imperative to consult an eye doctor for a dilated-eye exam immediately.

While approximately 98 percent of the people who have floaters have a harmless type of vitreous detachment, some 1% to 2% may have hemorrhage in the eye, infection (with inflammatory cells in the eye), a tear in the retina with pigment or retinal detachment.

If you have any of the following symptoms, you *must* see an eye doctor within twenty-four hours.

- Flashes of any kind
- Blurred vision
- New floaters
- Distortion in vision
- Cobwebs or veils in the vision
- Double vision (diplopia)
- A curtain descending over the vision

Following is a list of risk factors for flashes, floaters, and possible retinal detachment:

- Nearsightedness (myopia). The elongated, or nearsighted eye can be thought of as "stretched," making the retina thinner. This means that it's easier for the retina to become detached than it is in an eye that is not elongated or stretched.
- Uveitis (inflammation inside the eye).
- Previous eye trauma (injury).
- Intraocular infections.
- Spontaneous tearing of the retina.
- Previous intraocular surgery, especially cataract surgery and YAG laser surgery.
- PVD in the other eye (having it in one eye puts you at higher risk for having it in the other eye).

Diagnosis of Retinal Detachment

A direct ophthalmoscope is probably not adequate to diagnose serious posterior vitreous detachment, since it is not the only cause of floaters. Indirect methods—such as using a contact lens or a lens held very near the eye to look as far out in the retinal periphery as possible—are required. Most ophthalmologists are accomplished at looking for tears in the peripheral retina, since they are so common. If your ophthalmologist is uncertain of the diagnosis, consult a retina specialist, who can also oversee your treatment. If your ophthalmologist cannot see the peripheral retina well enough, he or she should refer you to a retina specialist immediately.

Once all of the retina is visible, the situation becomes evident. Even if there is no tear in the peripheral retina, follow-up dilated-eye exams should be performed again in three to four weeks, since the symptoms may signal an ongoing problem.

While this may seem like a lot of extra examinations, they are vitally important to prevent any tear in the eye from developing into a retinal detachment. Retinal tears often precede retinal detachment—in which the retina actually pulls away from the back of the eye—a much more serious phenomenon that can cause vision loss.

Treatment of Retinal Detachment

If a tear or hole in the peripheral retina is diagnosed early, it can be treated by either argon laser or freezing (if it's diagnosed early but is too large to be treated by laser).

If the retina becomes completely detached from the back of the eye (that is, if the retinal tear has not been diagnosed early enough to prevent detachment), a gas bubble can be placed in the eye for several weeks to encourage the retina to reattach to the back of the eye. The gas bubble expands after it is inserted inside the eye, holding the retina in place, while the gas itself is slowly absorbed. This therapy, however, can be used only if there is a single hole or tear and if not much fluid has accumulated between the retina and the back of the eye.

Scleral buckle surgery is the standard treatment for a detached retina, with the patient undergoing general anesthesia (instead of local), if appropriate. The success rate for retinal detachment surgery is high.

It's occasionally necessary to perform a *vitrectomy*, in which the vitreous fluid adhering to the retina is removed in conjunction with either the scleral buckle surgery or gas infusion.

Vision should not be diminished if the central portion of the retina (the macula) is not detached. Early diagnosis and referral to a retina specialist is crucial to preserving vision when a retinal tear occurs.

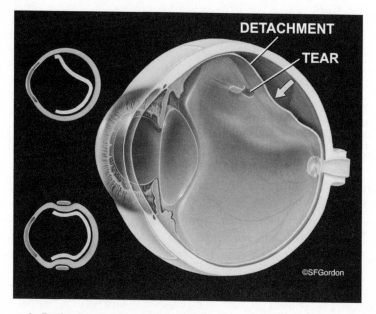

Figure 4. Retinal Detachment (the retina is detached; a tear is seen on the periphery)

Eye Emergencies and Ocular Trauma

Eye emergencies are true emergencies. Permanent vision loss—partial or total—can result from ignoring the signs of an eye emergency. Even if there's no pain in the eye, seek medical care immediately if you develop any of the following symptoms of an eye emergency:

- Swelling around the eye, particularly if it follows trauma or bug bite
- Sudden development of floaters
- Sudden development of flashes of light
- Sudden development of clouded vision
- Sudden development of blurred or wavy vision
- Pain, particularly if it follows abrasion or chemicals splashed in your eye, or in response to bright light
- Partial loss of vision (may be complete, incomplete, part of your visual field, or temporary)
- Sudden blindness (however fleeting). If you experience a loss of sight, but it returns within five minutes or even an hour, you have still experienced blindness, and that constitutes an emergency. Don't think

that because your sight returned, you are okay. It is an emergency until proved otherwise, and you must seek help immediately.

In action movies and television shows, a punch in the eye is often cause for laughter. In reality, however, it's no joke. Children need to understand that hitting someone in the eye can cause real and lasting damage. The consequences can be severe, causing grief to patients and families and too often resulting in loss of occupation, ability to read, watch television or movies, or drive a car. Auto and industrial accidents, assaults, and even warfare generate a tremendous amount of ocular trauma. It has been shown that 1 percent of the land mine explosions in Cambodia cause total blindness.

A 1997 study of emergency room records found that 2.9 percent of every 100,000 emergency visits were due to eye trauma. The study identified 2,939 cases of eye trauma, 635 of which were work-related and 638 were due to assault; most of these patients were male. The National Institutes of Health estimates there are up to 2.4 million cases of eye trauma in the United States every year, many of which require major surgery. According to the NIH, if surgery or other treatment is not obtained, blindness sometimes results. Alcohol is all too frequently associated with motor vehicle accidents that result in eye trauma.

Major sites and sources of ocular trauma include: sports, airbags, fireworks, exercise machines, toys, agricultural and industrial machines, and vehicles (cars, motorcycles, bicycles, lawn mowers). Corneal abrasion can result from being scratched by a fingernail, a dog or cat claw, a plant, or a piece of paper. Weapons (i.e., fingers, fists, guns, knives, and military accidents) and, worse yet, child abuse can result in eye trauma. We think of bruises and broken bones when we think of child abuse but, sad to say, abuse also includes severe trauma to children's eyes.

People who should take particular care to protect their eyes include those with keratoconus (a cone-shaped distortion of the cornea); those who've had previous eye surgery (for cataract, glaucoma, or a cornea transplant); construction workers; sports enthusiasts; and weekend hobbyists, who use saws, hammers, wood chippers, tools that spark, etc. Too often, a person who's doing "just one little job" around the house or yard doesn't put on safety glasses, thinking, "I don't need them." Always wear unbreakable polycarbonate safety glasses if you're in a situation in which your eyes can be hurt. It's just as important as wearing a seat belt in a car.

A newly identified danger posed by halogen lightbulbs (in addition to their being fire hazards) is their potential to cause corneal burns because they emit so much more UV light than regular lightbulbs. Sitting closer than six inches away from a halogen lamp can cause this temporarily blinding condition after only a few minutes. The first sign of this state, called *keratitis*, is clouding of the vision. Covering a halogen lightbulb with glass blocks nearly all of the UV light it emits and can help protect your eyes.

Trauma to the eye can result in:

- Orbital fracture (of the bones around the eye)
- Hemorrhage (bleeding) around the eye
- Subconjunctival hemorrhage (bleeding under the conjunctiva over the white of the eye)
- Eyelid laceration
- Lacerated tear duct
- Double vision (from eye muscle injury or cranial nerve injury from head trauma)
- A foreign body on the cornea or conjunctiva
- Corneal puncture (laceration), leading to scarring
- Inflamed eye (iritis or uveitis)
- Pupil distortion
- Blood in the front portion (anterior chamber) of the eye
- Cataract, lens dislocation, or artificial intraocular lens dislocation
- Intraocular foreign body
- Infection
- Glaucoma
- Vitreous hemorrhage, scarring, and contraction, which can lead to retinal detachment
- Facial paralysis and exposure (dislocation) of the eye

Prevention of Eye Trauma

To prevent most cases of ocular trauma, I recommend that you:

1. Wear polycarbonate eyeglasses during sports or any kind of activity like construction work that could result in your glasses being broken or your eyes being hurt.
2. Educate children about eye trauma.
3. Select sports activities carefully.
4. Avoid ballistic toys (like those that shoot missiles) and guns.
5. Use personal judgment and common sense.
6. Avoid bars after 11:00 P.M. If you're in a place where a lot of drinking is going on, and you detect a hostile change in the atmosphere, get out of there.

The pain and discomfort of eye trauma is extreme. If it happens to you, you may spend the rest of your life wishing that you had that moment back to undo the damage.

Treatment for Eye Trauma

Corneal abrasions and other eye traumas are usually treated with patching, antibiotic ointment, and pain relief (usually with NSAIDs). A bandage or medicated contact lens may be required in some instances to shield a corneal abrasion from being scraped by the eyelid during blinking.

If you get a foreign body in your eye—if a piece of dirt or metal blows into your eye on a windy day, for instance, or something falls into your eye when you're working under your car—try blinking rapidly to let your tears wash it away. Don't rub your eye! Rubbing an eye that has a foreign object in it can make the condition worse and possibly scratch the cornea. If blinking does not cause the tears to wash the object out of your eye, grasp your upper eyelid gently and pull it out (away from the eyeball) and down over the lower lid. Hold the upper lid in this position for a few seconds. This should cause even more tears to run out of the eye, and hopefully wash the foreign body out.

If neither of these techniques works and you can see the foreign object in your eye (an eyelash, for instance), hold your eyelids apart and, with a clean white handkerchief, try gently to brush the particle out of your eye. (You may want to ask someone else to help you do this.)

If you get a piece of metal or glass in your eye, you should seek emergency care immediately. If you are unable to coax any other type of foreign body out of your eye with tears or a handkerchief, call your eye doctor or go to a hospital emergency room (where there is an ophthalmologist on call) right away. If you think you have removed a foreign body from your eye but the pain or redness in the eye increases, call your eye doctor or go to a hospital emergency room immediately. Don't wait and hope it will just go away—a foreign object in your eye won't go away by itself. A piece of dirt, wood, or metal can scratch your cornea, potentially leading to scarring, infection, and vision loss.

Whenever you suffer any kind of eye trauma, it's important to start the healing process as soon as possible, so that secondary infections won't have a chance to develop. We're learning that eyes heal faster in the darkness and may do their fastest healing while we sleep, so if you have an eye injury, make sure you get adequate sleep.

I must repeat one final word of caution: If you suffer an eye trauma, even having a piece of dirt in your eye that you're unable to dislodge, seek medical help immediately. Don't wait. I've seen too many people who waited too long to seek care for an eye trauma, and were permanently damaged because of it.

Summary

Take care of your eyes and protect them from injury. Treat allergies early, using food, supplements, and appropriate eyedrops. Know the warning signs of an eye emergency—red eye, unrelenting pain, blurred vision, sudden appearance of flashes and/or floaters. Call an ophthalmologist, even at night or on the weekend, if you have any symptoms of an eye emergency. Manage headaches, even migraines, by getting to the source, and using exercise and common sense.

PART IV

PREVENTION AND TREATMENTS FOR COMMON EYE PROBLEMS

CHAPTER 6

The Cataract Epidemic

Myth: Everyone will develop cataracts if they live long enough.

Fact: It is possible to prevent, stabilize, and even reverse cataracts through nutrition and supplementation.

Cataracts are the leading cause of blindness around the world. Because of cataracts, more than forty-two million people worldwide have vision so poor they cannot read the big E on the eye chart. In the United States, cataracts constitute the major cause of vision loss, although, because of the generally high level of health care available to us, very few American cataract patients become blind. In fact, cataracts are among the most treatable causes of diminished vision.

Although cataracts can occur in people of all ages, they are generally seen in those with advanced age. By age 65, nearly half of all individuals begin to develop cataracts; the rate is even higher in women.

Patients often notice visual problems before their cataracts are diagnosed. For instance, people gradually realize they cannot read road signs when they drive, or that they need more light for close work. Golfers begin to have trouble following the ball; tailors have trouble threading needles.

Most of you have heard the word *cataract*, but don't know exactly what it means. It is not a growth over the surface of your eye. Instead, it is a cloudy haze (an opacity) that develops inside the normally transparent lens of the eye. Once the lens becomes cloudy, less light enters the eye and vision gradually diminishes.

The lens sits behind the pupil and the colored iris inside the eye. (See Figure 1 in Chapter 4.) In a healthy eye, the flexible, transparent lens focuses light onto the retina at the back of the eye. The retina absorbs the image transmitted by the light and sends it through the optic nerve to the brain.

You can think of the eye as being like a camera. The eye's lens is similar to a camera's lens, and the retina is like the film. The pupil of the eye resembles the camera's shutter, regulating the amount of light that enters. If your camera's lens becomes scratched and is no longer clear, you can't see through it properly. The same is true for the lens of the eye. If the lens in your eye becomes cloudy, you have a cataract. (Although people often speak of developing cataracts, each eye develops a single cataract. Only if both eyes are affected does a person have "cataracts." It's interesting to note that cataracts do not progress equally in both eyes in most people. If one eye develops a cataract, however, there is usually a cataract forming in the second eye.)

Dr. Abel's Tip

Cataracts and cataract surgery are not inevitable with age. It all depends on how you care for your eyes and yourself. Make deposits in your antioxidant bank account early and often to protect against cataracts.

The Anatomy of Cataracts

The lens is a very specialized filter for the eye. It has no blood vessels to bring it nutrients, but is nourished by the fluid, or *aqueous humor*, surrounding it. The lens also contains no nerves. Compared to other tissues in the body, it is a very dense structure. Some 33 to 35 percent of the lens is composed of a type of *crystallin proteins* that exist only in the lens.

A cataract begins to form when the crystallin proteins lose their shape and structure because of damage from free radicals. The crystallin proteins then clump together, causing the lens to become opaque rather than remain transparent.

The lens has several layers. It has an inner nucleus, which forms before birth, and to which layers are added throughout life. If you think of the nucleus as being the pit of a peach, it's easy to visualize the layers that surround it. Around the peach pit is the flesh, and surrounding the lens's nucleus is the fleshy part of the lens called the *cortex*. The peach has an outer skin, and so does the lens; its outer skin is called the *epithelium* (which is just another word for skin). The lens has another structure surrounding the epithelium called the *capsule*.

A cataract can form in the nucleus, cortex, or under the capsule of the lens. If the crystallin proteins clump together in the nucleus to form a *nuclear cataract*, the nucleus becomes very hard, and vision becomes hazy.

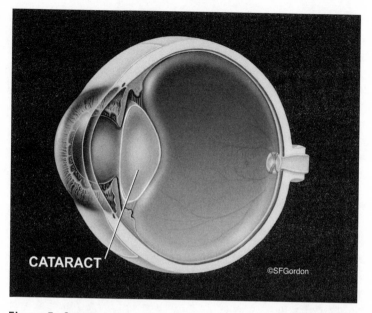

Figure 5. Cataract (clouding of the crystalline lens of the eye)

When the proteins in the cortex clump together, forming a *cortical cataract*, water droplets and gray clouds form in the vision.

A cataract can also form inside the capsular level. This type of cataract, called a *posterior subcapsular cataract*, is associated with diabetes, use of steroid drugs, and injury. It can also form after cataract surgery (which technically is also an injury to the capsule, since it is cut during surgery).

Cataracts develop in response to free-radical damage from many environmental sources, the most insidious being sunlight. It's essential to wear ultraviolet-filtering sunglasses to protect your eyes from sunlight's damaging effects.

Dr. Abel's Tip

The lens has no blood supply, so it depends on the eye's circulating fluids to bring it antioxidants to counter the free radicals created by smoking, sunlight, stress, and even redness or soreness in the eye. An increasing number of studies show that antioxidants not only penetrate the lens, but also lower the incidence and slow the progression of cataracts. Protect your eyes from cataracts by building up your antioxidant bank account.

You can also fight free radicals by building up your antioxidant bank account through diet or supplementation. I advise my patients that the most important step they can take to combat free-radical damage from all sources and protect against cataracts is to increase the amount of antioxidants they consume, through either diet or supplementation.

In the Middle Ages, sailors on long voyages often developed scurvy because they didn't have fresh fruits and vegetables and became deficient in vitamin C. People are more likely to develop cataracts when their diet is deficient in the essential nutrients glutathione and vitamin C and, to lesser degrees, vitamins A, E, and the Omega-3 essential fatty acids. In addition to these cataract-fighting antioxidants, the lens also needs the B vitamins, especially biotin and B_2 to decrease the incidence of cataracts.

The Symptoms of Cataracts

Gladys was remarrying at the age of 80, so a group of friends took her out to lunch to celebrate. At lunch, they tried, tactfully, to discover why Gladys was marrying again at her age. "I guess he's quite wealthy," one friend said, but Gladys replied that he was not. "He must be very good-looking," another friend commented, but Gladys said, "No, he's nothing special to look at." "Then he must be good between the sheets," a third friend finally suggested. "At our age? Of course not!" Gladys replied. "Why, then, are you getting married?" a friend finally asked. Gladys said, "It's simple. He's able to drive at night."

Loss of night vision is not the only symptom of cataract. Some others include:

- Seeing glare, especially at night
- Increasingly blurry or hazy vision, usually first noticed in distance vision
- Requiring more light for reading
- Glasses always seeming dirty
- Seeing halos around lights
- Fatigue when reading
- Inability to thread a needle or perform other fine actions
- Inability to judge distances or steps (poor depth perception)
- Development of so-called "second sight" in which the cataract grows in such a way that vision shifts, and either distance or near vision becomes clearer without glasses.

The Causes of Cataracts

Cataracts are caused by age, exposure to sunlight (ultraviolet and other types of radiation), injury, disease, prescription drug side effects, certain chemicals, diabetes and other diseases, smoking, heredity, poor nutrition, and poor digestion. Nutritional deficiencies cause cataracts to develop earlier and progress faster, as they do in underdeveloped countries. For instance, in impoverished urban areas of India, cataracts progress so fast that they require surgery at least ten years earlier than they do in the United States.

In every part of the world, people with poor digestion and chronic bowel problems have a fourfold higher incidence of cataracts. The reason is clear: they are unable to properly absorb the nutrients in the food they eat. Malnutrition and chronic diarrhea conditions substantially increase the risk of cataract formation. This is a major reason why I try to understand my patients' total health situation instead of just examining their eyes.

Now let's look at the causes of cataracts in more detail.

Even though cataract formation is not inevitable, *the aging of the eyes* contributes to cataracts. We know that the curvature of the lens changes as we age, which is why many older people require reading glasses. While cataracts generally develop in older people, however, they are not an inevitable result of the aging process. Research shows that good nutrition and supplementation can stop cataracts. Other ophthalmologists are starting to join me in suggesting supplementation and changes in their patients' diets as soon as cataracts are detected.

Cataracts can develop at any age, even in infancy, although this is unusual. If cataracts develop in infants, they can cause "lazy eye," *amblyopia*, so it's important to screen for the signs of cataract in newborns. Steroid drugs can cause cataracts in children, just as they can in adults. Any child who needs to take a steroid drug because of rheumatoid arthritis or asthma should be given the lowest possible therapeutic dose to prevent the development of cataracts.

Sunlight is definitely associated with the formation of cataracts. The invisible ultraviolet (UV) component of sunlight promotes free-radical damage in the lens. As I discussed previously in Chapter 4, the brighter the sun, the greater the UV radiation dose. The effects of radiation are cumulative throughout life—they add up as we go along. That's why skin cancers can develop four or five decades after major sun exposure. Cataracts are a similar symptom of overexposure to sunshine. Epidemiological studies around the world have indicated that people living at higher altitudes and in greater sunlight have a greater risk of cataracts each decade than control populations.

Changes in the Earth's ozone layer mean that more UV radiation is now reaching the surface. Therefore, the need to prevent cataracts will only increase. I advise all my patients who are exposed to reflected UV light from snow, on beaches, or in tanning salons to cover their entire eye area with ultraviolet-blocking sunglasses to prevent exposure to UV radiation.

Human beings are not the only organisms who suffer from the erosion of Earth's ozone layer. I remember being particularly struck by a late-1980s magazine article about the ozone hole over the southern hemisphere. The article noted that rabbits were developing cataracts, making many of them blind. You can be sure that if the rabbits are having problems, we are soon to follow!

Smoking is probably the most important lifestyle factor to be avoided. The Physicians' Health Study (an ongoing study of more than 50,000 doctors) has already documented a greater incidence of cataracts in men who smoke than in those who don't. Likewise, a study of 120,000 nurses over eight years found a positive correlation between smoking and cataract formation. An interesting exception were those women smokers who consumed large quantities of leafy green vegetables, which contains the carotenoids and vitamin C. Amazingly, they had the same low risk of developing cataracts as nonsmokers did. This again illustrates the importance of nutrition in preventing ill health in older age.

I've learned that cigarette smoke is rich in free radicals and other toxins, and it suppresses production of glutathione, a cell membrane protector that is an excellent free-radical scavenger and essential to eye health. You can protect your optic nerve and retina to a certain extent from cigarette smoke's toxins by taking B vitamins, especially B_{12}. It has also been recommended that smokers take an extra 25 milligrams of vitamin C for every cigarette smoked, because vitamin C helps neutralize the free radicals and poisons emitted in the smoke. I do not mean these suggestions as panaceas for the habit, even though I understand that smoking is highly addictive and very difficult to quit. Stopping smoking, however, is the only way to eliminate the risks posed to your vision by cigarettes' toxins. If you have suceeded in quitting the habit though, you should do everything possible to avoid secondhand smoke at home and in the workplace.

Photosensitizing drugs—which make people more sensitive to light—magnify the damage ultraviolet light causes to the lens. I advise patients taking such drugs to wear wraparound, UV-blocking sunglasses. (Opticians and optometrists can check the UV content of sunglass lenses if you're unsure how effective your sunglasses are.) Gout medications, cholesterol-lowering drugs, antibiotics, and diuretics are some of the most commonly prescribed photosensitizing drugs. If you are uncertain whether a drug you're taking has this effect, ask your physician or pharmacist. At least 200 drugs are known to have this effect.

One of my patients, a middle-aged executive, was on a cholesterol-lowering drug when he began to develop a cataract. I took him off that drug, dealt with his high cholesterol through diet and exercise, and prescribed a nutritional plan that resulted in his cataract being stabilized for eight years.

Make sure you continue to take the medications your doctor has prescribed for high blood pressure or high cholesterol, but also ask your doctor to monitor your situation carefully. Use these drugs to bring your condition under control and then, with your doctor's help and approval, switch to alternative methods of dealing with your health problems that will help protect your eyes. The eye care revolution is about blending mainstream and alternative regimens into a more comprehensive program that protects both your eyes and your total body health.

Steroid drugs are also associated with the development of cataracts. I repeatedly remind my patients that all drugs have side effects. Prednisone is recognized as a major cause of cataracts, whether it's applied topically (for skin disease), inhaled (for asthma), injected, or taken orally. Even steroid eyedrops, which are great for allergic conditions, inflammation of the eyes, and after surgery, can cause cataracts when used for long periods of time. We've known for more than twenty years that more than a limited amount of steroids after corneal transplant can cause cataracts even in young patients. So we must be mindful, both as patients and doctors, of the level and frequency of steroids used. Since steroids do not cure any condition but merely suppress certain symptoms, questions about their long-term usefulness for any disease should be addressed.

I cannot emphasize too strongly that taking steroids in any form—in an inhaler, by mouth, or even as a topically applied ointment—can result in cataracts. For example, I had a 49-year-old patient who was treating acne-like lesions on the right side of his forehead with a steroid cream. Within six months of starting to use the cream, he developed a cataract in his right eye. I've also had patients with asthma whose physicians prescribed a steroid inhaler without warning the patient that it could cause or worsen cataracts. Using other methods to control these patients' asthma nearly always stops the progression of their cataracts.

If you have an inflammatory disease or are receiving radiation for a tumor, please realize that the free radicals attacking the inflamed part of your body are consuming antioxidants that could otherwise protect your eyes. A person with inflammatory bowel disease, arthritis, or coronary artery disease is diverting antioxidants to those inflamed areas, thereby depriving the eye of much-needed nutrients. In these situations, the eye, which is under constant bombardment from light, becomes relatively deficient in the antioxidants that help block cataract formation, glaucoma, and macular degeneration.

Obesity is a major risk factor for cataracts as the ongoing Physicians' Health Study clearly demonstrates. People who are obese and who also smoke and drink are quadrupling their chance of developing cataracts. Obesity can lead to diabetes, a condition that also raises the risk of cataract formation.

One of my patients was an overweight man with high blood pressure and numerous other health problems directly related to his obesity. When I first saw him, he was taking two high blood pressure medications, using eyedrops to reduce the pressure in his eyes that was putting him at risk for glaucoma, and was developing early cataracts. At my insistence and that of his family doctor, he started exercising and changed his diet. Four months later, he had not only lost sixty pounds, he no longer required eyedrops or blood pressure medication. Five years later, he continued to have 20/20 vision in one eye and 20/25 (one line off in the eye chart) in the other.

Risk Factors for Developing Cataracts

• Excessive exposure to the ultraviolet rays in sunlight; lack of adequate UV-blocking capacity in sunglasses; not wearing sunglasses at all.
• Age.
• Smoking; exposure to secondhand smoke.
• Heredity.
• Poor digestion (characterized by gas, bloating, irregular bowel habits).
• Nutritional deficiencies.
• Poor education about health issues.
• Obesity and increased fat in diet.
• Excessive alcohol consumption.
• Chronic diseases affecting multiple areas of the body; that is, hypertension, arthritis, heart disease, diabetes, and others. While the medications used to treat these diseases can contribute to cataract formation, the illnesses themselves can also increase the risk of developing cataracts.
• Systemic medications which are often prescribed to treat chronic diseases on a long-term basis; many of these medications photosensitize the lens and skin.

- Inherited disorders.
- Head and eye injuries.
- Other eye conditions, including infections (like corneal ulcers) and inflammation of the eyes which requires treatment with cortisone eyedrops for extended periods of time.

Diagnosis of Cataracts

If eye examinations are done on a regular basis, the beginning of a cataract can be seen by an ophthalmologist or optometrist before it impairs sight. Once symptoms appear, the diminished or blurred vision caused by cataracts can have a tremendous impact on a patient's daily life, contributing to avoidance of night driving, increased risk of automobile accidents, difficulty reading or doing other detail work, inexplicable depression, falls, and even "false senility."

In treating my patients, I've learned that it's important to determine *why* people are depressed. I've often found that sight loss causes anxiety, depression, and low self-esteem. The caring eye doctor can identify vision loss as the cause of depression and address the situation. Depressed people are especially concerned about their inability to function. People with cataracts often feel that their lives are out of control. In many instances, I can actually help these patients significantly, sometimes by simply adjusting their glasses prescription. While this does not deal with the cataracts directly, it can improve a patient's quality of life immeasurably. Surgery is not the only remedy for dealing with cataracts.

Dr. Abel's Tip

Get a good, dilated-eye exam if you suspect you have cataracts or your family doctor has told you that you may be developing cataracts. Have your glasses prescription updated because you may actually see better (even if you have a cataract) just by having your glasses changed.

It's important to detect cataracts early, particularly the type called *posterior subcapsular cataracts.* Posterior subcapsular cataracts develop most often in association with diabetes or use of steroids, and can result in rapid vision loss. Sudden and progressive visual problems, such as glare, distortion, and blurry images are symptoms of this type of cataract.

Cataracts are usually detected when an ophthalmologist or optometrist examines the eye with a slit lamp and an ophthalmoscope. (See Chapter

4.) When the light of the ophthalmoscope is shone into a healthy eye, the doctor sees a "red reflex"—that is, the light reflected back is evenly red-colored. When a cataract develops, it appears as a dark silhouette within the red reflex.

It's easier and more reliable for your doctor to detect cataracts during a slit lamp examination when your eyes are dilated (i.e., when the pupil is made abnormally wide open with eyedrops). The slit lamp, a specialized microscope that allows the doctor to view the inside of the eye in detail, can detect even the subtlest cataractous changes.

I emphasize to my patients that function is more important than form— that the presence of a cataract is not cause for alarm if the patient can see well, function well, and understands that the cataract doesn't have to get worse because he or she has options to stop the damage from progressing.

Older people's vision diminishes naturally because the lens of the eye becomes slightly discolored throughout life from exposure to ultraviolet light. Not all discolorations or gradual opacifications, however are truly cataracts.

My father, for example, began to develop cataracts in 1978, when he was 68 years old. As soon as I noticed the changes, I put him on anti-oxidants (like the ones suggested at the end of this chapter) and advised him to wear sunglasses while playing golf or engaging in other outdoor leisure activities. Twenty-four years later, his vision was still 20/20. He was able to play both golf and tennis in the same day. It exhausted me to watch him!

As my father's case demonstrates, early cataract changes do not have to progress. There is much *you* can do to prevent vision loss from cataracts and other chronic conditions.

Modern Cataract Treatment: Surgery

I often find that a patient's glasses can be changed to improve his or her vision when a cataract first begins to develop. I also take advantage of this opportunity to recommend lifestyle modifications, dietary changes, and adding supplements. Just because you are told you have a cataract doesn't mean your vision is impaired by it. That is why, after fitting my patients with the best possible eyeglasses, I rely on them to tell me about their difficulties.

Despite my own and my patients' best efforts, cataracts sometimes become advanced, and I find that there is no way to restore good vision without surgery. Although frustrating, when these occasions arise I thank

God for the miracle of modern cataract surgery, which is very successful. One of the most gratifying aspects of ophthalmology is that I can help people medically, nutritionally, and with high-tech surgical methods if necessary. (For a detailed account of a cataract operation, refer to Appendix B.)

Because the surgical techniques available in the past were relatively unsophisticated, eye doctors used to wait until the cataract was very mature or "ripe" before performing surgery. Today's techniques have greatly improved, however, and it is no longer necessary for the cataract to reach an advanced stage before we operate. The patient must be involved in making the decision about when it's time to do surgery, which is why it's necessary for there to be an interactive relationship between patient and physician.

Many people think that cataract surgery is done with a laser. In fact, the FDA was slow to approve laser cataract machines because of their cost and lack of proven advantage. *Phacoemulsification* remains the currently used method. This technique, popularly known as *ultrasound,* has been used since the early 1970s, when it replaced the earlier approach of removing the whole lens *(intracapsular cataract extraction)* or washing out the center of the lens (called *extracapsular cataract extraction).* Phacoemulsification employs high-speed sound (ultrasound) to break up the hard center of the cataract. Once the cataract is broken up, it is extracted and a synthetic lens is implanted in the eye.

Dr. Abel's Tip

How should you decide when it's time to have cataract surgery? With your doctor's help, compare the quality of the vision you have in the eye that has a cataract, with your vision in the other eye. Some people actually like becoming more nearsighted as a result of the cataract (a common side effect of the condition) because it allows them to read without glasses. You, the patient, are the one who dictates the need for surgery. The so-called "ripeness" of a cataract is no longer an issue in scheduling surgery. If difficulty driving at night is the major problem caused by your cataract, consider taking bilberry supplements or eating blueberries to improve your night vision, or modifying your schedule. If you do need cataract surgery, make sure that your physician is experienced in phacoemulsification (the modern method of removing cataracts) and that he or she uses an artificial lens implant made of silicon or acrylic. Investigate all the pros and cons of the newer models of artificial lenses, such as multifocal lenses. While I generally advocate trying to improve your vision using natural means (like diet and supplementation) before having surgery, if your sight doesn't improve from using these methods within three months, it's time to consider having cataract surgery.

Confusion about cataract surgery being laser surgery arises because a YAG laser is used, months to years after the original surgery, to make a hole in the residual cataract capsule when the lens naturally becomes cloudy again (I'll explain why shortly). Doctors sometimes describe them-selves as "cataract/laser surgeons," further confusing the issue.

The lens of the eye has no feeling. Therefore, anesthesia applied in eyedrops, instead of through injection, can be used for cataract surgery. After the eye is numb, a small incision (one-eighth of an inch) is made at the edge of the cornea. An additional amount of 1 percent Xylocaine (a weaker anesthetic), is put into the eye, numbing the front of the eye completely. The pupil is dilated before surgery, so that the cataract can be seen clearly by the surgeon. If patients are on blood-thinning drugs such as Coumidin, they can continue to take them, since it is unlikely that any blood vessels will be injured during cataract surgery. Since the surgery is performed using anesthetic eyedrops instead of injections around the outside of the eye, patients no longer have bloodshot eyes or double vision following surgery, and are less likely to have experienced injury to the globe (the eyeball itself).

Over the years, the size of the incision made in the eye during cataract surgery has been decreased to about three millimeters (about an eighth of an inch) because artificial lenses have been developed that can actually be folded for insertion into the eye. These foldable lenses are made of newly developed materials, generally either silicon, acrylic, or collagin. (The silicon is not the same as that previously used in breast implants and, because the cataract's original capsule is retained, the implant is kept away from other tissues in the eye, reducing the possibility of a reaction to the new lens.)

My patients are often astonished at how painless and quick cataract surgery is. For example, I performed cataract surgery on Mrs. B., a very nearsighted patient who was extremely apprehensive about the surgery. After-ward, she was thrilled, telling me, "My husband looks years older, the colors of the clothes in my closet have sprung to life, and dust has appeared all over my house! I've always been a positive person, but now I'm ecstatic. I haven't seen this well in years."

Modern cataract surgery should cause no pain and no bleeding; it rarely requires stitches. You should be certain that your doctor is accomplished at performing the modern, ultrasound techniques. Don't be afraid to ask how many procedures he or she has done in the past year, how many are performed in the hospital or facility each year. Compare these records with those of other doctors and hospitals. Studies show that, the more procedures a surgeon does, the more successful the surgery usually is. Many hospitals and clinics report, or even boast, about how many of various types of procedures are done in their facility each year. That doesn't mean, however, that there's a problem if the doctor or hospital doesn't boast—just ask what their numbers are.

In addition to antibiotic eyedrops, vitamin supplements before and after surgery may speed healing and limit inflammation. Dr. Gary Price Todd, a pioneer in using nutrition to prevent and treat cataracts, recommends taking vitamins A, E, and C before and after cataract surgery. My patients have much to arrange before their eye surgery, and I find it is not an appropriate time to develop a new health and supplement regimen. Like Dr. Todd, I prefer to initiate a nutrition program before the date of surgery. I find that emphasizing protection of the other eye (the one with less cataract) is the best approach. The simplest recommendation is for the patient to take a good multivitamin with extra vitamin C. (See Table 8). During cataract surgery, I use the lowest available microscope illumination to protect the eye.

Cataract surgery is one of the most satisfying surgical procedures performed today—for both patient and physician—and can result in complete rehabilitation in a short period of time. It can be done under local anesthesia, at a charge of less than $1000 for the surgeon and $1000 or less for the surgical facility. (Of course, doctors and facilities in different parts of the country charge varying amounts; this is just an estimate.) The patient may be able to lift and bend after one day, and generally does not require sutures or an eye patch. Patients should be able to drive and even go bowling on the day following their surgery, depending on their personal circumstances. (It must be remembered that anything said here is simply a general observation, and cannot be specifically applied to your situation. You and your eye doctor will need to establish your specific needs and limitations following surgery.)

Possible Complications of Cataract Surgery

I have found that routinely using antibiotic eyedrops after surgery (and, in some cases, during surgery) can diminish postoperative infection and inflammation as effectively as injectible antibiotic does, without the side effects produced by injection. Perhaps one in a thousand patients develops an intraocular infection following surgery, which is a very serious situation. I instruct my patients to report any changes in their vision after surgery to me immediately.

Six months to several years following cataract surgery, about one-third of patients develop an opacification or cloudiness in the back capsule of the lens (the only portion not removed before implantation of the plastic lens). This occurs when cells migrate to the back capsule, trying to create new lens material there (a natural reaction) and instead creating a haze that interferes with vision.

Once the capsule begins to opacify, it will continue to do so at an increasing rate, so it's important to perform a laser procedure to open the capsule before vision is severely impaired. The YAG laser I mentioned earlier is used to open the capsule and clear the haze. The complications of YAG laser treatment are few; nicking the lens, inflammation, or glaucoma can result, but are not very common. Retinal detachment can occur very rarely, but it's important to be aware of this small possibility, as well as the possibility of increased floaters and flashing lights after laser treatment.

Other complications of cataract surgery include:

- Dislocated lens
- Irregular pupil
- Intraocular infection
- Corneal swelling
- Elevated internal eye pressure/glaucoma (usually short term)
- Retinal tear and detachment
- Corneal infection
- Chronic inflammation in the eye (iritis)
- Hemorrhage

Most of these complications happen infrequently because of our new surgical techniques. However, bacterial eye infection still occurs in one of every thousand patients and can cause loss of sight. I talk with my patients by telephone a few hours after their surgery and examine them in the office the following day to minimize the possibility of any postsurgical complications.

No surgical procedure offers so much quality-of-life improvement at such a low cost and in such a short time as cataract surgery does. Nevertheless, it is still a surgical procedure and there are risks—a good reason to prevent cataracts from developing in the first place.

Nutritional Methods of Preventing and Treating Cataracts

At a dinner party of my brother-in-law's, a retired psychiatrist mentioned that she was developing cataracts, and really didn't want to undergo surgery. When my brother-in-law told her that there were nutritional methods of stabilizing or reversing her cataracts, she had a very interesting series of reactions. At first, she was amazed. She'd never heard of any method except surgery for healing cataracts. Then she was skeptical. Were these nutritional methods scientifically valid? Her third reaction was most telling of all, because she asked, "What should I do?"

The first step is to increase antioxidant intake. The lens's major antioxidants are vitamins C, E, and A (or beta-carotene, its precursor). Numerous studies have demonstrated that high intake of these vitamins—or consumption of large amounts of fresh fruits and vegetables containing them (including green leafy vegetables, carrots, citrus fruits, and melons)—reduces the incidence of cataract formation. It has clearly been shown in animal studies that removing vitamin A (or beta-carotene), vitamins C, E, and the B vitamin riboflavin, causes cataracts to develop, and that replacing these nutrients caused the cataract to diminish.

A study published in the *American Journal of Clinical Nutrition* in 1991, examining the blood levels of several nutrients in elderly people with and without cataracts reached similar conclusions. Low levels of carotenoids (vitamin A-related compounds) and vitamin C in the blood were found to be associated with an increased risk of developing cataracts. Additionally, those individuals who consumed fewer than three-and-a-half servings of fruit or vegetables daily were at higher risk of developing cataracts than people who ate more fruits and vegetables.

Similarly, a study published in the *British Journal of Medicine* in 1992 examined the effect of vegetable consumption on incidence of cataract in more than 50,000 women over an eight-year period. The British study found that cataract formation was reduced 50 percent by eating five servings of spinach a week. Consumption of carrots, sweet potatoes, broccoli, or winter squash (beta-carotene-containing vegetables) had no effect on the rate of cataract development. (This was an unexpected finding, and hasn't been repeated, so don't stop eating your carrots and broccoli!)

Supplements also provide protection against cataracts. Dr. Jean Mayer at the USDA Nutrition Research Center on Aging found that women who take vitamin C for more than ten years have a markedly reduced risk of developing cataracts. Another study sponsored by the USDA measured the concentrations of vitamin A precursors (carotenoids and retinoids) and vitamin E (tocopherols) in the human lens and concluded that consumption of these vitamin supplements reduced free-radical damage (oxidative stress) and cataract risk. Additionally, the Physicians' Health Study found that male physicians who took multivitamins appeared to have a decreased risk of cataract.

A five-year epidemiological study found that vitamin E supplements alone could reduce cataract risk by as much as 50 percent. Riboflavin (vitamin B_2), pantothenic acid (vitamin B_5), selenium, and glutathione are also effective in neutralizing free radicals. These substances are promising enough in the fight against eye disease that more than twenty companies are now manufacturing vitamins for use against both cataract and macular degeneration.

Vitamins A and C have also been formulated for use as eyedrops in other countries. The question is whether they are absorbed at levels high enough to have an impact on cataract formation, which has not been studied.

Glutathione, a compound that is essential to making tissue enzymes and crucial in stopping free radical damage, is extremely effective at preventing cataract formation. Studies have shown that all lenses with cataracts contain a reduced amount of glutathione—one-fifteenth of normal—and the level of vitamin C is one-tenth of normal. It was originally thought that these deficiencies were a result of the cataract, but now it's suspected that the decrease in antioxidants precedes cataract formation.

Glutathione's precursor (cysteine) is found in eggs, garlic, avocado, asparagus, onion, and red meat. Your diet should include sulfur- or cysteine-containing foods, which also boost glutathione production in the body. (For more specific information about glutathione and its food sources, see Chapter 15.) Supplements that are glutathione-boosters include alpha-lipoic acid, melatonin, MSM, NAC and SAMe. Studies have shown that alpha-lipoic acid supplements can help some people avoid cataracts.

The B vitamin pantothenic acid apparently slows the clumping of lens proteins, and it is marketed as an anticataract eyedrop. Quercetin, a bioflavonoid available in supplement form, helps stop cataracts by blocking an enzyme (aldose reductase) that acts on sugars in a way that definitely causes cataracts.

Various enzymes—most notably, superoxide dismutase (SOD), catalase, glutathione peroxidase (an enzyme derived from glutathione, and methionine)—play key roles in scavenging free radicals and preventing tissue damage. These enzymes' effectiveness decreases with age, smoke, obesity, and sunlight; in addition, catalase and glutathione are destroyed with exposure to ultraviolet radiation. You can increase your levels of these enzymes through supplementation.

Polyunsaturated fatty acids are also present in the lens. A study that examined regional age-dependent differences in the lipid (fat) content of the lens suggested that the essential fatty acids may also be important in preventing or treating cataract.

Finally, estrogen appears to have a protective effect on the lens. Significantly more women, most of whom are postmenopausal, have cataract surgery than men. My son and I have completed a study of 10,758 people having cataract surgery over four years at the Wilmington Hospital, and 64 percent were women. This is a greater percentage than can be attributed to longevity alone, and I suspect that the lack of an estrogen-protective effect may play a role. Both the Beaver Dam and ECCDS Studies intimated that estrogen supplementation decreases the incidence of cataracts and macular degeneration in postmenopausal women.

Raloxifene, the latest in estrogen replacement therapy, appears to possess all the benefits of estrogen without estrogen's potentially cancer-causing effects on breast or uterine tissue. Because of its unique properties, Raloxifene is considered a specific estrogen-related drug. It (or a similar drug) may turn out to have benefits for all elderly people, both men and women. Natural hormonal therapy may be best.

All these nutrients prevent protein aggregation and cataract formation. The lens, the eye, and the whole body are constantly under stress, some of which is from our environment, our diets, our body's metabolism, and its very chemistry, and some of which we inflict on ourselves by not paying attention to our total mind/body health. We need, therefore, to consume a combination of nutrients, from both food and supplements (relying primarily on diet but using supplements as an insurance policy), that will help our entire being.

We need to think about prevention and treatment together. All cataracts are not the same, so each individual needs a specific nutritional program that takes into account heredity, age, and lifestyle.

My patient Jim, for instance, is a 53-year-old who had cataract surgery about fifteen years ago by another surgeon. When he became my patient, he asked me to implant intraocular lenses, which were not available when he originally had his surgery. During a routine examination, I asked him about his family history, and he confirmed that not only did his parents have cataracts, his 30-year-old daughter had already had cataract surgery, and his 29-year-old son had been told that he has cataracts. His son, Jim explained, was very interested in learning about alternative options to surgery, which I was happy to share. A situation like Jim and his children's is quite unusual, but if you have a family history of cataracts, it's important that you have your eyes examined regularly and that you take preventive measures designed specifically for your situation—especially since they will also be beneficial to your general health.

Possible Future Options

Dr. S. K. Gupta and colleagues have discovered that *pyruvate*, a normal tissue product, quenches free radicals and protects the lens against cataract formation. In animal studies, Dr. Gupta and his coworkers showed that oral pyruvate blocks the formation of cataracts when given prior to exposure to selenite, a substance that induces cataract formation. Pyruvate (in the form of eyedrops) also protects against chemically induced cataracts in rats. Although these studies were performed in animals, pyruvate has great promise because it is a natural medication. It's too soon to make recommendations about pyruvate until we have appropriate clinical studies, which I will be interested in reviewing when they are completed.

Some researchers have noted that they've seen cataracts improve with *bendazac* (which has anti-inflammatory properties), used either as eyedrops or as an oral medication. Young people who've had posterior subcapsular cataracts have improved, on occasion, with the use of bendazac. Interestingly, a form of bendazac (benzyl alcohol) is used as a preservative in European eyedrops. I am dubious about the effectiveness of this treatment.

A colleague in Wilmington, Dr. Anil Patel, a biochemist who has scoured India for the best herbal remedies, has devised a formula that appears to clear clouded lenses. Dr. Patel has obtained cataractous human lenses and improved their clarity by incubating them with different combinations of Ayurvedic (Indian) herbs to determine which herbs are able to reverse the condition. When the formula was used to treat twenty-six patients, one-third developed allergic reactions and quit the study, one-third had their cataracts stabilized, and one-third deteriorated. There appeared to be no systemic side effects. While this is clearly an experimental treatment and is still being studied, it may show promise.

Dietary Recommendations

Many of my recommendations for cataract prevention can also be used for cataract treatment. I recommend the following:

- *Fresh fruits and vegetables in a balanced diet.* Foods especially helpful in fighting and preventing cataracts are Brazil nuts (which contain vitamin E and selenium); carrots (which improve vision); the green vegetable purslane and the spice turmeric (high in vitamins C, E, the carotenoids, and Omega-3 essential fatty acids), raw sunflower seeds; and onions (which are high in the antioxidant quercitin). But the U.S. government recommended diet, consisting of five to ten vegetables or fruits each day, may not be available or affordable to everyone. Additionally, some people, because of health problems (like low stomach acid, which can result from taking antacids regularly, or bowel disorders), cannot absorb nutrients from food. Such people need to augment their diet with nutritional supplements such as antioxidants, while avoiding preservatives and junk foods.

• A *multivitamin*, one or two a day, preferably an eye-health-supportive multivitamin.

• *Vitamin A*, 10,000 I.U. daily. Studies have shown a 40 percent decrease in cataracts in women whose diet is rich in vitamin A. Check the amount of vitamin A in your multivitamin; it shouldn't contain more than 5000 I.U. if you are supplementing with extra vitamin A.

• A *B complex vitamin*, once daily. Multivitamins usually do not contain adequate amounts of B complex vitamins to be useful in a cataract prevention strategy (although certainly some is better than none at all).

• *Vitamin C*, 1000 mg three times daily. Studies have shown a 70 percent decrease in cataract risk in people taking vitamin C supplements. (The vitamin C dosage in these studies varies from 300 to 1000 mg/daily.) I personally take 2500 mg or more vitamin C a day. This antioxidant vitamin appears to minimize or delay the development of cataracts. If you aren't used to taking vitamin C, build up to taking more than 1000 mg daily gradually, because it can cause diarrhea. If you have this reaction, cut back the amount of vitamin C you are taking, and it will stop. Even 1000 mg vitamin C daily is useful in helping prevent cataracts, as studies have shown.

• *Vitamin E*, 400–800 I.U. daily. Studies have shown up to a 56 percent decrease in cataracts in subjects who take vitamin E supplements.

• *Quercetin* is a bioflavonoid that potentiates vitamin C activity. In laboratory animals, quercetin blocks posterior subcapsular cataracts caused by steroids and diabetes, and it should do the same in humans. In the future, I suspect that all eye doctors will probably prescribe quercetin routinely whenever they're forced to put patients on steroid eyedrops. An extra bonus is that quercetin seems to be helpful for allergies/hay fever.

- *Bilberry.* Like other bioflavonoids, bilberry may potentiate vitamin C. Its actions are not specific to the lens of the eye, but it is good for overall eye health, particularly night vision.
- MSM *(methanylsulfonylmethane)* is a form of sulfur that exists in high levels in all plants but is easily destroyed by processing (including cooking). Sulfur and sulfur compounds are essential to all life, just like oxygen. They contribute to the formation of *keratin* (found in hair and nails), help maintain protein structure and the immune system, and help process food into energy. Natural levels of MSM diminish with age, probably because of a decreasing ability to absorb nutrients in the gut. MSM is still the subject of research, but its properties are said to be anti-allergic; antacid; anti-arthritis; antiparasitic, anticancer, and helpful for eye conditions like conjunctivitis, red eyes, and eye injuries. MSM has been formulated into oral forms, skin lotions, and eyedrops, but there are no data supporting its effectiveness against cataracts.
- *Minerals* are coenzymes important to many systems in the body. I recommend magnesium (500 mg daily); selenium (50–100 mcg— don't take more than 200 mcg a day, because it can be toxic); zinc (30 mg or less); copper (2 mg); and manganese (2–5 mg).
- *Sunglasses* with UV- and blue-light protection.
- *Cessation of smoking.*
- *Awareness of medications* (i.e., steroids and photosensitizing drugs). Be sure to ask your doctor and your pharmacist, who may be very helpful.
- *Glutathione and Sulfur.* Eat avocado, onions, garlic, asparagus, and eggs. Supplements high in sulfur are MSM and alpha lipoic acid. Glutathione itself is not absorbed but is produced in the liver from precursors in fish and meats. Some practitioners suggest taking N-acetyl-cysteine (NAC) because cysteine is a major glutathione precursor. However, NAC is a pro-oxidant (the opposite of an antioxidant) in healthy individuals, so supplements should not be taken for long periods of time.

Cataracts are a major cause of blindness around the world, creating a great deal of human misery. They are a major disability in terms of lost wages and a major cost to governments in terms of lost manpower, as well as health care costs. Taking the specific steps I've outlined here to protect your eyes can help to decrease cataracts, but preventive techniques can be used even after receiving a positive diagnosis for cataracts to stop them from progressing. In my experience, most cataracts can be stopped from progressing if the factors that caused them are identified and reversed.

If you do need cataract surgery, it's a most successful, high-tech procedure that can be performed in minutes with excellent results. It is performed without sutures, without patches, without injection, at a reasonable cost, and with minimal convalescence. Nevertheless, as safe as cataract surgery is, like every surgical procedure, it does have some risk. Because there is less risk with nutritional management, I always suggest that path as the first step in stopping cataracts from progressing.

For a handy summary of my dietary and supplementation recommendations, see Tables 8 and 9. The suggestions you'll find there will not only help stop the progression of your cataracts (or help prevent you from developing cataracts), but will also improve the general health of your eyes and the rest of your body. You don't have to be sick or not see well to start protecting the health of your eyes and your entire body.

Table 8. Prevention/Alternative Treatment of Cataracts

Diet and Supplementation	Lifestyle	Water and Digestion
• Eat fruits and vegetables five times a day, especially: Spinach and corn (for lutein, or take 10–20 mg supplement daily at mealtime). Tomato-based products (for lycopene) Glutathione boosters: garlic, onion, avocados, eggs, asparagus, or take supplements. Increase Omega-3 fatty acid intake by consuming flaxseeds or flaxseed oil, purslane, fatty fish, and turmeric, or supplement with 500 mg twice daily at mealtimes. • Reduce the "bad fats" and packaged foods in your diet. • Decrease your consumption of alcohol; limit yourself to one glass of wine daily. • Supplement your diet with: Multivitamin (one or two daily) Vitamin A (10,000 IU daily with a meal) B complex vitamin (50–100 mg daily) Vitamin C (1000 mg three times daily, if tolerated) Vitamin E (400–800 IU daily with a meal) Include selenium	• Wear sunglasses and a hat to protect yourself from UV light. • Keep using your eyes reading, woodworking, needlework, or crafts, and hobbies, playing golf or other sports. • Stop smoking. • Keep learning about your condition. Read magazine and newspaper articles about research breakthroughs, new treatments, and dietary supplementation. • If you're a woman, you may want to consider estrogen replacement therapy, after weighing the risks and benefits; estrogen may confer some protection to the lens and retina.	• Drink eight glasses (8-ounce size) daily. • Control your weight; lose weight if you need to. • Take digestive aids if necessary. Try supplementing with Betaine (a weak hydrochloric acid) for one month. • Stop taking antacids.

Table 9. Additional Precautions

Other Diseases/Drugs	Whole Body
• Treat chronic diseases like asthma, high blood pressure, diabetes, elevated cholesterol, and heart conditions. • Treat other eye diseases with medications that don't increase cataracts. • Eliminate photosensitizing drugs, if possible. If it's absolutely necessary for you to take a photosensitizing drug, wear sunglasses outdoors, even on overcast days.	• Be extra conscious of the condition of your eyesight and any other symptoms you develop after being diagnosed with cataracts. • Take inventory of your general health. • Keep a calendar on which you record your medication and supplement regimens, so you can check when you started taking something new. • Exercise regularly. • Cover your eyes while in the sauna to protect them from the excess heat.

CHAPTER 7

Thief of Sight: Glaucoma

Myth: My eye pressure is normal, so I must not be at risk for glaucoma.
Fact: Glaucoma is now defined as a collection of diseases which cause optic nerve damage—and diagnosis is no longer based solely on whether an individual has elevated internal eye pressure.

One of my patients, a naturalized American who was born in India, has been treated for borderline but difficult-to-manage glaucoma. He's had a laser procedure and tried three different eyedrops because his intraocular pressure was very difficult to control. I suggested to him the possibility of using an Indian and Nepali herbal formula to control his eye pressure (along with other nutritional supplements, including magnesium and cod liver oil). He bolted upright in his chair, and said, "I cannot believe this, Doctor! My eyes do not cooperate with drops. I have red eyes. They weep. They are scratchy. My stomach is upset, and I have great trouble sleeping. I never heard of herbal therapies before in this country. My grandfather never would take me to Western doctors, until he had first tried herbal remedies." He then asked me, "When do I start this new therapy?" He has done very well reducing his glaucoma eyedrops by adding herbs, essential oils, and vitamins to his daily regimen.

Glaucoma is a complex condition caused by a group of diseases that damage the optic nerve and cause vision loss. Glaucoma has been recognized for centuries; in fact the word *glaucoma* comes from the ancient Greek word *glaucosis*, defined by Hippocrates as the "blue-green hue" of the affected eye. As the ancient Greeks used the term, it was not specific to glaucoma, but included other sight-robbing conditions like cataracts. It wasn't until the tenth century that Arabic physicians recognized that glaucoma is often—but not always—associated with increased pressure inside the eye. A complete description of glaucoma was not formulated until the nineteenth century, when the medical technology to provide a detailed scientific portrait of the condition evolved.

Most people (including eye doctors) used to think that glaucoma was defined entirely by increased internal eye pressure, which doctors call *elevated* intraocular pressure (IOP). Normal eye pressure falls between 12 and 21 millimeters (mm) of mercury, which is the standard measure of pressure. (Watch your local weather forecast carefully, and you'll notice that millimeters of mercury is also the scale used to measure weather-related barometric pressure.)

Even though we previously believed increased eye pressure and glaucoma to be inseparable, important clinical studies in the 1990s showed that a large number of glaucoma cases occur in the *absence* of increased eye pressure. Therefore, elevated eye pressure—which remains a key risk factor for the diagnosis of glaucoma—is no longer the sole criterion for diagnosing the disease.

As Alan Robin, M.D., of the Greater Baltimore Medical Center and the Johns Hopkins Hospital, explained in the December 1997 issue of *Ophthalmology Times*, glaucoma should be defined *not* by elevated pressure, but by optic nerve damage and its resulting vision loss. We still don't know exactly how glaucoma damages the optic nerve and destroys vision; its optic nerve damage appears to have numerous causes. One is increased eye pressure, which Dr. Robin called "an extremely important *risk factor*." Dr. Robin's new definition is supported by two very large studies of glaucoma—the Beaver Dam Eye Study and the East Baltimore Eye Survey—which found that about 40 percent of people with glaucoma have "normal," not elevated, eye pressure.

Dr. Abel's Tip

If you're told that you have glaucoma, learn your internal eye pressure measurement and what your optic nerves and visual fields look like. Ask to see a copy of your visual field test computer printout. Become a partner with your doctor in managing your treatment.

Incidence of Glaucoma

One percent of Americans currently have the commonest form of glaucoma, *chronic open-angle glaucoma,* and another 1 percent are at risk from high internal eye pressure or optic nerve disease. In other words, about three million Americans have some vision loss from glaucoma, and another two to three million are at risk of developing glaucoma. Matthew Wensor, M.D., and his associates in Melbourne, Australia, found that 1.7 percent of their patients had primary, open-angle glaucoma. The frequency increased with age, with up to 9.7 percent of people 80 years old and older having glaucoma. (Half of all these individuals had no idea they had the disease.) I can't emphasize too strongly how important it is to be tested annually (or more often, if your doctor recommends it) if you have any of the glaucoma risk factors. (See Table 10.) Glaucoma is truly a thief of sight.

People are more likely to be blinded by glaucoma than by cataract, even though cataract is more prevalent, because cataracts develop gradually and are less likely to limit people to seeing only the large letter E on the eye chart (the definition of blindness).

Glaucoma is particularly insidious, generally producing no symptoms in its early stage. The majority of glaucoma patients don't experience pain, eye inflammation, or even the visual abnormalities associated with the condition (like halos around lights). Changes in sight often occur first in the peripheral vision (the side vision), where they frequently aren't noticed. Furthermore, the second eye usually compensates for the damaged eye, since glaucoma is an asymmetrical disease and the two eyes generally do not have equal changes in vision. As a result, one eye's vision can deteriorate, unnoticed, for quite some time.

The basic problem in glaucoma is either poor drainage of intraocular fluids or poor circulation to the optic nerve. Many of these patients have other physical conditions, as demonstrated by a survey of 100 consecutive open-angle glaucoma patients in which most were discovered to be taking multiple medications. The number one other condition suffered by these patients was high blood pressure.

Anatomy

The eye is a fluid-filled sphere. The internal movement of the eye's fluid from its source of production (behind the iris) to its exit in the angle in front of the iris is important for the health of the lens and the cornea. (See Figure 6 for an illustration of how these parts of the eye relate to one another.)

The fluid in the eye must be under some pressure to keep the eyeball from collapsing, just as a basketball must be inflated to maintain its shape and buoyancy. If too much fluid is produced in the eye, or if it does not drain appropriately, the pressure inside the eye can become elevated, and optic nerve damage—and loss of vision—can result.

How easily the fluid exits the eye has an impact on eye pressure. The

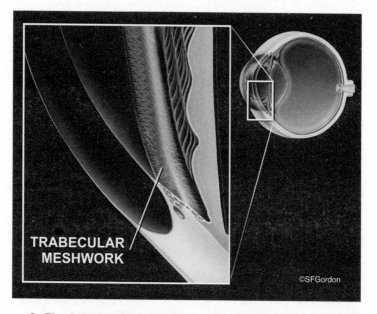

TRABECULAR MESHWORK

©SFGordon

Figure 6. The Anterior Chamber Angle (the aqueous humor fluid flows out through the trabecular meshwork)

fluid exits through a web between the cornea and the base of the iris. This web is called the *trabecular meshwork*. Think of it as resembling the meshwork covering the drain in your bathtub, which easily becomes clogged. From within the eye, the fluid exits through the trabecular mesh-work into the venous system, and travels down the jugular vein to the heart.

When this flow is impeded for any reason, the fluid backs up, and pressure inside the eye increases. The eye's drainage is blocked not only in glaucoma, but also in congestive heart failure and chronic obstructive lung disease. It can even occur as a result of breath-holding. This is another example of the interconnectiveness of all the systems in the body. The real culprit that starts the problem in the first place may be the heart or lung, but the eye sustains the damage.

One way the optic nerve is damaged in glaucoma is from lack of blood flow. Increased eye pressure is thought to damage the delicate capillaries around the optic nerve, which supply nutrients to the nerve fibers that enter the optic nerve from all parts of the retina. In other words, these capillaries nourish the nerves that carry images to the visual center in the brain and when that nourishment is cut off, so is vision. If no blood at all reaches the retina, sight can be lost completely.

Dr. Abel's Tip

An eye examination may be the key to diagnosing a serious eye disease, saving your vision, or even discovering a life-threatening condition. Make sure you get a complete eye exam every two years after the age of 40 unless you develop a glaucoma risk factor—in which case you should be examined every year.

Glaucoma: A Disease of Stress

It's clear that glaucoma is a disease of stress. When I talk to my patients about how stress can cause eye disorders, I explain that we actually have two involuntary nervous systems, the parasympathetic and the sympathetic systems. When we disturb the balance between them, we experience chronic stress. The *parasympathetic* nervous system controls the relaxation response and slows the heart rate; the *sympathetic* (or adrenaline) nervous system controls the anxiety response, speeding the heart rate and breathing.

There are circumstances in which each response is necessary, which is why we have dual nervous system wiring. If a mugger is chasing you down the street waving a weapon, you want your sympathetic (adrenaline) nervous system to go into high gear and get you out of there. After you escape to safety, however, you don't want your heart to continue pounding or to remain in a state of high anxiety. Then, your parasympathetic nervous system takes over, relaxing you, and slowing your heart rate and breathing.

With sustained imbalance between these two nervous systems, diseases like glaucoma can develop. We have always recognized that constant stress is not good for health. Decades ago, we assumed that stress could cause ulcers, but now we know they are caused by a bacterium named *Helicobactor pylori*. We also thought stress could cause heart attacks (and it is certainly a contributing factor). Nobody, however, thought about how stress might damage the eyes. It's extremely important to learn how to deal with stress, which we all experience, by using meditation or other stress-busters.

Stress makes us sick in many different ways. For instance, stressed people often hold their breath; carbon dioxide then builds up in their bloodstreams; the venous backflow in the head increases; fluid in the eye does not exit as easily as it does in a relaxed person; and, as a result, eye pressure can increase. This particular chain of events explains why people with chronic lung disease and asthma (or men wearing tight neckties) can develop elevated eye pressure at times. (They do not, however, necessarily go on to develop glaucoma.)

While we don't know exactly how the optic nerve is damaged by glaucoma, it is clear (as we've already discussed) that one feature common to all types of glaucoma is lack of blood flow to the retina and optic nerve. Starving the optic nerve results in retinal nerve cell death, enlargement of the optic cup, and loss of vision.

Classification and Characteristics

As we've discussed, elevated eye pressure is no longer used to define glaucoma. As many as 50 percent of people who experience elevated eye pressure at some time in their lives never develop optic nerve damage and its accompanying vision loss. And at least 25 percent of elderly people with damaged optic nerves never have elevated eye pressure.

An example of how elevated eye pressure and glaucoma do not always go hand in hand can be seen in the history of Barbara, a 70-year-old friend of my parents. After undergoing cataract surgery in both eyes, Barbara developed elevated eye pressure in her left eye. She was being cared for by a retina doctor in Philadelphia and by me in Wilmington. Although her physician in Philadelphia prescribed a common glaucoma medication that lowers eye pressure (one drop of Temoptic XE), Barbara's pressure on the date of her doctor's appointment was 22 mm in the untreated right eye and 24 mm in the treated left eye (normal eye pressure falls between 12 and 21 mm). The doctor told Barbara her eye pressure was too high, and that something needed to be done. Alarmed by her doctor's comments, Barbara asked if stress might be contributing to her condition. The doctor assured her that blood pressure and stress have no connection to eye pressure in people with glaucoma.

My experience has been quite the opposite, and numerous studies have also demonstrated that stress contributes to elevated eye pressure. Measurements such as eye pressure can change tremendously in a small period of time, because people can change a great deal in small periods of time. Eye pressure, like blood pressure, can change with weight and state of relaxation and/or anxiety—including the stress of visiting the doctor. At the time of this doctor's appointment, Barbara was in the midst of a number of very stressful situations, including coping with her husband's recent bypass surgery and her sister's health problems.

When I saw Barbara a number of days after her doctor's appointment in Philadelphia, her pressures were 19 mm in the untreated right eye and 15 mm in the treated left eye. Her eye exam, including her visual field test (which I'll explain later), was normal; in other words, the transient elevated pressure had not caused any optic nerve damage.

Barbara's case demonstrates how much eye pressure can fluctuate, depending upon the circumstances under which it is measured, and why having an elevated eye pressure at any given time is no reason to panic. It is simply a risk factor for glaucoma.

Executive glaucoma is another example of how eye pressure can change with circumstances. Men in ties and tight collars, nervous about their eye exams, can show a falsely elevated eye pressure because they are stressed and their blood flow is restricted by their clothing. So don't be uptight before your eye exam; loosen your collar, relax, and breathe deeply. You now know that intraocular pressure changes with circumstances, and I'm certain you would like it to fluctuate positively. You can participate in that positive development.

Glaucoma produces typical, easily recognized patterns of vision loss, and is classified according to the eye abnormalities that develop. There are six major types of glaucoma: (1) chronic, open-angle glaucoma; (2) angle-closure glaucoma; (3) secondary glaucoma; (4) low-tension glaucoma; (5) congenital glaucoma; and (6) glaucoma suspect.

1. The usual type of glaucoma in the United States is *chronic, open-angle glaucoma* (also called chronic, simple glaucoma). In open-angle glaucoma, there is plenty of room in the angle between the iris and the cornea for the eye's fluid to exit (see Figure 6). Glaucoma develops, it is thought, because the trabecular meshwork doesn't filter the eye's fluid very well. As many as 40 percent of patients with open-angle glaucoma have normal or low eye pressure and develop optic nerve changes and progressive visual loss without ever having elevated pressure.

2. A less frequent type of glaucoma in the United States (although it makes up almost 50 percent of this disease throughout the world) is *angle-closure glaucoma,* in which the base of the iris is too close to the cornea. Angle-closure glaucoma can be chronic, but it arises more often as a sudden attack with severe pain and visual halos. The pain can be so intense that the entire head aches and the patient feels nauseous and actually vomits. This is a true emergency.

3. The third type is called *secondary glaucoma,* because it develops secondary to other conditions, such as inflammation, injury, or blood in the eye. Secondary glaucoma may also be seen after the patient takes steroid medications (either orally or in the form of eyedrops). Fortunately, secondary glaucoma is easily diagnosed and monitored by most eye doctors; visits to a glaucoma specialist are only necessary when elevated eye pressure cannot be controlled.

4. The fourth type is *low-tension glaucoma,* which is thought to develop most often in elderly patients with diseases of poor circulation.

Since doctors are just beginning to realize how much glaucoma occurs in the absence of elevated eye pressure, it's important to know which conditions can mimic this type of glaucoma. Brain tumors, carotid artery blockage or aneurysm (swelling), certain hereditary optic nerve diseases, and toxic drugs or chemicals (especially methanol) can all produce optic nerve damage that may mimic glaucoma. *An eye exam may be the key to diagnosing one of these life-threatening conditions.* This is another example of how the eyes provide insight into the health of the rest of the body.

5. *Congenital glaucoma* is unusual, but can occur in the first few weeks to the first few months of life in one out of every 5,000–10,000 babies. Congenital glaucoma is extremely serious, and only aggressive surgery can blunt progression of the disease. (It is standard procedure to check for congenital glaucoma in newborns, so if you're having a baby, don't worry about this slim possibility. If you are concerned, just check with your doctor after your baby is born to make sure he or she examined the baby specifically to rule out this condition.)

6. The sixth form of glaucoma is *ocular hypertension,* which is also sometimes called *glaucoma suspect.* One-half of the patients I see have higher than normal eye pressure at some time, but never develop glaucoma. I follow these patients carefully, nevertheless, because it's impossible to determine who will eventually develop glaucoma. I offer them the opportunity to try some natural treatments, such as reducing stress and using supplementation. Some have high blood pressure, lung or heart disease, but have no other risk factor that might be raising their eye pressure. I'll tell you how to manage this type of situation a little later in this chapter.

Risk Factors

Most people don't realize that the commonest form of glaucoma—chronic, simple glaucoma—is a disease of stress. We all go to work and drive on the highway or ride the subway, but not everybody experiences the same amount of stress. Being under chronic stress is a *major* risk factor for developing glaucoma. All of the glaucoma medications currently used by ophthalmologists affect the body's adrenaline level, either stimulating or blocking it. Naturally produced adrenaline (also called *epinephrine)* produces stress, anxiety, and the "fight or flight" reflex. Anxiety, whether from internal or external causes, contributes to elevated eye pressure and, more importantly, may result in optic nerve damage.

Robert Ritch, M.D., director of the glaucoma service at the New York

Eye and Ear Infirmary, has described how anxiety affects his glaucoma patients. "You know, I had a patient whose wife died, and I couldn't control his eye pressure afterwards," Dr. Ritch notes. "I have another patient who's a trial attorney and whenever she's in trial, I can't control her pressure. When the trial's over, her pressure goes right down."

High blood pressure (hypertension) is clearly worsened by high anxiety, particularly in women. This condition was described as "white-coat hypertension" in a 1996 report in the *Journal of the American Medical Association*. Physicians should be aware that visiting the doctor can be very stressful and correct for that stress, for instance, by taking several blood pressure measurements throughout the office visit, or even suggesting that the patient buy a blood pressure cuff and measure pressure at home, under relaxed circumstances. The biochemical events that produce stress and high blood pressure also contribute to elevation of eye pressure. Low blood pressure also contributes to low internal eye pressure, which also isn't great—it can cause low-tension glaucoma.

Numerous conditions other than stress can raise internal eye pressure, including thyroid disease (hyperthyroidism), obesity, diabetes, emphysema, and cardiovascular disease. Digestive troubles may even play a role in causing glaucoma in some people. Therefore, you should be conscious about what you eat, and take supplements where relevant.

Dr. Abel's Tip

Remember that glaucoma is a disease of stress, and that relaxation can be your major contribution to treating your condition. Exercise, meditate, practice Tai Chi, take long walks, learn visual imagery, or sit quietly and think pleasant thoughts for ten minutes at a certain time every day. Eat meals slowly in a relaxed atmosphere to help improve your digestion.

Steroids—taken in the form of eyedrops, nosedrops, or inhalants—can contribute to the development of glaucoma, so their use must be managed appropriately. Sensitive people who are on long-term topical steroid therapy should be aware of this potential side effect.

Edeltraut Garbe, M.D., and her colleagues in Montreal, Canada, proved the correlation between taking steroid drugs and developing glaucoma. They did so by examining Quebec's health insurance database and cross-referencing the drug prescriptions of patients aged 66 and older with the rate at which they developed increased eye pressure or glaucoma. They found that those people who used inhalant or nasal steroids to treat asthma (and other conditions) for as short a time as three months had a significantly elevated risk of developing high eye pressure and glaucoma. Oral steroids—used to treat asthma, arthritis, lung disease, allergic reactions, and other chronic conditions—also increase risk for glaucoma.

I have seen this in my own practice, all too many times. A typical example was a woman whose internist had prescribed a steroid inhaler to treat her asthma. In response to the steroid, her internal eye pressure began to rise, so her eye doctor prescribed one of the most popular glaucoma eyedrops, a beta-blocker. Her eye pressure initially decreased, but her asthma worsened. Her internist then put her on systemic steroids to treat her asthma, but that made her eye pressure go higher. At this point, she came to me for a second opinion. I switched her to non-beta-blocker eyedrops, and recommended that she take as little cortisone as possible to control her asthma. I also recommended that she visit my Chinese doctor colleague in Wilmington, Delaware, who treated both conditions with herbs. She responded to the Chinese herbs, and is no longer on an inhaler or any other type of cortisone drugs. Her eye pressure continues to be under control.

If this horror story sounds unusual, unfortunately, it's not. This lady's drug-induced roller-coaster ride is all too common. An important part of the eye care revolution is to encourage people to use natural remedies whenever possible, so they don't suffer from the side effects produced by drugs. Conventional medications (usually eyedrops) should be used to get your glaucoma under control quickly. Meanwhile, steps should be taken to determine which alternative therapies (if appropriate for you) would be helpful.

Dr. Abel's Tip

Glaucoma is the leading cause of blindness in African Americans, who should be tested regularly for glaucoma beginning at the age of 35, especially if there is any family history of the condition.

If you are at risk for developing glaucoma, take that risk seriously. Glaucoma is the second-most important cause of blindness in the United States (after diabetic retinopathy), and the single most important cause of blindness among African Americans. If glaucoma is detected early and treated properly, blindness can be prevented. *There is no longer any reason for people to go blind from glaucoma!*

It is now thought that two or more risk factors have to interact for you to develop glaucoma. The risk factors are summarized in Table 10. Just having one risk factor does not imply that you might develop glaucoma. Having more than one, however, makes it evident that you are at risk.

Table 10. Glaucoma Risk Factors

• Being African American (more problematic for treatment because the iris contains a great deal of pigment; glaucoma is the leading cause of blindness among African Americans).
• Family history of glaucoma (means you probably are at risk).
• Extreme nearsightedness.
• Farsightedness, higher level and a risk of angle closure.
• Pigment dispersion (a syndrome in which the loss of pigment from the iris splashes onto the back of the cornea and into the trabecular meshwork).
• Pseudo-exfoliation (appears like dandruff on the front of the lens; approximately 20 percent of those who have it will develop progressively elevated eye pressure).
• Optic pallor (a pale optic nerve, which should be yellow to pink. This is a sign of nerve damage, which could be from any cause, including glaucoma).
• Optic cup asymmetry (i.e., optic cups of different sizes. Consider glaucoma first, carotid artery blockage second).
• Intraocular pressure greater than 21 mm (even more suspicious, greater than 24).
• Narrow anterior chamber angle (see Figure 6; this condition requires gonioscopy to be certain angle is still open; the pressure is usually normal if there is no attack of glaucoma).
• Nerve fiber defect (this is only determined by special testing; requires a follow-up every six to twelve months).
• Intraocular pressure asymmetry between the two eyes (especially when it is greater than 5 mm).
• Disc hemorrhage (can occur from straining, vomiting, being on aspirin therapy or other anticoagulants, but is more common in patients with glaucoma. A small hemorrhage on the disc may be normal in these conditions, but if none of them is present, it may be a sign of glaucoma).
• Branch vein occlusion (although rarely a cause, glaucoma may be secondary to this disease of poor drainage of blood from the eye).
• Peripheral vascular disease (not enough blood to the eye).
• Thyroid disease (prominent eyes, exposed to increased pressure from intraorbital swelling).
• Steroid use (elevates intraocular pressure mildly in approximately 16 percent of people on steroids; the elevation is more severe in postoperative patients).

Diagnosis of Glaucoma

Glaucoma is diagnosed by reviewing both the patient's risk factors and the outcome of his or her eye exam. Glaucoma is suspected in a patient with elevated eye pressure whose optic nerves look different from each other. The usual methods used to diagnose glaucoma are measurement of eye pressure, examination of the optic nerves, and a computerized examination of the visual field.

I don't rely on measuring eye pressure alone to assess glaucoma risk in my patients. I also perform a complete eye exam looking at the optic nerve and assessing the patient's angle (see Figure 6).

Again, you should have a complete eye examination every couple of years unless you: (1) have a family history of glaucoma; (2) have significant nearsightedness (myopia); (3) have corneal disease; (4) are diabetic; (5) are African-American; and/or (6) smoke a pack or more of cigarettes a day (or are around a significant amount of secondhand smoke daily). *If you have any of these risk factors, you should have a complete eye exam every year, to make sure you are not developing optic nerve damage.*

An eye doctor can see optic nerve damage through an ophthalmoscope. The optic nerve is a round area at the back of the eye; it is called the *optic disc.* Within the optic disc there is an indented region called its *cup.* The health of the optic nerve can be determined by noting the ratio of the size of the cup to the overall optic disc diameter. In healthy eyes, the two optic discs should be the same size, and the cup-to-disc ratio should not change much with age. An increase in the cup's size is a sign of optic nerve damage.

The visual field examination is very sensitive and detects the earliest changes at the edge of peripheral vision, where glaucoma first damages sight. The nerve fibers that supply the peripheral vision are most susceptible to starvation from lack of blood flow, one of the suspected culprits in glaucoma. Since the visual field examination is a computerized test, its results can be compared from year to year.

Other tests that help to diagnose glaucoma include: serial measurements of the eye pressure at different times of the day; digital photography; laser scanning of the optic nerve; and *gonioscopy,* during which a tiny contact lens with a mirror is placed on the eye. Digital photography and laser scanning of the optic nerve (and nerve fibers) are becoming state of the art.

Researchers are developing new ways of diagnosing glaucoma, including thermography and using scanning lasers to examine the eye's blood flow. While these new technologies are not yet available to everyone, they will make diagnosis and follow-up more precise.

Another new test soon to be available is short wavelength autoperimetry (SWAP). By having a patient look at a yellow screen on which the doctor randomly flashes blue lights of differing intensities, visual field defects can be recognized in early glaucoma patients. (The standard visual field examination now used, which uses black dots against a white background, is less selective for glaucoma.) These new developments will make glaucoma diagnosis and follow-up more precise when they become available.

Rest assured, however, that even if your doctor doesn't have all the latest gizmos, the computerized visual field tests now available are very sensitive tools for monitoring glaucoma, along with the doctor's watchful eye. Don't be afraid to ask your doctor, "Are there any changes in my condition?"

For the glaucoma risk group, ignorance can result in blindness. But you can take charge. Have your internal eye pressure checked at different times of the day (to control for factors like stress), and ask your ophthalmologist or optometrist for your pressure measurement.

Conventional Therapy

Eye doctors prescribe more drugs for glaucoma than for any other eye disease. These drugs (including eyedrops, which contain drugs in concentrated form) are absorbed in the body and can cause unexpected side effects. I will explain how some of the most-prescribed drugs work, and tell you what side effects you might experience if your doctor prescribes them for you.

Open-Angle Glaucoma Therapy

In most cases, I treat open-angle glaucoma with medication before contemplating surgery, but each patient's treatment is based on his or her individual situation. If a patient has early cataract changes, I would not use a *miotic* drug that causes the pupil to contract because these medications decrease the amount of light entering the eye—and light is already diminished because of the developing cataract.

Quite a number of antiglaucoma drugs are on the market, and can be used sequentially if the first medication prescribed is not effective. (See Table 11.)

There are three types of drugs that inhibit production of the eye's fluid: the *alpha agonists*, the *beta blockers*, and the *carbonic anhydrase inhibitors*. These medications interrupt different pathways in the adrenaline nervous system.

The beta-blocker drugs have been very popular glaucoma treatments since the late 1970s. Because they interfere with the nervous system pathway that governs heart rate and breathing, however, they can cause worsening of asthma and chronic lung disease, as well as lowering blood pressure and inducing heart rhythm abnormalities. Therefore, I reserve them for younger, healthier people, and watch for side effects in others, since it often takes years for them to develop. The side effects disappear when the drug is discontinued.

The beta blockers and carbonic anhydrase inhibitors (see Table 11) are the first-line drugs unless special circumstances exist (such as having a disease in which use of these drugs is contraindicated; having a narrow angle, or being allergic to the drug). Both work well over the long term in the treatment of chronic open-angle glaucoma and elevated internal eye pressure, but they work better when used together. Cosopt is a combination of timolol and dorzolamide, which reduces eyedrop administration and lowers intraocular pressure more than 30 percent. Additionally, timolol can upset the cholesterol ratio (HDL to LDL, i.e., "good" to "bad" cholesterol). Timolol and other beta blockers can worsen breathing in people with lung disease and asthma, and slow the heart in susceptible elderly people; Betalol is much less likely to have this effect on heart rhythm.

The alpha agonists (such as apraclonidine and Bromonidine), like the beta blockers, work by limiting the eye's fluid production. Alpha-agonist drugs, however, can produce serious allergic reactions in 10 to 30 percent of patients. They are useful in preventing acute pressure rises after laser procedures to the front of the eye. Patients taking them should be alerted to possible long-term side effects. Bromonidine produces fewer allergic reactions and is becoming a first-line drug. A recent study in twenty healthy eyes showed that apraclonidine (1 percent) can actually increase the blood flow to the retina. It remains to be seen how well this works in people with chronic glaucoma.

Pilocarpine, a parasympathomimetic drug (see Table 11), works by a different mechanism. It increases outflow from the trabecular meshwork (by pulling the iris out of the chamber angle and constricting the pupil and ciliary body). (See Figure 6.) This is especially helpful in treating narrow-angle glaucoma.

The antiglaucoma drug latanoprost deserves special mention because it is a hormone-like substance that lowers eye pressure so remarkably it comes in a strength of 0.005 percent in a vial containing only 2.5 cc's—about one teaspoon. Latanoprost is very powerful, but it is usually a second-line drug because of its expense. I have been told that the only side effect of latanoprost is that blue eyes can turn brown. Over the years, however, I've found that a number of patients experience eye pain and irritation while using latanoprost, which is one of the reasons the drug's manufacturer suggests using it at night. An inflamed iris and swelling in the retina are rare complications; both conditions were reversible. Latanoprost and similar medications must be used with care in postoperative eyes because it can lower eye pressure precipitously (which can be as dangerous as having increased eye pressure). *I can't emphasize too strongly that patients should evaluate how they feel after beginning any medication, including an eyedrop medication, and be constantly aware that all medications can have side effects.* Be sure to report all symptoms you suspect are drug-related side effects to your physician immediately.

Dr. Abel's Tip

Although there are many effective antiglaucoma drugs available if you need them, some produce unwanted side effects if they're used for longer than three months. Whenever you begin taking a new drug—including eyedrops—evaluate how you feel carefully, and note any new symptoms you develop and which old symptoms disappear as a result of treatment. It's often possible to use conventional eyedrops for glaucoma in quick, "pulse" therapy, while beginning a nutritional and supplementation program to treat it long term using natural means.

Oral carbonic anhydrase inhibitors (Diamox or Neptazane), as well as intravenous manitol (which is used for short periods of time to lower eye pressure before surgery) need to be used cautiously because they can change electrolyte balance. The family physician and any other physicians attending the patient should be informed when these medications are prescribed. Your family doctor should always be informed about your use of prescription eyedrops.

Angle-Closure Glaucoma Therapy

Angle-closure glaucoma usually requires a surgical or laser treatment such as *laser iridectomy.* (See Table 12.) This condition can sometimes be controlled for short periods of time with medications like pilocarpine eyedrops, beta-blocker eyedrops, alpha-agonist eyedrops (like apracloni-dine), or oral Diamox or Neptazane. Generally, these drugs are used until the eye pressure has been lowered enough so the ophthalmologist can see clearly to perform a laser iridectomy (using a laser to create a hole in the iris, so fluid can exit the eye properly). After the pressure has been relieved by the laser procedure, the drugs are cautiously reduced.

Occasionally, laser iridectomy does not cure angle-closure glaucoma patients because they also have a component of open-angle glaucoma. In this case, the patient may require treatment with medications used to treat open-angle glaucoma. In the rare case that the angle is still sealed shut after laser iridectomy and no fluid flows out of the eye, a nonlaser surgical procedure needs to be performed.

Some patients treated with blood pressure–lowering drugs like calcium channel blockers also experience a decrease in eye pressure, but this effect has not been confirmed in a large number of people. (Magnesium, by the way, is the natural calcium channel blocker, and is used successfully by me and other practitioners as part of a natural program to lower blood pressure.)

Carbonic anhydrase inhibitors (such as Diamox and Neptazane) lower internal eye pressure by decreasing fluid formation in the eye. These drugs are formulated as pills instead of eyedrops, however, and the folly of poisoning the body to get to the eye is obvious. To solve this problem, pharmaceutical manufacturers have created carbonic anhydrase inhibitors as eyedrops (Azopt and Trusopt), which appear to be quite effective but should not be used in people with corneal deterioration.

All drugs produce side effects, and you must certainly use your own judgment when taking a medication. Observe how it affects you. Only after prolonged studies, for example, did we recognize that the beta blockers sometimes exacerbate a rare muscle weakness disease called myasthenia gravis and can create impotence and loss of libido. By discontinuing a medication and watching the symptoms disappear, you can associate symptoms with medications or, for that matter, foods, herbs, or supplements. Conversely, by adding a medication (or herb, food, or supplement) and watching symptoms disappear, you can perceive its benefits.

Determining the benefit versus the risk helps physicians choose among various drugs (as well as between drugs and surgery) in treating their patients. In managing your own health, you should also be able to determine the benefit versus the risk of any proposed treatment or regimen. One way to do this is to keep a lifestyle calendar in which you note your general state of health, your diet (including supplements and drugs) and your daily activities.

A new class of antiglaucoma drug, called *glutamate antagonists*, is under development. These drugs, as their name implies, interfere with the action of glutamate, an essential amino acid required for conduction of nerve impulses in the eye and brain. Evan Dreyer, M.D., at the University of Pennsylvania, has found high levels of glutamate in glaucoma and cataract patients' eye fluid. Furthermore, the levels tend to correlate positively with the duration of glaucoma (that is, a higher level of glutamate in the eye is associated with having had glaucoma for a long time).

While glutamate is essential for sight, too much of this potent neurotransmitter is toxic to cells in the retina—it kills neurons and ultimately causes blindness. To allow glutamate to do its necessary job in the eyes, while making sure that any excess cannot cause damage, the new drugs target a very specific glutamate receptor. By binding to this receptor (and thereby preventing glutamate from binding to it), the glutamate antagonist medications will, it is hoped, stop excess glutamate from damaging the eye and causing blindness.

Because the ideal drug for treating glaucoma does not yet exist, researchers are attempting to invent it. The ideal glaucoma drug should: (1) lower eye pressure, if necessary; (2) be neuroprotective (to prevent nerve cell death in the retina and optic nerve); and (3) increase blood flow to the back of the eye.

Knowing what drug is best for you is a matter for discussion with your own doctor. Become conversant with your disease and the treatment regimen you are following, including the side effects of the drugs you're taking. Learn what kind of glaucoma you have (such as low-tension glaucoma, narrow-angle glaucoma, pigmentary glaucoma, or pseudo-exfoliation) and any variations that might be present in your case.

Table 11. Glaucoma Drugs and Their Side Effects

Drug	Possible Side Effects
Beta-blockers (eyedrops) • timolol (Timoptic, Betimol) • betaxolol (Betoptic) • levobunolol (Betagan) • carteolol (Ocupress) • metipranolol (Optipranolol)	dilated pupils slightly red eyes asthma and shortness of breath bradycardia (heart arrhythmia) congestive heart failure fatigue and reduced exercise tolerance impotence hair loss memory loss depression increased cholesterol and other blood lipids
Alpha-agonists (eyedrops) • apraclonidine (Iopidine) • bromonidine (Alphagan) • dipivefrin (Propine, a weaker agent) • epinephrine (Epifrin, the weakest agent in this group)	red eyes allergic conjunctivitis headache dry mouth tachycardia tremulousness hypertension allergic reaction Monoamine oxidase inhibitors (to treat depression) should not be used in conjunction with Iopidine and Alphagan (alpha-agonists).

Table 11. Glaucoma Drugs and Their Side Effects (cont.)

Drug	Possible Side Effects
Carbonic anhydrase inhibitors (eyedrops and tablets) • acetazolamide (Diamox, tablets) • methazolamide (Neptazane, tablets)	anorexia or weight loss fatigue or drowsiness increased urinary frequency kidney stones hair loss depression hypokalemia (lowers potassium) aplastic anemia (very rarely stops red blood cell production) paresthesia (tingling in fingers and toes) metabolic acidosis (changes the acidity of the blood) taste disturbance Stevens-Johnson Syndrome (a rare syndrome that affects all mucous membranes in an antibody-antigen reaction)
Carbonic anhydrase inhibitors (eyedrops) • dorzolamide (Trusopt, eyedrops) • Cosopt (a combination of dorzolamide [Trusopt] with the beta-blocker Timolol [timoptic]; eyedrops) • brinzolamide (Azopt, eyedrops)	metallic taste in mouth Use with caution in patients with sulfa drug (sulfonamide) allergies because it is a sulfa derivative and may cross-react. The combination should reduce the side effects of each individual drug. more comfortable than Trusopt
Prostaglandin analogs (eyedrops) • bimatoprost (Lumigan) • latanoprost (Xalatan) • travaprost (Travatan)	increase in iris pigmentation red eye intraocular inflammation (rarely) skin rash bronchitis arthralgia (achy joints) angina (chest pain)
Parasympathomimetics (eyedrops) • pilocarpine (Pilocar, Pilogel, Ocusert) • carbachol (Carbachol) • echothiophate (Phospholine iodide)	tearing (rarely) red eye (rarely) decreased night vision reduced accommodation (blurred vision) headache nausea diarrhea sweating Bronchospasm—asthma or wheezing increased salivation

One way to develop new neuroprotective drugs would be to reformulate old drugs used to treat other neurological conditions (like stroke or depression) so they can be used to treat the eye. Intriguing work on drugs used to treat depression (such as the serotonin agonists Prozac and Paxil) is being done by Neville Osborne, Ph.D., a professor of ocular neurobiology at Oxford University. In animal studies, Dr. Osborne has found that these substances lower eye pressure, are neuroprotective, and increase blood flow. Is it possible that glaucoma is actually depression of the eye—and that depression is glaucoma of the brain, that is, caused by poor blood flow to the brain? This could mean that drugs that are effective against glaucoma might also be effective against depression, and vice versa. It's interesting that glaucoma and depression may both result from unhandled stress, and may be improved by increasing levels of essential fatty acids and magnesium, as well as by meditation.

Laser and Surgical Treatments

If medical treatment of glaucoma is unsuccessful or inappropriate for some reason, laser or surgical interventions can be employed. Table 12 lists the various laser and surgical procedures that are currently available. In most situations, with the exception of congenital glaucoma or an attack of acute angle-closure glaucoma (which is a true medical emergency), medical therapy is tried first. In developing countries or where there are limited resources for purchasing medication, however, laser or surgical therapy is usually used first.

Whatever therapy is employed to control glaucoma, all patients require medical follow-up, because the patient is not able to determine whether the disease is controlled.

I cannot tell you which of these procedures would best correct your condition, but I generally recommend using peripheral iridectomy for all cases of angle-closure glaucoma. For open-angle glaucoma, I usually attempt medical treatment as the first option (including nutrition, supplementation and lifestyle changes), followed by a laser procedure (trabeculoplasty) if necessary, using surgery as a last resort, depending on specific conditions.

With the availability of all these options—medical, laser, and surgical— why are my colleagues and I not satisfied with conventional therapy for glaucoma? The answer lies in these therapies' side effects on the eyes or other parts of the body. Glaucoma does not develop independently from the rest of the body, as we have seen by examining the stress that can

Table 12. Current Laser and Surgical Procedures for Glaucoma

Type of Procedure	Information about Procedure
Laser Procedures • Argon laser trabeculoplasty	• Used for poorly controlled open-angle glaucoma patients, patients who are resistant or allergic to medication. The best results are obtained in brown-eyed people who have not had surgery.
• Argon laser peripheral iridectomy	• The laser makes a hole in the iris to allow fluid to go directly to the angle and deepen the chamber. Bleeding will not occur, because this laser cauterizes blood vessels.
• YAG laser peripheral iridotomy	• This laser in the infrared spectrum is far more powerful in opening the iris and works better in blue eyes. Minimal bleeding may occur but is easily controlled.
Surgical Procedures • Peripheral iridectomy	• The old technique for angle-closure glaucoma, now essentially replaced by lasers. It is performed with intraocular surgery to avoid angle-closure in the postoperative period.
• Trabeculectomy	• Removing a portion of the trabecular meshwork (the eye's drain) while leaving a scleral roof to allow fluid to filter out of the anterior chamber of the eye. This procedure is only 50 percent successful because of potential scarring.
• Trabeculectomy with mitomycin-C	• The anticancer drug mitomycin is applied briefly before the conventional surgery is performed to minimize future scarring. There's a small incidence of this procedure lowering the pressure too much, otherwise this would be the only one performed—in other words, it may work too well.
• Glaucoma tube shunts	• A small plastic tube attached to a tiny drainage bag is inserted inside the eye. This procedure is reserved for other surgical failures.
• Discocanalostomy	• A new, less invasive technique.

initiate it. All the interventions we've discussed treat the symptom, not the root cause, while alternative therapies strive to resolve the symptom by treating the underlying condition. If you have a family history of glaucoma, prevention is obviously the best medicine.

Alternative Therapies and Prevention

Total body wellness is the first goal of prevention. It's known that glaucoma patients have scored very low in a limited number of quality-of-life surveys, which means that either the characteristics of the disease or its treatment is making this group of people enjoy life less than other groups surveyed. Therefore, it's crucial to modify lifestyle, especially by controlling stress. Anxiety and stress increase production of cortisone and other natural chemicals that are toxic to the eye and brain.

I advise all my patients over the age of 40—and those of any age with special risk factors—to formulate a glaucoma prevention strategy. Periodic eye exams are a necessary part of that prevention strategy to diagnose glaucoma at its earliest stage, when vision loss can be stopped. Research is revealing specific genes linked to the development of glaucoma, so it's important to know your family history of eye disease.

Controlling risk factors that contribute to the development of glaucoma is also crucial to your prevention strategy. Conditions like high blood pressure (hypertension), obesity, thyroid disease, diabetes, and chronic obstructive pulmonary disease (emphysema) must be kept in check.

In our search to harmonize the eye and the body and provide greater health, we must examine options that are not only less invasive than conventional medical therapies but that will nourish the body and spirit as well. The health management concept originated by Dean Ornish, M.D. (author of *Dr. Dean Ornish's Program for Reversing Heart Disease* and *Love and Survival*), which includes food, exercise, and meditation, is a wise combination to consider as you make changes in your life (although Dr. Ornish's program, directed at heart disease, is stricter than what I propose here).

In addition to making lifestyle modifications, you must make sure you are consuming adequate amounts of protective nutrients to build up your antioxidant bank account. While certain amounts of the essential nutrients can be obtained from your diet, you will probably want to supplement your intake of crucial vitamins, minerals, and other substances if you are at risk for developing glaucoma.

Lifestyle Modifications

Exercise

The importance of exercise cannot be overstated. Thirty to forty minutes of walking every day is the equivalent of taking a daily beta blocker.

Michael Passo, M.D., at the Oregon Health Sciences University, found that thirty minutes of brisk walking four times a week reduced intraocular pressure 16 percent in all participants in his study and 20 percent in those with elevated eye pressure. A study of Finnish twins showed that leisure-time physical activity reduced mortality significantly, even after genetic and other family factors were taken into account. Walking, jogging, yoga, Tai Chi, Chi Kung, and riding a bike are all good ways to start improving bodily health. An outdoor activity is preferred to an indoor one, if possible, so that you can experience nature, which in itself is an aid to relaxation. Don't overdo it, however, by throwing yourself into a strenuous exercise program after months or years of being stationary. Take small steps toward long-term goals.

Relaxation

Begin by taking a deep breath. Few problems are really that bad. Breathe deeply, clear the mind, and think gentler thoughts. Think about how wonderful you are, and if that's too difficult, consider how important you are to your family and friends as well as to yourself. Chi Kung is a method of breathing exercises that the Chinese find very helpful in reducing stress. (The Chinese have developed treatments for glaucoma only relatively recently, since Chinese traditional doctors did not previously possess the ability to measure intraocular pressure. The Chinese strategy was to decrease excess fluid in the upper part of the body while normalizing blood circulation to the eye by relaxing the restriction of liver energy through various herbs. Interestingly, herbs that aid the liver will also help the eye.) Massaging the neck also reduces stress. Loosening the neck, freeing the mind, massaging the jaw joint (the TMJ) to improve blood flow and decrease constriction, stretching and exercising are all helpful, as is meditation.

An essential component in treating and preventing glaucoma is dealing with stress appropriately. Our two involuntary nervous systems, parasympa-thetic and sympathetic, must be kept in balance. They control the glands that regulate the production of hormones, creating either stress or relax-ation hormones. We need to counteract the effect of cortisone, for instance, through deep breathing, visual imagery, meditation, and exercise.

Stress not only affects the brain, it affects receptors in the eye. In treating or preventing glaucoma, we need to relax the body and improve blood and energy flow up the neck into the brain. The Chinese say, "Open the Three Gates to liberate energy." The Three Gates are the low back, high back, and neck.

Digestion

Proper digestion is crucial to the health of the parasympathetic nervous system. The production of the intrinsic B_{12} factor (which nourishes nerves) requires the production of normal digestive juices and the absence of *helicobactor pylori*, the bacterium recently implicated as the cause of most ulcers. If you don't produce enough stomach acid to digest your food, you may develop what appears to be stubborn indigestion or acid reflux and food sensitivities. You can even develop memory problems, mood swings, poor bowel habits, and feel sleepy or sluggish all the time. If you have these symptoms and suspect a poor supply of normal digestive juices may be to blame, ask your physician to test your stomach acid, begin taking digestive enzymes, and increase the amount of fiber in your diet. It's rare to have too much stomach acid after the age of 35, so stop taking antacids (unless you have a hiatal hernia, in which case antacids should be taken after a meal when you're ready to lie down). Antacids are actually the opposite of what many older people need.

Despite our new high-tech devices, we still need to use common sense to determine if disease is present and decide what to do about it. If an eye condition is diagnosed, patients should be full participants in making treatment decisions, and should get a "report card" with each visit to chart their progress in assisting with their own treatment. Glaucoma treatment is a participatory event. You can act on your own behalf as long as you take your medications and work with your physician to make informed decisions.

Dietary Recommendations

Diet

Protect your liver (which protects your eyes) by eating a plant-based diet. Make sure you consume plenty of foods containing potassium and magnesium (which will probably require supplements, since it's difficult to obtain adequate amounts from food). Don't add extra salt to your food; excess salt can raise blood pressure and internal eye pressure. It can also reduce the stores of potassium within your body.

Water

Drink water to dilute the toxins in your body. Water has many values, which include hydrating your kidneys (so they don't rely on the liver to do their work); helping in fat metabolism; and diluting and draining the body of toxins. Agreed, you may be going to the bathroom a lot, but when the color of the urine changes from orange to clear, you'll know you're excreting as many toxins as possible. Water also hydrates the stool, which has a beneficial effect for glaucoma patients. Normally, drinking six to eight glasses of water a day is useful, although it occasionally temporarily raises intraocular pressure. Nonetheless, its value outweighs potential risk. You may not be able to drink eight glasses of water each day, but start increasing your intake gradually. Our cells cannot afford to be dehydrated, and consuming adequate amounts of water helps to reduce joint and back pain, too.

Alcohol

Alcohol is not water. In general, moderate your alcohol use. One or two glasses of wine in the evening can be good for eyes and for insomnia, but a greater quantity of wine (and hard liquor) should be avoided. (I recommend that my patients minimize or eliminate hard liquor.) Wine, especially red wine, can contribute to the health of body and eyes if consumed in moderation (one glass a day), because it contains important nutrients. Those nutrients include: anthocyanins, the red pigment in grape skin (and other fruit skins); flavones, which decrease capillary fragility; proanthrocyanins (also called OPCs), a newly discovered class of powerful antioxidants; resveratrol, an OPC with antioxidant and anti-estrogen activities (now available as a supplement); amino acids, the building blocks of proteins; tannins, plant extracts used as astringents; small amounts of vitamin C (which disappears with complete fermentation of the wine); high levels of rutin, a bioflavonoid that's thought to reduce capillary fragility; and the B vitamin thiamine, which appears to have positive effects on Alzheimer's disease and other mental conditions.

Wine may have anticancer properties because it contains transresveratrol (a form of the antioxidant resveratrol), catechins (which, like tannins, have astringent properties), and other antioxidants. Additionally, alcohol (in the form called phenol) dissolves fat, one reason it can be helpful in dissolving the fatty plaques that clog arteries. Studies are beginning to demonstrate the value of moderate amounts of wine in preventing (and possibly reversing) eye disease. For instance, Thomas O. Obisessan, M.D., M.P.H., found that two glasses of wine daily (red or white) actually halved his study subjects' risk of developing macular degeneration.

Cholesterol

Treat your elevated cholesterol naturally, if possible, with supplements that are also good for the circulation: essential fatty acids, vitamins E, A, C, garlic, *Ginkgo biloba*, L-arginine, alpha-lipoic acid, bilberry, lutein, lycopene, and zeaxanthin. Try eating oatmeal for breakfast every morning to lower your cholesterol before you consider taking cholesterol-lowering drugs, which have many unwanted side effects.

Self-Monitoring

Note days when you don't feel well—or can't see well—and what you ate, drank, and did in the preceding days. When you add (or subtract) a drug or supplement, note it on your lifestyle calendar, and evaluate its effects in thirty to sixty days.

Supplementation Recommendations

Essential Fatty Acids

Omega-3 essential fatty acids: 500 mg daily. Supplements derived from fish oil, microalgae, and certain plant foods (like flaxseed, borage, evening primrose and currant oils) provide these essential nutrients. Most Americans' diets don't include sufficient amounts of these substances that are so protective to the eyes. The Inuits of Alaska, for instance, have traditionally had a low incidence of glaucoma because of the high fish oil content of their diet. Transfats, which displace the essential fatty acids in the body, are often found at higher concentrations in the diets of people with glaucoma and high internal eye pressure.

The essential fatty acids are important in maintaining the health of the rest of the body as well. They are required for healthy cell membranes (to keep blood vessels from leaking); for proper brain functioning (50 percent of the fats in the brain, retina, and adrenal glands are the essential fatty acid DHA); and for visual acuity. Essential fatty acids improve circulation (by making the lining of blood vessels smoother and thinning the blood). They also improve the flexibility and permeability of cell membranes and protect the retina's photoreceptor cells (the rods and cones). In the elderly, essential fatty acids decrease stress while increasing the activity of the adrenal corticosteroids. Essential fatty acid deficiency can decrease visual acuity. The two major types of essential fatty acids are the Omega-3 and Omega-6 fats. While it was initially thought that we should consume, by supplementation if necessary, equal amounts of both these essential fatty acids, research has shown that the standard American diet is very high in Omega-6 fats and extremely depleted in Omega-3 fats. This imbalance between Omega-6 and Omega-3 essential fatty acids appears to contribute to the development of a large number of chronic illnesses, including allergies, learning disabilities such as attention deficit disorder and dyslexia in children, arthritis, autoimmune diseases, some types of dementia, hyperactivity, and some vision problems.

The Omega-3 essential fatty acids increase immunity, coat the gastrointestinal tract, increase the slipperiness of platelets (i.e., decrease platelet adhesiveness or the tendency to form blood clots), and improve circulation. Omega-3 fatty acids may also lubricate the trabecular meshwork, allowing fluid to exit more easily. Giving cod liver oil (which is high in Omega-3 essential fatty acids) to rabbits lowers intraocular pressure, so obviously mother knew best when she told you to take your cod liver oil. A daily dose of 500 milligrams of essential fatty acids is safe for most people, although individuals with bleeding conditions or who are on anticoagulants should not increase their essential fatty acid intake except on the advice of their doctors.

The Omega-3 essential fatty acids come from both animal and plant sources. The major source of the Omega-3 essential fatty acid DHA (docosahexaenoic acid) is fish, which is why it is often called "fish oil." Its best sources are cold-water fatty fish (salmon, tuna, mackerel, cod, herring, sardines, and trout) and eel. If you buy fish oil capsules, it's important to make sure they're fresh and have been refrigerated, since they easily go rancid. Carlson makes an excellent Super DHA; for vegetarians there is a supplement containing microalgae-derived DHA called Neuromins™. (Note other supplement manufacturers in the Resource Guide. For more information, see my book *The DHA Story*.

Vegetable sources of Omega-3 fats include walnuts, canola oil, flaxseeds and flaxseed oil, and green leafy vegetables. The high Omega-3 content of green vegetables is one of the reasons that nutritionists advise us to eat five to nine servings of fruits and vegetables every day.

Essential fatty acids can be purchased in either liquid or pill supplement form. Neuromins™ DHA, or fish oil, can be purchased separately from the other essential fatty acids, generally in capsule form. Essential fatty acid supplements should be taken with a meal and a fat-soluble vitamin, like vitamin E.

Vitamins

Multivitamin: one or two daily. A study of visual changes performed at five Veterans' Administration hospitals found that a daily multivitamin (designed to help the eyes) stabilized macular degeneration, while the macular degeneration in a group of veterans who received a placebo worsened. It also slightly decreased the incidence of cataract formation in these veterans in a study that was performed before lutein (which protects against cataracts) was added to the vitamin's formula.

Vitamin A: 10,000 IU daily. Vitamin A (or its provitamin, beta-carotene, and the other carotenoids) protects retinal receptors. Vitamin A is often included in adequate amounts in multivitamins. The toxic dose of vitamin A is 30,000 IU per day over a long period of time, so don't go overboard with this supplement. Many people take this supplement in beta-carotene form, because it's impossible to overdose on beta-carotene. I generally take "preformed" vitamin A.

Lutein/Zeaxanthin (6–10 mg daily): Two of the carotenes, lutein and zeaxanthin, are concentrated in the macula and found in the aqueous humor. It's important to know that lutein and zeaxanthin compete with beta-carotene, as well as vitamins with A and E, so adequate amounts must be consumed for them to be effective. Along with vitamin E, lutein protects against damage caused by blue light, stabilizing the pigment layer underneath the retina. It is especially helpful to take lutein at night when the eyes are healing. Spinach, collard greens, and eggs have very high levels of lutein, but I recommend taking a supplement of lutein daily.

B vitamins: a B complex vitamin containing 50 or 100 mg of all the B vitamins. The B vitamins include thiamin (B_1), riboflavin (B_2), pyridoxine (B_6), B_{12}; niacin, pantothenic acid, biotin, and folic acid. Choline and inositol are unofficial members of the B vitamin family, and are often included in B vitamin complexes. Most multivitamins, however, will not contain enough B vitamins, which is why a B complex vitamin is important. B vitamins help maintain the myelin that protects nerves, the fatty acids around nerves, and the retinal receptors. B_{12} is necessary for optic nerve function, and supports the myelin sheaths that protect nerve fibers. B_{12} also protects the optic nerve from cyanide toxicity, which can result from alcohol use and smoking. B_6 (50–100 mg daily) also helps the essential fatty acids attached to nerves. Even biotin and inositol have been found to have some role in retina function. Folic acid (400 mcg daily) decreases levels of homocysteine, a compound now recognized as a major contributor to arterial blockage (including blockage of the retinal arteries), as well as the development of heart disease, hardening of the arteries (atherosclerosis), and osteoporosis. Folic acid needs adequate amounts of B_{12} and B_6

to decrease homocysteine. If you take oral B_{12}, it's generally advised to take 2 mg a day for one month, and then 1 mg daily thereafter. The methylcobalamine form is the most effective. Taking B_{12} sublingually (under the tongue) is the most efficient way to provide B_{12} other than by injection. A company located in Phoenix, Arizona, named KMI, also manufactures a B_{12} spray that is absorbed from the mouth in seconds and so does not require digestion. I recommend this product highly, at least on a once-a-week basis. I use either sublingual B_{12} or the B_{12} spray periodically to make sure I am absorbing adequate amounts of this essential vitamin.

Blood levels of B vitamins are reduced by stress, alcohol, smoking, diuretics, and numerous diseases. Since they are water-soluble, the B vitamins are not stored in the body, and need to be replenished daily.

Vitamin C: 1000 mg three times daily. Research published in early 1998 from Manchester, England, suggests that taking over 500 mg vitamin C a day requires some thought, but the bulk of the evidence on vitamin C is very supportive of taking higher levels, since it is water-soluble and is excreted easily in urine. I take this much vitamin C myself. If you haven't been taking vitamin C regularly, build up to this amount slowly. If it gives you diarrhea (which it sometimes does), cut back your dose until you no longer have diarrhea.

Vitamin D: 400–600 IU daily. This vitamin is especially important for preventing osteoporosis in the elderly. We make vitamin D in our bodies when we are exposed to sunlight, so it's necessary to supplement if you don't get fifteen to thirty minutes of moderate sunlight (early morning or late afternoon) every three or four days.

Vitamin E: 400–800 IU daily. Vitamin E protects cell membranes, and is the most effective vitamin in preventing the formation of the cholesterol plaques that clog arteries, leading to heart attacks and strokes. In animal experiments, early retinal degeneration (like that seen in macular degeneration) is influenced by the availability of vitamin E and the carotenoids; if these nutrients are not available, the retina deteriorates faster. Dietary deficiency of vitamin E has been shown to lead to the development of *drusen* in the retina (i.e., deposits of metabolic waste that lead to macular degeneration and vision loss), loss of photoreceptor cells (the rods and cones), and accumulations of lipofuscin (a pigment that signals degeneration in nerve, muscle, heart, and liver cells). Vitamin E helps to protect against cataracts, heart disease, and cancer. It is most effective when taken in conjunction with selenium; both vitamin E and selenium work with essential enzymes. When you are buying vitamin E, be sure you look for the natural form (which will be noted on the bottle label).

Amino acids

L-arginine: 500 mg daily. L-arginine dilates blood vessels more potently than nitroglycerine, and may have no other long-term effects. This is not a first-line treatment, because L-arginine (which is found in chocolates) may actuallly stimulate herpes and should not be consumed in conjunction with nitrates or Viagra. That's why men who eat chocolate live longer.

Bioflavonoids

Bilberry: 100 mg once or twice daily. Bilberry is a type of European blueberry containing anthocyanins, which retard the breakdown of vitamin C. (It's good to take them together.) Like vitamin C, bilberry increases collagen cross-linkage, thereby strengthening capillary walls and stopping capillary leakage. Bilberry is good for night vision, especially in glaucoma patients, and is helpful for diabetics.

Ginkgo biloba: **15 drops twice daily.** A selective cerebrovascular dilator, *Ginkgo biloba* dilates blood vessels in the brain, improving blood flow. I recommend one pill (or drops in liquid) twice a day; make sure your supplement contains 24 percent ginkgosides. *Ginkgo biloba* is derived from the ginkgo tree and has long been used in Chinese medicine. It smoothes the internal lining of blood vessels and increases blood flow to the brain. Ginkgo has a mild blood-thinning effect that, unlike aspirin's, lasts only about twenty-four hours.

Minerals

Magnesium: at least 500 mg daily. Magnesium is the natural calcium channel blocker, lowering blood pressure by dilating and relaxing blood vessels. It stops vasospasm (which is a cause of sudden death), and helps control the tendency to develop high blood pressure. Patients with high blood pressure are also candidates for high eye pressure, and magnesium is useful for treating both. Take your magnesium at night, on an empty stomach, and it will be less likely to cause diarrhea (a possible side effect). Magnesium labeled *chelated* is less likely to cause diarrhea. Patients with kidney failure should consult their treating physician before taking magnesium or any supplement. If you supplement with calcium, take it at a separate time from when you take magnesium.

Zinc: up to 30 mg daily for adults; up to 15 mg daily for children. Zinc assists retinal function. In the elderly, zinc deficiency decreases vision, taste, and smell. Zinc supplements should not be taken with copper, iron, calcium, or fiber (which bind the zinc and make it unusable)—even though most multivitamins include them all. (Check the contents of your multivitamin.)

Copper is inhibited by zinc, so if zinc supplements are used, 2 mg of copper should be taken daily.

Chromium: 200 mcg/daily. Chromium makes insulin more effective at getting sugar into cells.

Selenium: 50–200 mcg daily. Selenium works very effectively with vitamin E and glutathione and also lowers cholesterol.

Enzymes

SOD, catalase, and glutathione peroxidase may play important roles in the treatment and specific reactions in the trabecular meshwork. Specific dosage recommendations are not available, but researchers have found that the concentrations of proteins and the vital tissue enzyme SOD in the trabecular meshwork decline with age. Do we need more? I suspect we do. But these can be made in the body; a good diet and healthy liver are prerequisites.

Other Suggested Supplements

Alpha-lipoic acid: 250 mg twice daily. This antioxidant is both fat- and water-soluble, and can be taken at night (before bedtime) when the eye is being repaired by rest. It should be used for severe glaucoma only under a doctor's supervision.

Garlic: 1000 mg aged garlic with meals, or as a regular dietary ingredient. Garlic increases immunity and arterial dilation, neutralizes some carcinogens, may lower cholesterol (although some studies dispute this finding), and delays clotting.

Herbs

Herbs have been used in both Western and Eastern medicine over the centuries.

Coleus forskohlii is an herb from India used in Ayurvedic medicine that lowers eye pressure. A number of herbs like forskohlii have been shown in studies in the United States to be effective in lowering eye pressure and blood pressure over the short term. Forskohlii may lose its effect over a six-month period of time, so be sure to have your eye pressure reassessed every three months. Since its effect is temporary, however, I now rarely use this herb.

Trifola is a combination of herbs that normalizes the liver and stimulates the parasympathetic nervous system. Trifola was formulated by Dr. Mana in Nepal, who uses it to treat glaucoma. Dr. Mana is a Buddhist priest and the twenty-first generation of herbal physicians in his family. His fruit-derived herbal preparation—which is based on the triphala combination but includes other ingredients—relaxes the bowel, acts as a laxative, lowers blood pressure, reduces stress, and after one month, appears to produce an average reduction of 20 percent in intraocular pressure. This effect was originally observed to wear off fairly quickly in some individuals, but that appears to have occurred because its supply was not constant and patients were going on and off it. Its effect is variable, so it should be monitored by your eye doctor. Take 2 grams twice daily. (See Resource Guide for further information.)

Marijuana: Although touted as an effective treatment for glaucoma, marijuana is really only minimally effective and has too many side effects for responsible people to recommend or use (not to mention its status as an illegal substance under Federal law).

Oregano: James Duke, author of *The Green Pharmacy*, reports that oregano acts an antioxidant.

Silymarin: the flavonoid in milk thistle, increases the glutathione content of the liver.

Skullcap is another liver-supportive herb.

Some herbs that are used by Chinese medical practitioners (but generally not by other herbalists) include the following. Note that these herbs should be taken in individual dosages not to exceed 400 mg twice daily or as a total formula of 2 grams twice daily.

Pueraria (1 percent solution): Chinese doctors have found that this herb enhances blood circulation.

Aloe pharbidis (2–4 grams daily), in combination, acts as a laxative.

Cnidium, citrus, capillaris, and corydalis have been shown to increase retinal blood flow.

Xiao yao san (a powder) contains a combination of herbs that relieves the constricted liver.

Herbal treatments have been successful in a number of my patients. Gladys, for instance, is a very intense, middle-aged woman who has primary open-angle glaucoma. Over the years, she's taken multiple medications and had laser treatment on both eyes as well as surgery in one eye. When she and I began discussing possible alternative therapies, she was taking two medications and her eye pressure was not under control. At the time, she had a pressure of 29 in one eye and 27 in the other (normal being 21 or less; as a matter of fact, a safe number for her would really be in the mid-

teens). Using Dr. Mana's formula*—Trifola—her eye pressure went down to 21 in each eye and stayed there. At that point, I got her to stop taking the drugs completely. I then added back one of the conventional prescription eyedrops. The eye pressure dropped again to 17, which was much safer for her. In addition, she had been concerned about a bad taste in her mouth due to one of the eyedrops she was using. This went away, enabling her to continue using it. She felt more relaxed, and a blotchy area in her vision in the operated eye improved. The swelling in her retina, called central serous retinopathy (which is seen in some patients between 20 and 50 with "type A" personalities—that is, it's associated with stress), which had not responded to other treatments over the past year, was relieved by these herbs. Gladys still needs to take conventional eyedrops to lower her pressure further, but the addition of Eastern to Western medicine has stabilized her peripheral vision and may be a way for her to avoid further surgery. This is the beauty of using complementary medicine—using conventional and alternative medicines together.

If your eye pressure, like Gladys's, is difficult to control, start a stress reduction program today. Try a simple guided imagery exercise. Sit quietly for five minutes, close your eyes, and imagine energy washing over your body as waves of light. Make this habit as regular as brushing your teeth. Remember, you clean your teeth to keep them free from disease. Using meditation helps to clean your body from stress, keeping your body free from disease.

Finally, remember, if you or a loved one has glaucoma, do not despair. Keep these facts in mind:

- Many patients with increased intraocular pressure do not develop glaucoma. Elevated eye pressure does not lead inevitably to optic nerve damage or vision loss. In fact, the Baltimore Eye Survey established that only one in ten people with high eye pressure will go on to develop glaucoma.
- There is no universally accepted cutoff between "normal" and "high" eye pressures.
- Glaucoma probably has a vascular component, since it occurs more often in people with vascular diseases. If you have a vascular disease such as diabetes, high blood pressure, or coronary artery disease, you should consider using *Ginkgo biloba* and other bioflavonoids to improve your circulation.

---

*To obtain Dr. Mana's formula, which has been standardized updated, call Alan Tillotsan, Ph.D. at 302-994-0565 or you can e-mail him at alanT3@aol.com.

Become an active participant in managing glaucoma. Learn what your eye pressures and your optic nerve cup-to-disc ratios are. Ask for a copy of your visual field. Choose ophthalmologists and optometrists with whom you can be a partner, so you can get a report from them to know how you're doing. *You are the key to your own success.*

Table 13 summarizes my recommendations for the prevention and alternative treatment of glaucoma.

Table 13. Prevention and Alternative Treatment of Glaucoma

Diet and Supplementation	Lifestyle	Water and Digestion
• Avoid refined foods, harmful fats, and artificial sweeteners. • Increase your essential Omega-3 fatty acid intake by consuming flaxseeds or flaxseed oil, purslane, fatty-rich fish, turmeric, and fish oil or Neuromins™ DHA; or supplement with 500 mg Omega-3 fatty acids twice daily with meals. • Increase your consumption of fruits, vegetables, and whole grains. • Decrease your consumption of alcohol, diet sodas, and caffeine. • Supplement your diet with: Multivitamin as directed B complex vitamin (50–100 mg daily) Sublingual vitamin B_{12} Vitamin C (1000 mg three times daily) Vitamin E (400–800 IU daily, taken with a meal) Magnesium (500–1000 mg daily) Vitamins A and D (unless in multivitamin) Zinc (30 mg daily for several months) Copper (2 mg daily while taking zinc) garlic (one odorless pill daily) alpha-lipoic acid (200 mg daily) *ginkgo biloba* extract (to improve circulation; 15 drops twice daily) *Coleus forskohlii* Dr. Mana's formula (Trifola) DHA (500–1000 mg daily) Lutein (6–10 mg daily)	• Exercise regularly. • Learn to relax; use meditation and deep breathing. • Stop smoking. • Keep using your eyes. Use eye exercises and acupressure to keep them feeling comfortable. • Massage your TMJ, temples, and neck three times a day.	• Drink eight 8-ounce glasses of water daily. • Increase the amount of fiber in your diet. • Encourage regular bowel habits. • Eat slowly, in a relaxed setting, so you can digest your meal properly. • Take digestive aids if necessary. Try supplementing with Betaine (a weak hydrochloric acid) for one month.

Table 14. Further Ways to Prevent and Treat Glaucoma

Other Diseases/Drugs	Whole Body
• Manage chronic diseases like asthma, high blood pressure, diabetes, elevated cholesterol, and heart conditions. • Avoid drugs that narrow and jeopardize the eye's angle. There are 130 drugs that have this effect. Check with your ophthalmologist. • Watch out for drugs, like steroids, that increase internal eye pressure in open-angle glaucoma. • If you suffer from obesity, try to lose weight. Exercising regularly, as suggested for other reasons, will help you in this difficult effort.	• Use diet, exercise, and supplementation wisely for maximum health. • Be extra conscious of the condition of your eyesight and any other symptoms you develop after being diagnosed with glaucoma. • Keep a calendar on which you record your medication and supplement regimes, so you know when you started taking something new and how it affected you. • Get a copy of your visual field examination and/or optic nerve map for comparison.

CHAPTER 8

Starvation of the Retina: Macular Degeneration

Myth: There is no treatment for macular degeneration— your vision will continue to decline, robbing you of ability to see well, but you will not become completely blind.
Fact: Macular degeneration does not have to progress— you can take steps to save and even improve your vision.

A lovely older lady, Miss L., consulted me because she feared that her macular degeneration was worsening. Now 84 years old, she'd experienced a number of problems with her eyes over the years, including having elevated eye pressure for forty-five years. Following cataract surgery, her intraocular pressure returned to a normal level, so she was no longer at risk of developing glaucoma, but she was still concerned about her mild macular degeneration. Miss L. feared that her condition was progressing because she was having trouble seeing. During my examination, I discovered that part of Miss L.'s problem was that her glasses kept slipping down on her nose. She also needed new eyeglasses prescription. The combination of adjusting her glasses' fit and correcting her vision returned her eyesight to 20/25 in one eye and 20/30 in the other—very good indeed for an 84-year-old. I reassured Miss L. about her macular degeneration by recommending some nutritional steps she could take to keep her eye disease from worsening (I will describe these steps in the pages ahead).

Age-related macular degeneration (sometimes abbreviated AMD) is the leading cause of blindness in the United States among people age 65 or older. Macular degeneration develops after a lifetime of damage to the delicate center of the retina, called the *macula*. People with severe macular degeneration lose the ability to drive, read, and even to recognize faces. Although early macular degeneration can usually be prevented from progressing, there is no treatment for advanced macular degeneration; the loss of sight it produces is currently irreversible. By 2030, experts predict that 40 million Americans will have developed age-related macular degeneration unless widespread prevention measures are instituted. According to 1996 Medicare data, at least 14 million Americans show some evidence of macular degeneration.

While too many ophthalmologists will still tell you that nothing can be done to slow or halt the vision loss resulting from macular degeneration, I'm going to share with you a specific nutritional and supplement strategy to prevent macular degeneration from ever beginning or progressing. I'm not alone in my focus on prevention here either. Increasing numbers of eye doctors are now beginning to investigate nutritional means of trying to stop this tragic disease.

Quite simply, the macula, the central portion of the retina, is very responsive to free-radical-fighting antioxidant nutrients. These nutrients are readily available in our diets and through supplementation. They include the B vitamins, the carotenoids (which are related to vitamin A), vitamins C and E, plant-derived flavonoids (like quercitin, *Ginkgo biloba*, and bilberry), selenium, zinc, and taurine. A study performed at the National Eye Institute (part of the National Institutes of Health) showed that, in many cases, diet and supplementation can delay or even stop vision loss due to macular degeneration (see chapter 23 for more information).

Since macular degeneration is a painless condition, it usually develops gradually, stealing sight with little warning. However, it can also occur as an acute condition that leads to a rapid loss of vision in one or both eyes. Macular degeneration generally develops first in one eye—but once it develops there, the second eye is at risk. Obviously, the conditions within your body that allowed macular degeneration to develop in the first eye— such as poor digestion—will probably affect your second eye. Your response should be strong and clear. Use a diagnosis of macular degeneration as an opportunity to improve the health of your eyes and your body.

Anatomy

The macula is the very center of the retina where the most detailed vision occurs. It is one of the most metabolically active tissues in the body. Although the macula occupies only about 2 percent of the visual field, it contains approximately one-quarter of the cone cells (photoreceptor cells), and it is represented in about half the brain's visual areas.

The cone cells (which are specialized for daytime vision; the rods being specialized for night vision) are very tightly packed together in the macula. Each cone cell in the macula has its own nerve fiber that communicates directly to the brain, which is why the macula transmits the most detailed sight of any part of the retina. In the peripheral areas of the retina, in contrast, several photoreceptor cells share a single nerve fiber.

In addition to having the greatest concentration of cone cells, the macula has a very high density of yellow pigments. These protective pigments, derived primarily from two carotenoids (lutein and zeaxanthin), neutralize ultraviolet light damage to the retina, filter dangerous wavelengths of blue light, and stabilize the pigment layer beneath the retina.

It's not understood exactly what causes macular degeneration, but it develops when the retina and the layer of cells underneath it, called the *retinal pigment epithelium* (RPE), both begin to deteriorate. Lack of proper nutrition can hasten this deterioration. Destruction of the macula imperils central vision and, once the macula has deteriorated, there is no treatment to restore sight.

The RPE (the pigment layer under the retina) nourishes the macula as well as removing the metabolic waste from the photoreceptor cells (the cones). One theory of macular degeneration suggests that, as we age, the RPE no longer possesses sufficient levels of antioxidants to remove the metabolic waste. As the waste accumulates, it harms the macula and leads to the development of macular degeneration. This is only one reason why I continue throughout *The Eye Care Revolution* to urge you to eat antioxidant-rich foods, as well as to supplement with antioxidants. In terms of macular degeneration, these dietary changes can help protect you against a blinding condition we currently have no medical treatment for.

There are two forms of macular degeneration. The common, "dry" (or *atrophic*) form of macular degeneration occurs in about 90 percent of cases. It develops slowly and while it doesn't usually cause blindness, it can cause a significant amount of vision loss. In dry macular degeneration, tiny white deposits called *drusen* accumulate in the retina. Drusen are believed to be waste products that accumulate because of a lack of antioxidants (in the RPE, as we discussed above) to clear the waste from the eye (see Figure 7). The Salisbury Eye Evaluation (a.k.a. Visual Impairment and Function Status in Older Persons) found that drusen are more common in Caucasians than in African-Americans, and there is no significant difference between the sexes.

In about ten percent of macular degeneration patients, blood vessels under the retina begin to grow new offshoots that burrow and bleed into the retina. This results in the scarring or destruction of the macula and RPE, and causes sudden, rapid loss of vision. The "wet" or "exudative" form of macular degeneration is this severe, rapid-onset, blinding form. While detection of drusen by your eye doctor can be the first signal that

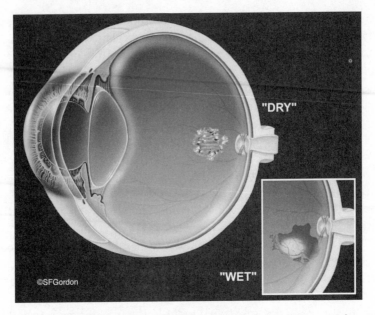

Figure 7. Macular Degeneration (dry form is more common; wet form with hemorrhage and potential scarring seen in inset)

wet macular degeneration is developing, the condition progresses rapidly when blood vessels in the retina become leaky, proliferate, and/or hemorrhage.

Remember: Macular degeneration develops in one eye at a time, with the other eye only at risk. A five-year study, however, found that macular degeneration developed in the second eye at a rate of 8.8 percent per year, indicating that the risk of macular degeneration developing in the other eye increases with time.

Dr. Abel's Tip

Ninety percent of people with macular degeneration have the dry form. Do not accept being told "Nothing can be done," especially in the early stages. Take inventory and start to heal your entire body, because the health of your whole body is related to the health of your eyes.

Symptoms of Macular Degeneration

The symptoms of macular degeneration are blurry vision, fading of color perception, normally straight lines (like telephone poles, sides of buildings, or lines of type on a page) appearing crooked, or a dark or empty area appearing in the center of vision. To test your own vision for possible early signs of macular degeneration, refer to the Amsler Grid diagram in this chapter.

If you notice any distortion in the Amsler Grid, macular degeneration has already been present for some time. Know that macular degeneration can also develop after twenty-five years or more of exposure to risk factors like smoking, poor digestion, and exposure to sunlight without sunglasses.

Dr. Abel's Tip

If you are a postmenopausal woman, have light-colored irises (blue or hazel), elevated cholesterol, high blood pressure, heart disease, osteoporosis, a family history of macular degeneration, are a smoker over the age of 50, take multiple medications, and/or have been told that you have drusen or loss of pigment, take immediate action. Begin a nutritional program, and load up your antioxidant bank account. Block UV and blue light (from sunlight) with sunglasses and/or orange glasses (which block the blue light and improve contrast). Have periodic eye examinations.

Causes of Macular Degeneration

Although we don't know precisely what causes macular degeneration, or what triggers its development, some of the leading suspects are:

1. *Free-radical damage* from ultraviolet and blue light from sunlight passing through the crystalline lens. These free radicals are enhanced by smoking, chronic fatigue, and decreased immune competence, which underlines the importance of building up your immune system. Stress and environmental toxins consume many antioxidants and therefore may contribute to macular degeneration as well as other eye diseases.

2. *Nutritional deficiency*, particularly of zinc, taurine, essential fatty acids, the B vitamin complex, and antioxidants, especially lutein, zeaxanthin, and other carotenoids.

3. *Increased blood vessel growth*. The presence of the newly identified *vascular endothelial growth factor* appears to initiate the blood vessel growth that causes damage in both macular degeneration and diabetic retinopathy.

4. *Genetics*. A gene that encodes a retinal rod photoreceptor protein, ABCR, has been found to be defective in a rare hereditary form of macular disease called Stargardt Disease. In the future, a test that detects a faulty *ABCR* gene could help to determine which individuals

are at high risk of developing macular degeneration, and alert them to begin taking preventive measures immediately. This is another reason to know your family history.

5. *Poor circulation and shallow breathing.* Good circulation and proper breathing are required to deliver enough oxygen and other nutrients to tissues (including the macula) and remove toxins. Deep breathing also decreases stress.

6. *Liver congestion.* Nutrients aren't properly processed if the liver is clogged or not working efficiently.

7. *Digestion.* A reduced amount of stomach acid can lead to poor digestion, as can an imbalance of the good intestinal flora and too many toxins in the colon. Antibiotics are notorious for upsetting this balance. A deficiency of stomach acid, which is common among older individuals, results in less absorption of many essential nutrients. It can result in a lack of antioxidants and a reduced ability to fight free-radical damage in the eye. What's good for the digestion is good for the macula. Remember, it takes only twenty minutes for the nutrients (or toxins) you eat to reach your eyes, and certain eye diseases correlate with dietary deficiencies. Macular degeneration is a disease of poor digestion.

Natural Alternatives to Antacids

Having low stomach acid doesn't help digestion, so stop taking your antacids. There are plenty of natural substances that aid digestion, including:

- Plant-derived digestive enzymes (lipases, amylases, proteases, cellulases) available in supplements. Fresh pineapple and papaya have bromelain, which can also help digestion.
- Animal-derived digestive enzymes (elastases), which are available as supplements.
- Microbe-derived digestive enzymes (from lactobacillus or acidophilus cultures, which can be obtained from sauerkraut, yogurt, and supplements).
- Fiber, both soluble and insoluble.
- Natural betaine and other forms of hydrochloric acid (to make up for deficient stomach acid). Many elderly people make decreased amounts of stomach acid and bile, and so cannot absorb vitamins B_{12}, C, or the fat-soluble vitamins.
- Aloe vera, licorice root, comfrey root, ginger, and garlic all have anti-inflammatory effects on the gut.

> **Dr. Abel's Tip**
>
> Macular degeneration is a disease of starvation, especially of the good fats (like DHA and the other Omega-3 fats) that coat the retina cells. Fat-soluble vitamins and enzymes, working with the good fats, protect against the constant free-radical formation caused by sunlight. Improve your digestion and increase the Omega-3 essential fatty acids in your diet.

Fiber and Beneficial Bacteria

Make sure you're eating an adequate amount of fiber-rich foods like cooked oats, which contain both soluble and insoluble fiber. Soluble fiber promotes normal bowel function, and insoluble fiber decreases toxicity in the colon, among their other functions.

Be certain you're consuming adequate amounts of "good" bacteria, which help fight infection as well as aiding digestion. There are many good books about probiotics, the science of your colon.

Protection Against Leaky Gut Syndrome

Just as it's important that blood vessels not develop leaks, the health of both the gastrointestinal system and the immune system depend on the lining of the intestines remaining intact. Some of the same dietary deficiencies that contribute to leaking blood vessels are also associated with *leaky gut syndromes,* or *intestinal permeability defects.* Overuse of painkillers and alcohol, trauma, aging, infection, and nutritional deficiencies can all result in this syndrome, as can candida (yeast) overgrowth. Once the lining of the gastrointestinal system is damaged, food is not properly digested; instead, it ferments in the colon, causing gas and pain. Leaky gut syndrome appears to contribute to the development of autoimmune disorders like inflammatory bowel disease, rheumatoid arthritis and lupus; food and chemical sensitivities; and bacterial infection (septicemia). Supplements that can help heal intestinal permeability defects include glutamine, a deficiency of which results in intestinal damage; gamma-linolenic acid (GLA), an essential amino acid that acts as an anti-inflammatory agent; acidophilus, the "good" bacteria (which, by the way, you cannot get from eating frozen yogurt); vitamin A, which supports the intestinal lining; N-acetyl-D-glucosamine (NAG), which promotes the formation of a healthy gut lining; phosphatidylcholine, which protects the gastrointestinal lining from chemicals; and gamma-oryzanol, an extract of rice bran oil that is a potent antioxidant.

Overgrowth of bacteria or yeast in the gastrointestinal system can lead to bloating, gas, pain, constipation, or diarrhea, and the development of another bowel disorder called *gut fermentation syndrome.* Our usually friendly gut microorganisms grow out of control when we use antibiotics or antacids too frequently, don't produce enough stomach acid, or undergo surgery. Gut fermentation syndrome can also occur as secondary infections in diabetics or people with parasites. Reduce the refined sugar in your diet, increase your garlic intake, cut down on processed wheat products, and use phosphatidyl inositol (PI, a form of lecithin) and lactobacillus supplements between meals to prevent this overgrowth of intestinal organisms.

Poor digestion results in starvation of the eye and the rest of the body over many years before the joints ache, the heart skips a beat, and the small print looks wavy. Take steps now to prevent these conditions from affecting you.

Dr. Abel's Tip

The macula has a powdery yellow pigment that absorbs dangerous blue light and UV wavelengths. This fat-soluble pigment is rebuilt by lutein and zeaxanthin, found in green leafy vegetables, eggs, and corn, so eat plenty of these vegetables.

Risk Factors for Macular Degeneration

- Age (over 60 or twenty-five years of exposure to the other risk factors)
- Family history of macular degeneration
- Light blue, green, or hazel eyes (usually found in Caucasians)
- Farsightedness (hyperopia)
- Aphakia (a condition that develops when a cataract was removed years ago and an artificial lens was not implanted)
- Pseudophakia (a condition that develops when a cataract was removed, before 1984, and an intraocular lens without a UV blocker was placed in the eye)
- Presence of drusen (white spots on the macula)
- High blood pressure (hypertension)
- Postmenopause (for women)
- Cigarette smoking (increases risk two or three times in both sexes)
- Diet high in fat and cholesterol and elevated blood cholesterol/triglyceride levels

- Hardening of the arteries (atherosclerosis) and/or heart disease
- Reduced gastrointestinal nutrient absorption
- Excessive alcohol consumption
- Lack of exercise
- Free-radical damage from UV light (people who work outdoors)
- Diabetes
- Obesity

Diagnosis of Macular Degeneration

Only an eye exam can diagnose macular degeneration before you lose any vision. The drusen, the white deposits under the retina, do not generally *cause* vision loss but indicate the beginning of macular degeneration. Drusen only cause vision loss when so many accumulate that they run together or when the pigment in the macula becomes scattered so that there is not enough of it to absorb light or neutralize free radicals. When the pigment becomes this scattered, new blood vessels can penetrate the retina. This causes a loss of central vision.

The methods generally used to diagnose macular degeneration are:

- Amsler grid, a test with which everyone should become familiar. (See Figure 8.)
- Ophthalmoscopy with slit lamp examination using special high-magnification lenses.
- Fundus photography (photographs of the back of the eye, i.e., the retina).
- Fluorescein angiography (to determine if the wet form of macular degeneration is present and treatable).
- Computer-enhanced indocyanine green video angiography (for cases in which fluorescein angiography does not visualize the blood vessels under the retina well, usually because they are hidden under scars or by blood in the retina).
- The MaculoScope focal ERG (a concentrated, electroretinal test that can determine early macular changes even in individuals with near-normal vision).
- Macular pigment density testing. Max Snodderly, M.D., at the Schepens Eye Research Institute in Boston, has developed a macular pigment density test using flickering blue and green lights. The test evaluates vision sensitivity and should provide not only earlier detection of macular degeneration, but also an early warning system about the need for nutritional therapy. Currently, less expensive models are being evaluated.

- Serum carotenoid levels (an ancillary test). Such testing has been done in several large clinical studies, but may be of most value in conjunction with other nutritional tests (hair, stool, blood) to determine the adequacy of your diet and gastrointestinal tract absorption.

Conventional Therapy for Macular Degeneration

The usual therapy for macular degeneration taught to newly trained ophthalmologists is—none.

It amazes me that so many of my colleagues do not recognize the abundance of evidence, both scientific and anecdotal, showing that proper diet and supplementation can prevent and stabilize macular degeneration. Patients are still told that their macular degeneration will probably increase; that they'll lose most, if not all, of their sight.

Those statements are no longer true. If nutrition and supplementation help prevent vision loss in macular degeneration, and does no harm, let's use them! The wait for "official" medical confirmation via controlled studies of nutritional therapy may just be the kind of professional caution that too many patients simply can't afford.

Before looking at alternative therapies, however, let's examine the conventional treatments for macular degeneration, such as they are.

Surgical Treatments for Macular Degeneration

Laser photocoagulation surgery has been used for decades to stop retinal bleeding in wet macular degeneration. While laser photocoagulation can arrest the decline in vision, it is effective only when performed in the early stages of the disease.

Furthermore, we are learning that new blood vessels grow back after laser treatment 50 percent of the time. Since only 13 percent of patients with macular degeneration can be treated with laser photocoagulation, only about 7 percent of patients are treated successfully by this method. In other words, laser photocoagulation cannot be used in or is not effective in 93 percent of patients.

There are also important concerns about damage to the retina from laser photocoagulation, which can destroy healthy macular cells as well as the underlying blood vessels that are its targets. I recommend that patients increase their levels of supplemental antioxidants immediately prior to laser therapy to try to protect against this damage.

Experimental Surgical Treatments

Macular degeneration surgery is an active area of research because of the aging of the American population and the projected increase in the number of people with this condition. Therefore, numerous research centers are investigating experimental surgical techniques.

A novel technique has been developed by Robert Machemer, M.D., professor of ophthalmology at Duke University Medical Center in Raleigh-Durham, North Carolina. This technique detaches the retina and rotates it so that the macula is positioned in a different area of the retina, where the underlying RPE has not deteriorated. While there is still a damaged area in the RPE, it no longer supplies the center of the macula, so central vision is restored.

Peter Gouras, M.D., professor of ophthalmology at Columbia University's Edward S. Harkness Eye Institute in New York City, is investigating transplantation of healthy RPE cells to replace those that have been damaged. To be successful, it must be performed before vision has deteriorated too far.

Henry J. Kaplan, M.D., and a team of researchers from Washington University in St. Louis, have developed a surgical method for treating macular degeneration. The method arose from experiments in monkeys. Dr. Kaplan surgically removed the layer of RPE cells, which had been damaged by a fungal infection. When the damaged layer of cells was removed, a new layer of RPE cells actually grew back, restoring sight. This was an astonishing finding, since scientists had not previously realized that this very delicate layer of cells could regenerate itself. Dr. Kaplan advises that this form of surgical treatment is likely to work only on patients whose layers of RPE and photoreceptive cells (i.e., rods and cones) have not been damaged, and who've had macular degeneration for less than a year.

In the past, radiation was investigated as a way to destroy new blood vessel growth in eyes, but it made no sense because it damaged healthy retinal cells. This research has been discontinued.

Dr. S. Chou invented a silicone chip to provide "artificial" vision for patients with retinitis pigmentosa. This may become an option for those with advanced AMD.

Experimental Drug Treatments

An experimental treatment that employs photoactivated drugs (drugs that respond chemically to light) in conjunction with lasers is under investigation in Canada. Julia Levy, Ph.D., of the Vancouver-based QLT

Photo Therapeutics Inc., developed the experimental treatment after her mother's vision was severely affected by macular degeneration. This treatment, a photosensitive substance named QLT (which is extracted from cow parsley) is administered intravenously to patients. This substance can destroy certain types of tissue (including the unwanted blood vessels that develop in macular degeneration) when it is activated by light. In this instance, lasers are used not as surgical tools, but to activate QLT, which then destroys the targeted tissue. The QLT treatment is still experimental, but anecdotal reports suggest it can restore some vision within as little as twenty-four hours. Another study using a photoactivated drug to treat macular degeneration, the Verteporfin in Photodynamic Therapy (VIP), is being evaluated in multiple hospitals and clinics across the U.S. and is now reasonably widely available. Several further studies are looking at this method of treating the wet form of macular degeneration.

The infamous drug thalidomide—implicated as the cause of catastrophic birth defects in the 1950s—has been found to have properties that might be useful in treating numerous conditions, including leprosy, cancer, and macular degeneration. Thalidomide works by a process called *anti-angiogenesis*—preventing the growth of new blood vessels. Other anti-angiogenesis compounds are currently being studied as potential cancer therapies, since tumors require new blood vessels to nourish their growth. The children born to mothers who took thalidomide during pregnancy had stunted or missing limbs because embryos require new blood vessel generation to grow arms and legs. Thalidomide may work the same way in macular degeneration, stopping damage to the macula by preventing the growth of new blood vessels. This effect is still under investigation, and thalidomide, because of its tragic history, is a very tightly regulated drug.

There is no standard medical, pharmaceutical therapy for macular degeneration. Vitamin manufacturers, however, have formulated eye vitamin packages specifically to prevent cataracts and macular degeneration. This is one situation in which the salesperson who calls on the doctor is delivering a product with great benefit and very little risk. Enlightened ophthalmologists are also telling patients to quit smoking, decrease sun exposure, and be alert to adverse drug reactions.

Prevention/Natural Therapy

Whole foods, which contain multiple phytonutrients, appear to confer greater protection against macular degeneration (and other eye diseases) than do vitamin supplements. We should depend primarily on whole foods to meet our nutritional needs, since they contain combinations of nutrients (some of which we haven't yet discovered), and use vitamins and supplements as an insurance policy. Studies show that consuming foods rich in carotenes (especially lutein and zeaxanthin)—as opposed to taking vitamin pills—seems to have the greatest effect on inhibiting the development of macular degeneration.

One study comparing people with advanced macular degeneration to control subjects found that high levels of the carotenes lutein and zeaxanthin *in the diet* were most strongly associated with a reduced risk for macular degeneration. In particular, eating increased amounts of spinach or collard greens was highly associated with a decreased risk of developing macular degeneration. People who obtained high amounts of vitamin C from food sources also appeared to have a lower risk, but those who took supplements of vitamins A, C, or E showed no benefits. I still advise my patients to take vitamin A, C, and E supplements, however, because most people just don't obtain enough of these nutrients from their diets.

Lutein obtained from food (corn, spinach, kale, collard and mustard greens), in addition to protecting against macular degeneration, also protects the rods and cones from free-radical damage caused by UV light. Like the other carotenoids and vitamins A, D, E, and K, yellow lutein is a fat-soluble nutrient that requires a small amount of cholesterol to be transported to the retina. (See page 384.)

Lycopene (which is abundant in tomatoes) is another carotenoid that appears to be important in preventing macular degeneration. Studies have shown that very low blood levels of lycopene are associated with its development.

I realize it's not always possible to obtain the required amounts of nutrients from food sources (or to absorb them, particularly for older people), so there *is* a place for supplementation in developing vision-preservation strategies. In the January 1997 *Townsend Letter for Doctors & Patients*, Charles Krall, O.D., F.A.A.O., described a program of nutritional supplementation utilizing forty-one antioxidants, minerals, and herbs. Within six months, as Dr. Krall found, this supplement program improved the visual acuity in six out of ten patients with macular degeneration. "This study supports the potential efficacy of a nutritional program to retard the usual deterioration that occurs with macular degeneration," Dr. Krall concluded.

While whole foods nearly always provide more balanced nutrition than individual supplements do, I must emphasize again that patients with macular degeneration already have nutritional deficiencies. They generally require supplementation as well as an improved diet.

Some specific nutrients that help to protect against the development of macular degeneration and may help, in some cases, to retard its progression are the following:

- *Vitamin C.* Present in very high levels in the eye, which protects against free-radical damage from UV light. This is one reason I take 2500–3000 mg of vitamin C every day.
- *Vitamin E.* Highly concentrated in the retina, prevents lipid peroxidation (deterioration of fats), and protects against free-radical damage from UV light.
- *Carotenoids.* Form the "yellow spot" that indicates a healthy macula, and help nutrients to pass from the blood vessels under the retina to the cone cells, and debris to pass from the cone cells out to the blood vessels, which clear them from the eye. (An added benefit to increasing dietary carotenoids, especially lutein and zeaxanthin—from spinach, kale, mustard greens, and turnip greens—is that studies have shown an association between increased carotenoid consumption and prevention of heart disease.)
- *Flavonoids.* Substances found in a wide variety of plants (especially blueberries and grapes), flavonoids are powerful antioxidants that help improve the eye's adaptation to darkness (night vision) and appear to improve or retard progression of macular degeneration. Wine, particularly red wine, contains fairly large amounts of these flavonoids (from the grapes and grape skins) and studies suggest that moderate wine consumption can lower the risk of developing macular degeneration. Flavonoids, particularly bilberry, are widely available in supplement form.
- *Taurine.* This amino acid from protein, found in high levels in the retina, is thought to protect against both ultraviolet light and toxic substances. The amino acid glutamine may also be important.
- *Glutathione.* People with macular degeneration and other eye conditions, like cataracts, have a significantly diminished level of glutathione, found in avocados, asparagus, eggs, and garlic.
- *Garlic.* In food or as a supplement, garlic is known to increase immunity and arterial dilation, which is helpful in supplying the eye with nutrients.
- *Superoxide dismutase (SOD).* An antioxidant enzyme, SOD is significantly decreased in macular degeneration.
- *Zinc.* Found in high concentrations in the eye, especially the retina and its underlying tissues, zinc helps bind the protective pigment layer of the retina to the underlying tissue. Also required by central nervous system neurons, zinc is thought to be important in forming connections between nerve cells.

- *Magnesium.* The natural calcium channel blocker, magnesium reduces vasospasm in blood vessel walls and helps dilate small blood vessels like those found in the eye.
- *Selenium.* Present in very high levels in the eye, it protects against free-radical damage from UV light.
- *Ginkgo biloba.* This extract from the *ginkgo biloba* tree appears to prevent or reverse some symptoms of aging, such as depression, memory loss (even in Alzheimer's disease), and atherosclerosis (hardening of the arteries), as well as macular degeneration; stimulates blood flow.
- *Wine.* One or two glasses of wine in the evening can be good for eyes and for insomnia. Be aware, however, that too much wine can cause sleeplessness—more is not better. Wine can contribute to the health of body and eyes if consumed in moderation (one to two glasses a day), because it contains important nutrients, including anthocyanins, the red pigment in grape skin (and other fruit skins); flavones, which decrease capillary fragility; proanthrocyanidins (also called OPCs), a newly discovered class of powerful antioxidants; resveratrol, an OPC with antioxidant and anti-estrogen properties; amino acids, the building blocks of proteins; tannins, plant extracts used as astringents; small amounts of vitamin C (which disappear with complete fermentation of the wine); high levels of rutin, a bioflavonoid that's thought to reduce capillary fragility; and the B vitamin thiamine, which appears to have positive effects on Alzheimer's disease and other mental conditions. Wine may have anticancer properties because it contains transresveratrol (a form of the antioxidant resveratrol), catechins (which, like tannins, have astringent properties), and other antioxidants. Additionally, alcohol (in the form called phenol) dissolves fat, one reason it can be helpful in dissolving the fatty plaques that clog arteries. Research studies are beginning to demonstrate the value of moderate amounts of wine in preventing (and possibly reversing) eye disease. For instance, Thomas O. Obisessan, M.D., M.P.H., found that two glasses of wine daily (red or white) actually halved his subjects' risk of developing macular degeneration.
- *Sunglasses.* Protect your eyes from the sun. Wear wraparound sunglasses to protect your eyes from UV light. It is also worthwhile for a macular degeneration patient who has lost some vision in one or both eyes to have special orange lenses that block blue light.
- *Chelation.* In the 1950s, Norman Clarke, Jr., started to use chelation with EDTA (ethylene diamine tetracetic acid) to treat battery factory workers who were suffering from lead poisoning. This chemical

compound has the ability to bind metals (such as lead, iron, copper, and calcium) and draw them out of the body through the kidneys. The technique was later applied to removing calcium from clogged capillaries and arteries to improve circulation, memory, alleviate angina pectoris (chest pain), avoid amputation in borderline cases, and reduce the risk of heart attack. Chelation therapy has been reported by admirers as being very successful in selected cases, whereas conventional physicians require further controlled studies before adopting the technique. Physicians who utilize chelation note that it's a safe complementary therapy and not a replacement for traditional medical care.

I have personally known several people who told me they'd had chelation treatments to avoid bypass surgery. Each said that he or she felt better and was functioning well; all had changed their diets and lifestyles, discontinuing harmful practices like smoking. Mineral supplementation is necessary in people who undergo this procedure, however, since many minerals are removed during chelation therapy.

I've also talked with macular degeneration patients treated with chelation by the popular Robert Atkins, M.D., author of *Dr. Atkins' Vita-Nutrient Solution*, who said they had improved their vision as a result. Several other patients whose course of treatment I agreed to follow had coronary heart disease and macular degeneration. They were given chelation therapy with intravenous vitamins and minerals. Not only did their vision improve, they also had a decrease in the number of drusen in their eyes. As a traditionally trained Western doctor, I always place my patients' safety first when they suggest trying unproved therapies. In this case, however, I recognize that chelation therapy may turn out to be beneficial for macular degeneration patients, but it remains as yet unproven.

Supplementation Recommendations

Multivitamin: one or two capsules as directed with meals.
Vitamin A: 10,000 IU daily.
Beta-carotene: 5000–10,000 IU daily.
Lutein: 6–20 mg daily.
Vitamin C: At least 1000 mg daily, and as much as 3000 mg if you can tolerate it without getting diarrhea. (If you develop this side effect, cut back.)
Vitamin E: 400 IU daily.
Magnesium: 500 mg daily (if you don't have kidney disease).

Bilberry: 100 mg twice daily.

Ginkgo biloba extract: 15 drops once or twice daily.

Garlic: 1 odorless capsule (100–1000 mg, depending on tolerance) daily.

Essential fatty acids: one tablespoon of flaxseed oil daily. (Be sure to keep your flaxseed oil refrigerated.)

Fish oil DHA (or microalgae-derived DHA): 500 mg daily, or twice daily if you're not taking flaxseed oil. Less should be taken if you're on a blood-thinner like coumadin or aspirin, so consult your physician. (Be sure to refrigerate fish oil capsules.)

Make sure your diet or your vitamins also include adequate amounts of:

Selenium: 50–200 mcg daily

Taurine: 200 mg daily

Chromium: 200 mcg daily

Zinc: 30 mg or less daily

Digestive enzymes: as required

The Big Picture for Macular Degeneration: Further Recommendations

• Have regular eye exams.

• Learn whether you have drusen, the earliest sign of macular changes due to aging.

• Know your risk factors: What drugs are you taking? How many of the drugs you're taking make your eyes more sensitive to light? (Ask your doctor or pharmacist.)

• Wear UV-blocking sunglasses.

• Protect your eyes from heat when taking a sauna.

• Eat a diet rich in fruits and vegetables, essential fatty acids (including DHA from fish, fish oil capsules, or Neuromins™ DHA microalgae capsules, and Omega-3 fatty acids from plant sources like flaxseed oil or from supplements). Recognize that a diet that is good for your heart will also protect your macula. Always work on building up your antioxidant bank account. Eat spinach often (five times a week, if possible), fish two or three times a week (preferably fatty fish), increase the fiber in your diet, don't allow your fat intake to exceed 30 percent of your diet, avoid supermarket oils (like corn and other "vegetable" oils), which may be rancid and contain preservatives and transfatty acids.

• If you've been told that you have macular degeneration, test yourself regularly with the Amsler Grid. (See Figure 8.) Try to find out if macular pigment density testing is being performed anywhere in your area (in 1998, it was being done only at the Schepens Research Institute in Boston).

- Get regular exercise.
- Develop regular sleeping patterns.
- Decrease caffeine consumption.
- Eliminate smoking.
- Have one large glass of red wine in the evening if tolerated and recommended by your doctor.
- Eliminate unnecessary medications. High blood pressure medications deplete essential minerals and water-soluble vitamins, and may actually accelerate macular degeneration.
- Remember that there are low-vision aids to help you if you have macular degeneration in both eyes. There are many optical devices to enlarge the visual image, as well as other resources like talking books and large-screen monitors; see the Resource Guide or call your state Ophthalmology or Optometry Society to learn how to see better.
- Try natural bulk, which you'll find in whole grains, especially oats, If that does not work to regulate your bowels, try laxatives for a limited time only. If you eat correctly, you should not need laxatives.
- Relax! Learn to use meditation and visual imagery, or other methods of relaxing that work for you.

For a summary of my recommendations for the prevention and treatment of macular degeneration, see Table 15.

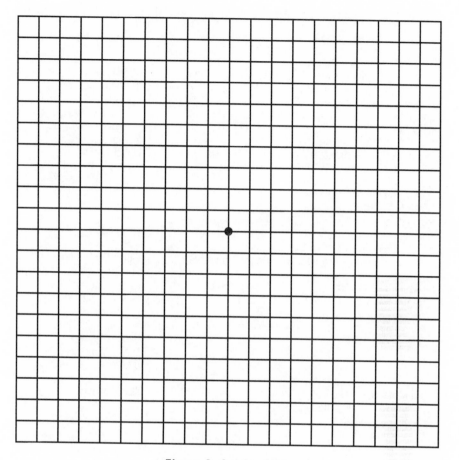

Figure 8. Amsler Grid

This checkerboard-patterned square has parallel vertical and horizontal lines. You should look at the central dot with one eye covered, and note the pattern of the lines. If any of the lines in any direction are missing or wavy, mark it in with a pencil or make a note. This Amsler grid can be used to determine if there is a disorder of the optic nerve or macula; in particular, it is an excellent way to follow degeneration to see if it is stable or progressing. Feel free to photocopy this grid to test your vision. Use a separate grid for each eye.

Table 15. Prevention and Alternative Treatment of Macular Degeneration

Diet and Supplementation	Lifestyle	Water and Digestion

• Decrease your consumption of alcohol, diet sodas, and caffeine.
• Increase your Omega-3 fatty acid intake by consuming flaxseeds or flaxseed oil, fatty-rich fish, fish oil or DHA 500 mg twice daily, with meals.
• Increase your consumption of fruits, vegetables (especially spinach and corn), and whole grains.
• Avoid refined foods, harmful fats, and artificial sweeteners.
• Supplement your diet with:
  a multivitamin (which should include a good amount of vitamins A and D)
  B-complex vitamin (50–100 mg daily)
  sublingual vitamin B_{12} (1–2 mg daily)
  vitamin C (1000 mg three times daily, if tolerated)
  vitamin E (400–800 IU daily with meals)
  magnesium (500–1000 mg at bedtime)
  zinc (30 mg daily for several months)
  copper (2 mg daily while using zinc)
  garlic (one odorless pill daily, 1000 mg)
  CoQ10 (60–120 mg daily)
  Ginkgo biloba extract (15 drops twice daily)
  lutein (12–20 mg daily)
  zeaxanthin (.5–1.0 mg daily)
  the amino acid taurine (which could be in your multivitamin)
  enzyme therapy
	• Learn to relax; use meditation, deep breathing, and visual imagery.
	• Make sure you're getting an adequate amount of sleep.
	• Stop smoking.
	• Keep using your eyes. Use eye exercises to keep them feeling comfortable.
	• Wear sunglasses and hats outside on sunny days. Be extra vigilant if you've had previous eye surgery. Avoid tanning booths.
		• Drink eight 8-ounce glasses of water daily, but not with meals.
		• Increase the amount of fiber in your diet. Encourage regular bowel habits.
		• Supplement with N-acetyl choline (NAC) and phosphatidyl choline to improve digestion.
		• Eat slowly, in a relaxed setting, so you digest your meal properly.
		• Take natural digestive aids if necessary. Try supplementing with Betaine (a weak hydrochloric acid) for one month. (Ask your doctor to test your stomach acid.)

Table 16. Further Ways to Prevent and Treat Macular Degeneration

Other Diseases/Drugs	Whole Body
• Manage chronic diseases like heart disease, high blood pressure, elevated cholesterol, diabetes, osteoporosis, and indigestion. • If you suffer from obesity, try to lose weight. Exercising regularly, as suggested for other reasons, will help you in this difficult effort. • Many supplements have blood-thinning effects; have your blood clotting time checked if you're on coumadin or aspirin.	• Be extra conscious of the condition of your eyesight and any other symptoms you develop after being diagnosed with macular degeneration. • Remember, your eyes and total body health are interrelated. Eat correctly. Exercise. Follow good health procedures. • Keep a calendar on which you record your medication and supplement regimes, so you know when you started taking something new. • Test yourself regularly with an Amsler grid. • Exercise regularly, and work on improving circulation in the lower limbs. • Have a massage once in a while to improve circulation in the whole body. • Educate your children and other family members about macular degeneration.

CHAPTER 9

Diabetes: Is Blindness Inevitable?

Myth: Eventually, many diabetics will go blind.
Fact: The percentage of diabetics who lose sight is small.

Diabetics do not have to go blind. Here are some simple tips that will allow most diabetics to preserve their vision, so they can continue to read, watch television, and even drive throughout their lives.

The current explosion in the number of people developing diabetes is directly related to our modern diet and lifestyle, but diabetes has been recognized by physicians for centuries. The term *diabetes* was coined from the Greek words meaning "siphon" and "to run through" by ancient Greek physician Aretaeus, and literally means "the chronic excretion of an excess volume of urine."

Excessive urination does not cause diabetes, of course—it is just one symptom. Diabetes results when our bodies aren't able to process sugar properly. Sugar is vital to health, but its level in the blood must be carefully controlled. Our bodies control the blood's sugar level by having the pancreas produce insulin. Insulin breaks down sugar so it can enter cells and provide them with energy. If all the sugar in your body is just floating around in the bloodstream, your cells are being deprived of their major source of energy. When we don't make enough insulin or our insulin doesn't work properly, sugar isn't absorbed as it needs to be, and diabetes develops.

When cells are starved of their energy source, as they are in diabetes, very serious conditions can result. Sugar is the main energy source for the brain and enters it freely, unlike most substances, which are prevented from entering the brain by the blood-brain barrier. Any decrease in the brain's sugar level can have a grim effect on people's level of alertness and coherence. You've probably heard horror stories about diabetics having blood sugar levels so low they are incoherent and unsteady on their feet. These are only two of the dangerous symptoms that an unregulated blood sugar level can cause in diabetics. When the brain is deprived of sugar for long enough, a potentially fatal diabetic coma can result. Fortunately, we've made such important strides in managing diabetes that this is a very rare occurrence today.

The main way that diabetics can control their sugar levels is through diet. Proteins, fats, and complex carbohydrates are all required for good nutrition and to generate energy. Over the past few decades, nutrition experts have recommended that we eat a diet containing differing percentages of each of these foods (complex carbohydrates, fats, and proteins), but the pace of nutrition research is so rapid that these dietary recommendations are continually changing.

Dr. Abel's Tip

Don't let diabetes control you. Use a diagnosis of diabetes as an opportunity to take control over your life.

I can tell you something absolutely certain about diet: People were never meant to eat so much refined sugar. In nature, only honey and maple syrup have high levels of sugar, and honey, at least, contains multiple vitamins and nutrients meant to nourish young bees. (You also must limit the amount of honey you consume, because it can have the same effect in the body as excess sugar.)

Our whole civilization has changed because of our use of sugar for its taste, appearance, medicinal value, preservative value, and even association with religious holidays. Every culture that adopts a high-sugar diet, however, suffers similar damage to health, as dentist and researcher Dr. Weston Price has documented. Being "good" and being "sweet" have become synonymous. When we want to be good to ourselves, we eat sweets.

Our forefathers' diet was very high in starch (grains), or in meat that had been fed naturally raised grass. In our modern diet, however, as much as 10 percent of the food we consume can be simple sugars. This is taking a toll on our health at earlier and earlier ages. The most direct results are decreased immunity, increased chance of infections, and altered metabolism of sugar (which can result in diabetes). The increasing number of cases of diabetes reflects the evolution of our diet to include high levels of hydrogenated and saturated fats and refined sugars; vegetable foods grown on soil depleted of minerals and nutrients; meat from animals fed scraps and waste from other animals and artificial foods spiked with antibiotics and hormones; and our habit of eating on the run (i.e., stress).

Diabetes has two causes: (1) the body produces too little insulin or (2) the insulin produced does not work properly. Type I diabetes (previously called "juvenile diabetes") develops when the body produces too little insulin, and generally starts in childhood. One cause of childhood diabetes is thought to be an abnormal reaction to a remote infection which creates antibodies that attack the pancreas, destroying its ability to produce insulin. Another possible cause is an autoimmune reaction; in other words, we make antibodies that attack our own insulin and stop it from working. The cause of childhood diabetes (Type I) is not really known. Since they lack adequate insulin, people with Type I diabetes must give themselves insulin injections every day.

Type II diabetes, also known as adult-onset diabetes, develops over many years. The amount of insulin produced by people who develop Type II diabetes gradually decreases over their lifetimes. Fortunately these patients are able to take oral medications that encourage insulin production.

Nearly 6 percent of Americans, or 15.7 million people, have been diagnosed with diabetes, according to the Centers for Disease Control and Prevention, and many others have diabetes and are not aware of it. All American minorities, with the exception of Native Alaskans, have a prevalence of adult-onset diabetes that is two to six times greater than that of Caucasians. When the rate of diabetes among senior citizens is examined, the numbers are awesome. The ultimate cost among working-age as well as retired individuals is so high that our health care management systems are buckling under the strain.

The length of time a person has diabetes is an important factor in the development of complications, including diabetic eye disease (diabetic retinopathy). After twenty years of having *untreated* diabetes, approximately 90 percent of childhood diabetics and up to 75 percent of adult-onset diabetics develop vision loss, according to the World Health Organization. In fact, blurred vision may be the first symptom of diabetes in an undiagnosed person. Many such individuals do not know that they have diabetes and therefore, are not alerted to the possibility of eye complications.

Diabetes can affect many different tissues of the body, but we also have many methods of treating its symptoms. All too often physicians only advise patients about the usual treatments: pills, insulin injections and, in the case of eye patients, laser therapy and surgery. But there are other, often gentler, methods of avoiding and correcting problems associated with diabetes.

Risk Factors for Diabetes

Every person is different; any one of the risk factors mentioned here, whether labeled "major" or "minor," may be the one that's important to you. These are the risk factors most closely associated with people who have or are going to develop diabetes.

Major Risk Factors

- High blood sugar (hyperglycemia); primary in diabetic eye disease.
- Elevated "bad" hemoglobin levels (hemoglobin A1-C; the normal level is below 7 percent).
- Obesity—an indicator of dietary imbalances.
- High cortisone levels; either natural cortisone, from the adrenal gland (cortisol is part of the adrenal gland's response to physical or emotional stress and has a way of affecting metabolism and elevating blood sugar), or cortisone administered for the treatment of another condition such as arthritis, chronic lung disease, asthma, collagen vascular disease, or immune conditions. While cortisone can suppress inflammation, it has a significant effect on the metabolism of sugar and the development of diabetes.

Minor Risk Factors

- Elevated blood pressure. The severity of eye disease increases as the arteries narrow in hypertension. There's also a condition called Syndrome X, in which diabetics, after a number of years, develop high blood pressure because of the clogging of the small arteries, which requires the heart to pump harder, increasing blood flow and blood pressure in response.
- Heredity (not only genetic factors, but the continuation of old family dietary habits).
- Previous pancreatic disease, such as alcoholism.
- Infections that affect the pancreas.
- Psychic stress; this causes a breakdown in nutrition and increased risk of infection.
- Long-term smoking, which causes thickened eye artery linings.
- Lack of exercise.

> **Dr. Abel's Tip**
>
> Clean out the pantry. Do not use sugar for your sweets. Instead of an artificial sweetener, use a natural one like Stevia or D-xylose. Avoid, *and I mean really avoid,* all synthetic artificial sweeteners, because they can increase your chances of neuropathy.

Symptoms of Untreated Diabetes

Untreated diabetes produces three main symptoms: (1) increased thirst (polydipsia); (2) increased hunger (polyphagia); and (3) increased urination (polyurea).

I have found that the commonest complaint of people who are diabetic but who have not yet been diagnosed is blurred vision. It's amazing to me how often physicians do not recognize blurred vision as a signal that the patient may be diabetic. If you have blurred vision, remind your doctor that diabetes may be a possible cause, especially if you are thirsty all the time, drinking more water, and urinating more frequently. Elevations of blood glucose will cause frequent urination. As a result, people become very thirsty (an effect of the high blood sugar level), and are constantly drinking and urinating, which continues the cycle.

A high blood sugar level can also be considered a symptom of diabetes. Laboratory tests reveal high blood sugar both after fasting (not having eaten for several hours) and after meals, as well as too much sugar in the urine. The blood sugar level is rarely higher than 160 mg per 100 cc of blood (shortly after a meal) or lower than 60 mg per 100 cc (during fasting).

As the diabetic condition worsens, by-products of fat metabolism called *ketone bodies* are secreted into the blood to provide another source of energy; however, they make the blood too acid, which can result in coma and death. This is increasingly rare in the United States, and usually happens only in people with untreated diabetes, or in those whose diabetes is under very poor control.

Other symptoms of diabetes include hunger, fatigue, itching, visual disturbance, and skin infections. Visual disturbance can result from increased sugar in the fluid areas of the body, including the eye. The sudden development of nearsightedness in an adult, for instance, can be a symptom of diabetes. This can also happen to children, so pay special attention to children's complaints about their eyes and vision.

The secondary symptoms come from complications in different organ systems. The target areas of diabetes are the kidneys, heart, circulatory system, eyes, and nerves.

Many diabetics develop eye problems over time. Most diabetics who've had the disease for twenty years have some level of eye disease (retinopathy). Only about half these individuals, however, develop seriously impaired vision. Blindness occurs in only about 6 percent of diabetics with eye disease.

Blindness is largely preventable, if the entire care team—including the patient—is active and diligent. Early detection and careful follow-up are crucial. Because we have yet to develop adequate screening or personal management strategies to help diabetics deal with their disease, it's vital for you to read about diabetes with the idea that you can command it— it does not have to command you.

High blood pressure (hypertension) can accelerate the development of heart and eye disease in diabetics. Diabetics with hypertension should take all possible measures to control it, including stopping smoking. Smoking increases the changes in the small blood vessels that hasten hardening of the arteries, including the arteries in the eye. In other words, smoking worsens diabetes and its many complications. I cannot make this point strongly enough. Smoking absolutely increases your risk for many eye diseases, including diabetic retinopathy.

Nerve damage can create pain, especially in feet and hands (neuropathy), in untreated diabetics. I have found that artificial sweeteners (like aspartame) increase the chance of this nerve damage developing in diabetics; this condition can be reversed by increasing water consumption and decreasing the number of soft drinks (especially diet drinks containing artificial sweeteners) consumed daily. I suspect that much of the neuropathy blamed on diabetes itself is actually caused by artificial sweeteners, but this has not yet been proved in clinical trials.

I urge my diabetic patients to make every effort to prevent heart disease since, as diabetics, they already have circulatory problems. A newly identified risk for heart disease is an elevated level of homocysteine, a compound that accumulates in the blood when too much saturated fat is consumed. High homocysteine levels may turn out to be even more important than high cholesterol in predicting heart disease risk. Homocysteine appears to clog veins and arteries, which leads to heart attacks, strokes, and eye disease. The good news is that homocysteine levels can be controlled by consuming the vitamins folic acid (from citrus fruits, tomatoes, vegetables, grains, or a 400 mcg supplement), B_6 (from chicken, fish, liver, eggs, soybeans, oats, and unmilled rice), and B_{12} (found in animal products, peanuts, and walnuts).

> **Dr. Abel's Tip**
>
> Control your blood sugar, and keep a copy of your highest and lowest blood sugar measurements, because both shock the system and are toxic to cells. This is a situation in which your high antioxidant level will help support the retinal capillaries.

Diabetics need to manage their insulin through testing serial blood or (less likely) urine levels. If you have diabetes, you'll learn more about this from your physician, nursing coordinators, and nutritional advisers. If you are diabetic, it's important to relate the results of a glucose blood test to your previous meal. Test your blood, watch your food, make diabetes a wake-up call for the rest of your life or your loved one's life.

Eye Symptoms of Diabetes: Diabetic Retinopathy

Diabetic retinopathy, the eye disease that develops in diabetes, is caused by changes in the cells that line blood vessels (the *mural cells*), which are normally leakproof. When mural cells begin to diminish in number, the blood vessels leak small amounts of blood into the eye, causing tiny hemorrhages and exudates (yellow spots in the retina). This is called background diabetic retinopathy.

If the blood vessels do not supply enough oxygen to the eye, the body responds by growing new blood vessels. These new blood vessels can also cause loss of sight (a condition called proliferative diabetic retinopathy), because they are fragile and tend to leak blood into the eye. Bleeding into the vitreous humor (hemorrhaging into the eye) may clear by itself, or it may cause scarring and lead to the development of a serious condition called *retinal detachment.*

Macular edema, another type of diabetic retinopathy, occurs when the macula swells because of excess fluid leaking from below the retina.

Background diabetic retinopathy is an early form of the disease that should serve as a warning sign to protect the eyes from further deterioration. Background diabetic retinopathy should also be seen as a sign that blood vessels throughout the body are being damaged.

Diabetes can decrease the sensitivity of the cornea, which is important for people having contact lenses fitted or undergoing corneal surgery. Cataracts can develop as a complication of diabetes, particularly in older people. Besides the usual type of cataract (a nuclear cataract), high sugar can cause a posterior subcapsular cataract. The incidence of eye (and other) infections is slightly higher in diabetics.

All the problems caused by diabetes may not result from the blood sugar level itself, but from swings in the blood sugar level (high to low) and the breakdown of the immune system that those swings cause. The body is stressed by both very high and very low levels of blood sugar, and the shock to cells kills them slowly. I encourage diabetic patients to build up their antioxidant bank accounts to stabilize their immune systems, preserve the cells in the retina, and protect the cells inside the blood vessels.

Because the retina is so metabolically active, diseases like diabetes may be obvious in the eye before they produce symptoms elsewhere in the body. Your eyes reflect your general medical condition. You may never have any eye problems, but if you are a diabetic, it's very important to have an annual, dilated-eye examination. This is part of taking charge of your own health and understanding how to manage your disease. Demand explanations from your doctor as well as his or her participation—your vision is too crucial to your life to expect any less from your physician.

Dr. Abel's Tip

Be very vigilant about any skin infections you develop. Because diabetics often have poor circulation, infections that are exceptionally difficult to heal can become established in even minor cuts, especially on the feet and legs. Try to avoid developing *any* infections, and treat any infection you do develop thoroughly and vigorously.

It's important to remember that low blood sugar, or *hypoglycemia*, is another part of the wide spectrum of diabetes. Hypoglycemia can occur in people who don't handle sugar well, and it can occur in people who eventually become diabetic. Just because you're hypoglycemic, however, doesn't mean you will eventually become diabetic. If you suffer from hypoglycemia, take control of your life now by following some of the suggestions I present here.

Diagnosis

Diabetes is diagnosed by measuring blood sugar levels. Two fasting blood levels above 126 mg per 100 ml of blood confirm a diagnosis. After a meal, blood sugar can rise as high as 200 mg/100 ml of blood; the fasting blood sugar level (after 12 hours or longer without eating) should be between 60 and 110 mg/100 ml of blood, although it increases slightly with age. As the diabetic condition worsens, by-products of fat metabolism called *ketone bodies* are secreted into the blood to provide another source of energy. Ketone bodies make the blood too acid, however, which can result in coma and death; so it is important to test blood acidity as well.

Laboratory testing of blood sugar is crucial. As an ophthalmologist, I make it a point to remind others (patients and physicians) about the need for such testing. Following the blood levels of hemoglobin A1-C is also important. High blood sugar increases the amount of this type of hemoglobin; less than 8 percent is preferred.

How quickly diabetes and its complications progress is associated with glucose control, the duration of the diabetes, and the frequency of timely, dilated-eye exams. A dilated-eye examination is important to recognize who is at greatest risk for developing diabetic eye disease; a basic eye exam is often inadequate. Findings of decreased vision can sometimes often be determined by testing color vision and contrast sensitivity in a dilated exam.

Dr. Abel's Tip

Get to know your body and how you feel. Close your eyes and, while breathing deeply, try to feel each toe and each finger. Since circulation problems usually affect the feet first, you will develop better sensation. Aim to achieve your optimal weight. Exercise regularly, and closely monitor how you feel so that you intuitively know whether your blood sugar is up or down. Guess your blood sugar at every opportunity.

As we discussed in Chapter 4, a complete eye exam includes several elements: a slit lamp examination; a check of the eye's internal pressure; and a panoramic viewing of the retina through a dilated pupil. (Don't forget to bring someone with you to drive you home following your eye exam, because your vision will be blurred after your eyes are dilated.)

Fluorescein angiography can also be very important in diagnosing diabetic eye disease. In this test, a harmless vegetable dye is injected into the blood vessels. The test shows whether there is any leakage from the blood vessels into the retina. Color fundus photography is helpful as well to indicate vascular abnormalities. Using these two tests, it's possible to pinpoint areas of concern.

I also make sure my diabetic patients have their blood pressure, hemoglobin, urine protein, and lipid profiles measured; that they receive self-management education, medical nutrition education, and education on self-monitoring glucose; that their tobacco status is evaluated; and that they receive a counseling referral, when necessary. Finally, I always encourage them to keep their medical appointments, since they should be followed by their eye doctor, family doctor, and any other necessary specialists.

Management

A report in the March 1997 issue of *Diabetes* revealed that diabetic clinics take better care of patients with diabetic eye disease than do general medical clinics. In other words, the clinic physicians—who tend to be specialists like diabetologists, endocrinologists, medical residents, podiatrists, optometrists, and ophthalmologists—tend to be more sensitive to potential eye problems.

The gatekeeper approach to managed care used by many HMOs shifts patient care from specialists to generalists. This is a terrible development. Even though health maintenance organizations (HMOs) save money by limiting visits to specialists, in the long run, better care will save money by catching diseases early. We need to teach family doctors when to refer patients to specialists to avoid costly complications, and teach diabetic patients, in particular, to demand proper eye care.

The American Diabetes Association and the National Committee for Quality Assurance (NCQA) have launched programs to assure that people with diabetes get the quality of care necessary to prevent or delay complications. There is also an organization called HEDIS (Health Plan Employer Data and Information Set) which scores HMOs in terms of how good they are at making sure diabetics have regular dilated-eye examinations. You can check out your HMO by getting in touch with this organization.

All diabetics need dilated-eye examinations annually. More frequent examinations are needed if you have signs of proliferative retinopathy (diagnosed by either observation or photography).

It's interesting to note that in Iceland the incidence of blindness from diabetic retinopathy has dropped dramatically, apparently due to the fact that every screening center has an ophthalmologist to perform the appropriate laser therapy (argon laser photocoagulation) immediately. Because there is no delay in referring the patient to an ophthalmologist, the disease is less likely to progress, preventing blindness in many cases.

Traditional Management

Management of diabetic retinopathy is the same as that of diabetes in general: tight control of blood sugar markedly reduces the chances of developing eye disease, as well as all problems related to long-term diabetes.

I urge my diabetic patients to develop a stable and healthful diet. I also emphasize that treating obesity is extremely important.

Traditional management of diabetes includes:

- *Annual dilated-eye examinations.* Vision loss is often a late symptom of diabetes, and early signs of diabetic eye disease may be difficult for the general physician to recognize. It's important for diabetics to consult an ophthalmologist or optometrist whose knowledge about diabetes is up-to-date.
- *Periodic eye photography for those at greatest risk.*
- *Laser photocoagulation,* which stops the bleeding into the eye (for macular edema or proliferative retinopathy). This treatment can reduce the likelihood of visual loss by 50 percent, as has been shown by many long-term studies, but is more effective when performed before visual loss has occurred.
- *Removing damaged fluid from the eye (vitrectomy).* This procedure may restore some vision in patients whose disease is too advanced for photocoagulation. Ultimately, vitrectomy only cleans out the involved fluid and makes it possible to perform photocoagulation. Even photocoagulation, however, is just treating a symptom and not the cause.
- *Drug therapy.* Drug therapy for diabetes—including insulin therapy for those who do not respond to the oral medications—is important. There are new classes of oral agents under development that seem able to stimulate a patient's production of insulin, even in cases where it was not thought possible. One of these drugs, Piaglitazone, seems to stimulate insulin production even in juvenile diabetics. The oral drugs are not forms of insulin; they cannot, therefore, be used as substitutes for insulin.
- *Diet.* Caloric management—especially avoiding simple sugars—is helpful in diabetes. (Ask any diabetic what happens after he or she consumes a food like ice cream, candy, or even fruit.) The American Diabetic Association has created several diets, and I recommend them to my diabetic patients. There is ample evidence to show that these diets are helpful in controlling serum level by controlling daily calories as well as the balance of fats, carbohydrate, and protein. Though there are new drugs that show promise in treating obesity, they must be approached with caution. At this point, it is far safer to rely on nutritional balance in conjunction with lifestyle adaptation and exercise.

Alternative Management

One threat to vision in diabetic eye disease is the growth of new blood vessels in response to a lack of oxygen. A new group of therapies counteract the *angiogenic factors* that cause blood vessels to grow. (These new therapies employ *anti-angiogenic* factors.) Genistein from soy, for instance, is well known as an anti-angiogenic agent. It has been recommended for patients who are at risk of developing breast cancer, which also depends on the growth of new blood vessels. Likewise, genistein is wonderful for patients who are at risk for diabetic retinopathy. An antitumor compound called *squalene* that works as an anti-angiogenic factor has been developed from sharks. Squalene may retard tumors. The actual product that contains squalene is called Shark Liver Oil. (See Resource Guide.)

Dr. Abel's Tip

Diabetics will have better sugar control on a mostly vegetarian diet.

The essential fatty acids—especially the Omega-3 and Omega-6 fatty acids—are very helpful in fighting free-radical damage. An essential fatty acid is one which is not made by the body; therefore, we must consume it from food sources. These fatty acids have multiple actions, including lining cells, stimulating immunity, decreasing platelet stickiness, and fighting free-radical damage. Retinal photoreceptors—rods and cones, the cells that allow vision to occur—break down in the presence of light, and the essential fatty acids protect against the free radicals produced by light. Numerous studies have shown that addition of essential fatty acids to the diet can help prevent or improve diabetic retinopathy and improve vision in general. Japanese researchers have suggested that Omega-3 and Omega-6 fatty acids help prevent blood vessel disease, which may be why these essential fatty acids can prevent and treat diabetic eye disease.

Diabetic neuropathy improves on a vegetarian diet, which does not mean every diabetic has to become a vegetarian. I don't emphasize this too strongly, but we can learn from nature. For instance, there aren't too many animals who are diabetic in the wild, and most animals eat plants. This shows that decreasing animal fat and increasing plant-derived protection in our own diets can be helpful. Diabetics who are overweight need to restrict their calories. The American Diabetes Association points out that vegetables like spinach, broccoli, asparagus, cabbage, celery, and string beans—all of which are high in complex carbohydrates, and thus smooth the absorption of sugars into the blood—can be consumed in nearly unrestricted amounts (but hold the Béarnaise sauce!). Whole grains, like brown rice, have the same effect on blood sugar absorption. Consumption of saturated fats should be limited, and greasy fried foods should be avoided by diabetics. At all costs, avoid artificial sweeteners, including saccharine and aspartame; they may contribute to neuropathy.

The first problem to address in treating diabetic eye disease is bleeding in the eye (capillary leakage). Therefore, we should identify agents that build up blood vessels.

• First and foremost is vitamin C, which makes collagen and keeps capillaries strong. We can see that by looking at scurvy, a disease that results from lack of vitamin C. The British sailors who were first diagnosed with scurvy had bleeding gums because their blood vessels were very fragile. Their capillaries broke down because they didn't have any fresh vegetables or fruits—main sources of vitamin C—with them on long sea voyages. I recommend 1000 mg of vitamin C three times a day, but vitamin C works even better if taken with bioflavonoids like quercetin. Over the years there have been numerous studies that indicate a relationship among diabetic retinopathy, capillary leakage, and bioflavonoids.

Dr. Abel's Tip

Your antioxidant bank account is extremely important in avoiding diabetic retinopathy. Leaky capillaries are the equivalent of scurvy of the retina. Therefore, in addition to other antioxidants, you should take daily high amounts of vitamin C and quercetin. Add bilberry as well if you find it helps your night vision.

• Quercetin is one of the most powerful bioflavonoids. It can be bought as a supplement, and is also found in the skin of apples and in red onions. The bioflavonoids in plants are nature's way of counteracting the toxicity of the sun and protecting the fruit and its seeds from free radicals. Bilberry, which comes from the plant *Vaccinium myrtillus*, is very helpful in improving night vision and capillary stability. A good bioflavonoid supplement program is 100 mg of bilberry twice a day in addition to 1000 mg of quercetin daily, along with vitamin C (1000 mg three times a day). Pine bark has been used in the treatment of diabetic retinopathy in France and Germany, countries which are more sympathetic to the use of naturopathic remedies, and European researchers report that this supplement has restored sight among diabetics. This remedy has not been tested in the United States.
• Antioxidants in general are very important, including vitamin A (beta-carotene), vitamin E, and a multivitamin (in addition to vitamin C, quercetin, and bilberry). The B vitamins stabilize nerve function and prevent nerve pain (neuropathy). They also have a role in keeping the essential fatty acids inside nerve cells. Vitamins B and C are water-

soluble and their levels can be decreased by diuretics (which cause more frequent urination), blood pressure medications, exercise, and excessive urination due to any cause.

• Certain minerals are also important; for instance, levels of magnesium and potassium need to be maintained. Magnesium is the natural calcium channel blocker. It lowers blood pressure and provides increased blood flow in hands and feet. Patients who have migraine headaches, tingling in the hands and feet, cramps in the calves at night, and irregular heart beats (atrial fibrillation) need more magnesium.

• Italian investigators found that giving bilberry to patients with diabetic eye disease resulted in less bleeding in the eye. Bilberry also improves night vision.

• German researchers found that *Ginkgo biloba* is helpful in treating chronic cerebral retinal insufficiency syndrome, a condition that causes vision loss in elderly patients. Significant improvement was seen after treatment with 160 mg daily of *Gingko biloba* extract. *Ginkgo biloba* has also been found by German scientists to improve vision in patients with other blood vessel–related eye diseases. Researchers in the United States have found that ginkgo appears to improve memory in some patients with Alzheimer's disease, suggesting that it increases blood flow to the brain, which is intimately connected to the eye.

• A class of antioxidants called pycnogenols (or OPCs) helps people with diabetic retinopathy by protecting against the breakdown of protective fats.

• Alpha-lipoic acid is a natural antioxidant that lowers blood sugar, and supplementation with it can be helpful to diabetics. Alpha-lipoic acid helps regenerate levels of other antioxidants like vitamin E and glutathione, as well as supporting nerve function, which is especially helpful for patients with diabetic neuropathy.

• The Chinese prescribe herbs to stop internal bleeding and absorb leaked blood. San qi, a ginseng-like compound, is taken regularly by Chinese athletes to decrease trauma-related bleeding. I referred three patients who'd had multiple laser therapy and still experienced bleeding to my Chinese medical colleague for treatment with Chinese herbs. These patients' bleeding stopped completely, even the bleeding in one patient who'd already had seven ineffective laser procedures. After he was put on san qi, along with other herbal medications, his bleeding stopped completely. An organization named the National Commission for the Certification of Acupuncturists (the phone number is listed in the Resource Guide) will recommend a Chinese doctor in your area.

The development of these new therapies is a sign that researchers are beginning to investigate compounds that are active in nature and bring those substances to the pharmaceutical table. You don't have to wait for drugs to be developed to benefit from this new approach. Soy, for instance, is readily available and can supply genistein through your diet. Four ounces of tofu (a soy food) contain 21,000–24,000 micrograms of genistein. Soy supplements are also available, and you can take two to four grams daily.

Other herbal preparations may also be helpful in controlling eye bleeding, as medical journals are beginning to note. An article in the *Annals of Ophthalmology* in 1992 described *Morita luaha*, an Ayurvedic (Indian) herb, that showed a beneficial effect in stopping damage from bleeding and preventing recurrence of diabetic eye disease. The internationally acclaimed product Yu Xiao San, the sixth-most popular health food in Japan, has been found effective in lowering blood sugar. According to the manufacturer's claims, Yu Xiao San restores the function of the pancreas. I don't know enough about this compound to recommend it here, since it is untested in the United States. Its apparent success in Japan, however, emphasizes the need to evaluate new products as alternatives both to blindness and to interventional therapies. While all these remedies need more controlled study, they give hope to the countless number of diabetics who are desperate for solutions. As there is no one therapy that works for everyone, some understanding of the options available to you may do you a world of good.

My Recommendations

Diabetes is increasing in our population due to the poor quality of our immune defense systems and because of what we eat. I urge my patients to make every effort to have a balanced diet and an appropriate lifestyle that includes exercise, stress reduction, and adequate levels of water; you should try to build up to eight glasses daily. My particular recommendations to diabetics seeking to avoid eye disease include: frequent monitoring of blood sugar levels; adequate blood sugar control, using supplements and diet to reduce the need for either oral or injected drugs; avoiding refined sugars and flour wherever possible and reducing cholesterol and other lipids through dietary management; being sure to have a dilated-eye examination once a year—more often if indicated; control of blood pressure, as well as monitoring of physical and emotional stress; cessation of smoking; and supplemental nutrition.

Supplemental nutrition is absolutely vital in protecting a diabetic's eyes. My specific recommendations include the following:

1. *Vitamins*
   - Multivitamin, as indicated.
   - Vitamin C, 1000 mg 3 times per day.
   - B vitamin complex, 50–100 mg per day.
   - Vitamin E, 400 IU per day, along with 200 mg coenzyme selenium per day.
   - Vitamin A, 5000 IU per day.
2. *Bioflavonoids*
   - Quercetin, 1000–1500 mg per day as an antihistamine and aldose reductase inhibitor (to avoid diabetes-induced cataract).
   - Bilberry, 100–250 mg per day (or grape seed extract or pine bark extract); other anthocyanins are useful, but perhaps not as effective.
3. *Minerals*
   - Chromium, 200 mcg per day (chromium lowers blood sugar).
   - Magnesium, 500 mg per day (magnesium is the natural calcium channel blocker).
   - Manganese, 5–15 mg per day.
   - Zinc, 15 mg per day.
4. *Essential fatty acids.* To protect nerve fibers, take a combination of essential fatty acids, plant and/or fish fatty acids in a 500 mg dose twice a day with meals.
5. *Alpha-lipoic acid.* Take a maintenance dose of 250 mg per day following an initial dose of 500 mg per day under a doctor's supervision; alpha-lipoic acid appears to lower blood sugar and therefore to reduce the need for insulin or oral medications.
6. *Gemnema sylvestri*, 50 mg per day, and *fenugreek*, 15 mg per day. These Indian herbs should be taken under a doctor's supervision.
7. *Phosphatidylinositol* (PI), derived from dietary phytates or phytic acid (inositol hexaphosphate), is essential for many important reactions in the body. Phytates are found in high-fiber foods like cereals, legumes, and vegetables. PI (the form in which phytates are incorporated into cell membranes) plays a role in starch digestion, and is inhibited by high blood sugar levels. It's involved in cell membranes, important enzyme reactions, and lipid synthesis in the liver. In fact, inositol (the *I* in *PI*) is considered a member of the B vitamin family like choline. PI or inositol is recommended by some practitioners

for managing diabetes, renal disease, and the respiratory distress syndrome seen in infants.

My most important advice to diabetics is this: Take charge of your life. You can avoid losing your vision. If you smoke, stop. If you are overweight, restrict your calories and begin exercising (after consulting your physician). Get rid of the excess sugar you're consuming. Work on building up your antioxidant bank account, which will protect your eyes from all kinds of free-radical damage, including damage from the ultraviolet light in sunlight. Wear sunglasses when you're outside. If you are going to add new foods, vitamins, or herbs to your daily regimen remember to tell your doctors; these may cause fluctuation (up of down) of your blood sugar levels.

Remember, it is only a very small number of diabetics who lose their eyesight because of their disease. You *can* take control of your life and your disease to lower the chance that you will be one of them.

Tables 17 and 18 provide a summary of my recommendations regarding diet, lifestyle, and supplements.

Table 17. Prevention/Alternative Treatment of Diabetes

Diet and Supplementation	Lifestyle	Water and Digestion
• Eat a mostly vegetarian diet strong on high-fiber vegetables and whole grains. • Increase your Omega-3 fatty acid intake by consuming flaxseeds or flaxseed oil, purslane, fatty fish, turmeric, fish oil or Neuromins™ DHA; or supplement with 500 mg twice daily with meals. • Avoid artificial sweeteners; use Stevia or D-xylose instead. • Decrease your consumption of alcohol, which is fermented sugar. • Decrease your consumption of diet sodas and coffee. • Avoid refined foods, harmful fats, and supermarket oils. • Supplement your diet with: a multivitamin with vitamin A B complex vitamin (50–100 mg daily) sublingual vitamin B$_{12}$ (1–2 mg daily) vitamin C (1000 mg three times daily, if tolerated) vitamin E (400–800 IU daily at mealtime) lutein (6–10 mg daily) zeaxanthin (.5–1.0 mg daily) magnesium (500–1000 mg at bedtime) chromium (50–200 mcg daily) selenium (50–200 mcg daily) zinc (30 mg daily for several months) copper (2 mg daily while taking zinc) vanadyl sulfate (20 mg daily for two weeks, then 2 mg daily) quercetin (1000 mg daily) bilberry (100 mg twice daily) garlic (one odorless pill daily)	• Stop smoking. • Gradually begin an exercise program while monitoring your blood sugar carefully. • Keep a blood sugar–level chart; anticipate highs and lows, and try to figure out what causes them. • Recognize that diabetes is not an embarrassment; it's a fact of life. • Note how herbs and supplements like chromium and gemnema can help you regulate your blood sugar.	• Drink eight 8-ounce glasses of water daily, but not with meals. • Increase the amount of fiber in your diet. Encourage regular bowel habits. • Supplement with N-acetyl choline (NAC) and phosphatidyl choline to improve your digestion. • Eat slowly, in a relaxed setting, so you can digest your meal properly. • Take digestive aids if necessary. Try supplementing with Betaine (a weak hydrochloric acid) for one month.

Table 17. Prevention/Alternative Treatment of Diabetes (cont.)

Diet and Supplementation	Lifestyle	Water and Digestion
alpha-lipoic acid (200 mg twice daily) phosphatidylinositol (PI) the herb Gemnema CoQ10 (60–120 mg) *Ginkgo biloba* extract (15 drops twice daily or 160 mg in pill form in individual doses)		

Table 18. Further Ways to Prevent and Treat Diabetes

Other Diseases/Drugs	Whole Body
• Manage chronic diseases like high blood pressure, atherosclerosis, elevated cholesterol, osteoporosis, and indigestion. • If you suffer from obesity, try to lose weight. Exercising regularly, as suggested for other reasons, will help you in this difficult effort. Drinking lots of water will also help you approach your ideal weight while flushing toxins from your body. • Be especially vigilant in avoiding infections in cuts, particularly on your feet and legs; these can become extremely serious in diabetics. • Avoid cortisone, which elevates blood sugar. Likewise, minimize stress, which produces cortisol. • Manage depression. I've found that people who don't feel well don't eat well.	• Be extra conscious of the condition of your eyesight and any other symptoms you develop after being diagnosed with diabetes. • Take inventory of your general health. • Keep a calendar on which you record your medication and supplement regimens so you're aware of when you started taking something new. • Work on improving circulation in your lower limbs through specific exercises (ask your doctor or physical therapist). • Have a massage once in a while to improve circulation in the whole body. • Have an annual dilated-eye exam. This is mandatory.

CHAPTER 10

Second Chances: Cornea Transplants

Myth: You have to be able to see well to be a cornea donor.
Fact: Being near- or farsighted does not affect your cornea, and you can be a donor even if you have refractive error. There are never enough cornea donors to save the sight of everyone who needs a transplant.

• *Annette had cornea transplants more than ten years ago on both eyes. Her vision was very good just after I performed her transplants, but slowly her nearsightedness (myopia) and extremely curved corneas (keratoconus) returned. This was a very unusual situation. Interestingly, Annette's increasing nearsightedness and gradually curving corneas paralleled the way her keratoconus had developed in the first place. Annette reacted to her deteriorating vision by changing her glasses prescriptions fairly often for several years following her cornea transplant, no doubt hoping that she wouldn't need to undergo surgery again. But finally, it became clear to both of us that the cornea transplant would have to be repeated. Prior to her second cornea surgery, I talked to Annette about other health conditions that might be contributing to her corneal deterioration. Annette finally mentioned that she had mitral valve prolapse, a defect of one of the valves that regulates blood flow inside the heart. In mitral valve prolapse, the mitral valve becomes floppy and prolapses, or falls forward making it incapable of opening and closing to regulate blood flow properly. When I asked why she hadn't told me before, Annette said it had never occurred to her. Knowing that she had both corneal disease and mitral valve prolapse made Annette's situation much clearer. Since keratoconus and mitral valve prolapse both involve floppy collagen tissues, the problem that causes one may very well cause the other. If I had known years earlier that Annette had mitral valve prolapse, I would have had an important clue in dealing with her keratoconus. This is why I encourage my patients to discuss their entire health situations with me. Annette underwent successful repeat corneal transplant surgery in both eyes, and is now taking two grams (2000 mg) of vitamin C daily to prevent future changes in her corneas. (I'll explain exactly how vitamin C protects the cornea later in this chapter.) After my experience with Annette, I now recommend 2000 mg daily of vitamin C to all my keratoconus patients, whether they are going to have corneal transplant surgery or not.*

• *In my office one afternoon I encountered a woman patient in her late 40s whom I'd treated for dry eye complaints only a few weeks previously. Her dry-eye symptoms were a result of a cornea transplant which I performed for her. It's especially important for patients who've had cornea transplants to treat dry eyes (a common aftereffect of the surgery) immediately, and to avoid developing repeated dry-eye symptoms by ensuring a good tear film. Although she was accompanying another patient that day and did not have an appointment herself, she rushed up to me and said, "I have to tell you that, after you encouraged me to treat my dry eyes with diet and nutrition, I began eating lots of fresh vegetables, and even juicing with carrots and other vegetables several times a day. Now my dry eyes and cornea irritation are completely gone!" I asked if she were still using eyedrops to moisten her eyes. She said no—she had wanted to see if the nutritional therapy alone was making her eyes better. It was! She added, "Be sure to tell all your cornea transplant patients what you told me about treating dry eyes with diet and nutrition."*

The cornea is the transparent outer portion of the eye through which light enters. Because it is curved, the cornea also helps the lens focus light. The cornea covers the iris (the colored portion of the eye) and is a tough outer protective coat that can endure a fair amount of manipulation—rubbing and even minor injuries—without damage. Once the center of the cornea becomes irrevocably damaged, however, the only remaining option to restore sight is to perform a cornea transplant.

More than two million cases of corneal disorders are reported in the United States every year. Sixty-two percent of all reported eye injuries involve the cornea, and approximately 50,000 corneal transplants are performed each year in the United States. This procedure has become incredibly successful in the past few years because of advances in surgical techniques and eye banking. Corneal transplantation is considered to be the most successful of all transplant surgeries.

Anatomy

The cornea is the most powerful refracting, or focusing portion of the eye: the lens performs about one-third of the focusing of light, but the cornea performs almost two-thirds of the focusing. (The tear film provides a little focus power, which we generally don't notice until it's disturbed. When the tear film is not intact, it breaks up the clarity of the focus.) Figure 1 shows you where the cornea is in relation to the rest of the eye.

The cornea has five layers: (1) a surface *epithelium* (the outermost layer); (2) its basement membrane, which separates it from the inner layers; (3) the *cross-linked collagen* (which makes up 90 percent of the cornea, is clear, and focuses light); (4) the internal *endothelium*; and (5) its own basement membrane. The cornea is compact, dehydrated (because both the epithelium and endothelium pump water out of the cornea to keep it clear), has no blood vessels to get in the way of vision, and contains plenty of nerves. In fact, corneal sensation is so exquisite it can detect hot and cold as well as pain.

The cornea, like the lens of the eye, is a dry, firm, refracting surface which has to rely on circulating fluids (tears and aqueous humor) for much of its nutrition. And therein lies its vulnerability. If the entire body is not nourished properly, the cornea will not be nourished properly either, and so will be less able to respond to injury or infection.

The front surface of the cornea (the surface epithelium), which can be scratched or injured with minor trauma, grows back quickly and heals rapidly, even in the elderly. On the other hand, the endothelium (which is composed of only one cell layer) rarely reproduces in adults, and may undergo progressive deterioration in some diseases as well as following an injury.

The corneal collagen is made of glycine, proline, and hydroxyproline. Ascorbic acid—which is vitamin C—is the nutrient necessary for making hydroxyproline. People who develop warpage of the cornea (one of the problems that leads to cornea transplantation) are usually deficient in hydroxyproline, which implies they are also deficient in vitamin C. Therefore, one of the first recommendations I make to people with corneal disease is to consume more ascorbic acid (vitamin C). I suspect that adequate vitamin C might help some patients avoid having to undergo corneal transplant surgery altogether, but that has not been demonstrated in any scientific studies.

It's possible that vitamin C eyedrops like the ones used in Japan (but is not yet available in the United States) could even "freeze" the cornea in a certain state, preventing further deterioration. Jonathan Wright, M.D., of the Clinical Nutrition Center in Tacoma, Washington, makes up his own vitamin C eyedrops from buffered vitamin C. He reports success in treating allergies and viral infections as well as irritated eyes. Such eyedrops would no doubt be useful in all surgical procedures in which an incision is made in the cornea (including cataract surgery and refractive surgery to correct eyesight) and, of course, in cornea transplants.

Dr. Abel's Tip

Since it is so exposed, the cornea is easy to injure, examine, and repair. To protect your eyes, treat the cornea as you treat the headlights of your car—you wouldn't want to bump them into the wall every time you park. Additionally, chemical burns and high-risk accidents are largely avoidable—if you think ahead and consciously protect your eyes from potential injury.

Symptoms Signaling a Possible Need for Corneal Transplantation

If corneal infections and injuries are treated promptly, they often improve without causing scarring. If not treated immediately, or if the center of the cornea is damaged by injury or infection, scarring and loss of vision can result. I can't stress enough how important it is to see an eye doctor immediately if you have an eye infection or injury.

The symptoms of a corneal injury are pain, redness, tearing, and blurred vision. If the injury is not treated, the damage may become progressive. Even with prompt treatment, there still may be a scar that causes distortion of vision to such an extent that it becomes difficult to read, drive, or even walk unassisted (although that is a rarer situation).

Although, as I've described, the cornea is a hardy and resilient tissue, it sometimes becomes damaged beyond repair by disease or injury. A number of conditions can eventually necessitate corneal transplantation.

Bacterial infections can result in ulcers that cause irreparable damage to the cornea. Many of these infections are entirely preventable, because they are due to abusing extended-wear contact lenses or even soft contact lenses. If you wear soft contact lenses, follow the instructions given you by your eye care professional carefully, and *do not wear them longer than the recommended time*, because you will risk developing a vision-threatening infection if you do. The organisms usually responsible for these infections are the *pseudomonas, staphylococcus*, and *streptococcus pneumoniae* bacteria. (*Staphylococcus* also causes the dangerous staph infections you can pick up in the hospital.) Table 19 lists the antibiotic eyedrops used to treat bacterial infections.

Bacteria are described as being "gram positive" or "gram negative." If the bacterium possess a cell wall, it is gram positive (which describes how

Table 19. Antibiotic Eyedrops for Bacterial Infections

Antibiotic	Gram Positive	Gram Negative	Used to Treat
Sulfonamides (sulfa drugs)	±	±	Conjunctivitis
Bacitracin	±		Eyelids
Erythromycin	+		Eyelids; necessary for corneal disease
Bacitracin/Polymyxin	±	+	Eyelids
Bacitracin/Polymyxin/ Neomycin	+	+	Cornea (neomycin is a common allergen)
Chloramphenicol	+	+	Rarely used because of side effects
Tetracycline	+		Rarely available
Gentamycin	+	+	Cornea (first choice)
Tobramycin	+	+	Cornea (first choice)
Trimethaprin/Polymyxin	±	+	Conjunctivitis
Ocufloxacin	+	+	Cornea (first choice)
Ciprofloxacin	+	+	Cornea (first choice)
Levofloxacin	+	+	Works on a twice-daily basis
Moxifloxacin	+	+	(instead of four to five times a day), which is easier for patients to deal with.

it responds to a type of stain called a gram stain). In the past, different antibiotics were used to treat gram-negative and gram-positive bacteria, but newer antibiotics are broader spectrum and can treat both types.

At the present time, fluoroquinolones are our mainstay, being the best eyedrops with broad-spectrum (both gram-positive and gram-negative) activity. Gentimycin and Tobramycin are also very good. These antibiotics are very effective against one of the more dangerous bacteria, *pseudomonas*. Antibiotic resistance is developing from overuse of common antibiotics, and some common gram-positive organisms, such as *staphylococcus* and *streptococcus*, are becoming resistant to the most specific antibiotics. Therefore, we need to develop antibiotics from new groups such as streptogramins, oxazolidinones, macrolides, and the peptide antibiotics to cover all the bases. We also need to be cautious in our application of antibiotics and may even have to revisit prophylactic therapy in eye surgery—that is, treating people with cataracts or cornea transplants with broad-spectrum antibiotics at the time of surgery and for a week afterwards to insure they don't develop infections. Using antibiotics as we have in the past has protected individuals, but because of the natural evolution of organisms, may have jeopardized our greater community.

Dr. Abel's Tip

Treat corneal infections rapidly and vigorously, whether they're caused by the ubiquitous herpes virus or are bacterial. Soft contact lenses may contribute to corneal infection. If you have had a bad experience with contact lenses and do not want to wear glasses, you should consider undergoing the LASIK procedure to correct your nearsightedness instead of relying on soft contact lenses.

Corneal ulcers can also be triggered by infectious agents like the *Herpes simplex* virus, trachoma (caused by an organism called chlamydia), fungi (in tropical climates), and parasites (like acanthamoeba, which contaminates stagnant water and can contaminate soft contact lenses). When the ulcers caused by these infectious agents heal, scar tissue can form, clouding vision. Vitamin A deficiency (more common in less-developed countries) also delays healing. In tropical or impoverished countries, infections like river blindness, trachoma, and others we don't see in the United States are major causes of corneal scarring and blindness, if corneal transplantation is not readily available (which it isn't for most people in these countries). There are specific therapies for almost all of these infections, and the damage can be neutralized by instituting treatment as soon as possible. The old adage "an ounce of prevention is better than a pound of cure" is certainly applicable here.

Dr. Abel's Tip

The cornea is weakened in keratoconus (warpage of the cornea), and often melted by enzymes in rheumatoid arthritis patients. Vitamin C (which helps make the cross-linked collagen in the cornea) will help corneal ulcers to heal.

Congenital cloudiness of the cornea is sometimes present at birth and can have a hereditary component. In these cases, corneal transplants are performed as soon after birth as possible, so that the child's vision can develop normally. Such a condition is instantly obvious to the physician, and plans to correct it can be instituted immediately.

Other inherited corneal conditions, called *dystrophies*, that affect vision, tend to occur at an early age, in the center of the cornea, and in both eyes. Dystrophies can develop in the epithelium, the stroma, or the endothelium of the cornea. The most common is Fuch's endothelial dystrophy, which may be passed on in family lines and is a leading cause of corneal transplants. When the endothelium deteriorates, fluid seeps into the cornea, and its crystalline structure becomes spongy (a condition called *corneal edema*).

Corneal edema is a common cause of corneal transplantation, not only in people with dystrophies, but also in older individuals who have undergone previous eye surgery, usually cataract surgery. The old-style intraocular implants (twenty years old or older) used after cataract surgery, or a previous, complicated cataract surgery may cause the cornea to deteriorate. (Fortunately, our technology and surgical techniques have progressed so much that the new implants don't cause this type of complication.) Corneal edema, in which fluid collects in the cornea and causes it to become cloudy, should be managed aggressively, before the cornea deteriorates completely and a cornea transplant must be performed. If a transplant is necessary, most surgeons prefer to wait until the eye is "quiet," or not inflamed, to perform the surgery. There are medical treatments for corneal edema, but a cornea transplant—particularly if corneal edema develops following cataract surgery—is sometimes necessary.

Injury can result in a need for corneal transplantation. The cornea can become cloudy after penetration of the eye by a sharp object, or even after the eye has been hit hard. Trauma is a terrible and unnecessary cause of lost vision. One percent of the landmine injuries in Cambodia, for instance, have caused blindness in both eyes. Other injuries—like severe abrasion or laceration of the cornea—and complications of refractive surgery (to correct nearsightedness) can on rare occasions severely damage the cornea. Chemical burns can also destroy corneal tissue, harm vision, and necessitate a corneal transplant. If you work with chemicals, do woodworking, chop wood for a fireplace, or engage in other activities that could result in damage to your cornea, be sure to wear protective glasses or goggles. (See Chapter 4.)

Keratoconus is a disease that causes the cornea to become "pointed," which distorts vision. It often begins in the late teens or young adulthood, and is slowly progressive. Mild keratoconus may appear at any age, and the eye doctor will recognize it by the patient's fluctuating vision and frequently changing eyeglasses prescriptions. Only one patient out of ten with keratoconus requires a cornea transplant, since it can generally be managed successfully with contact lenses. There is a very infrequent complication of keratoconus in which the cornea stretches so much that it rips and becomes suddenly swollen (that is, corneal edema develops). As in other cases of corneal edema, we wait until the eye is quiet before performing a cornea transplant. If you or someone you love requires a cornea transplant to treat keratoconus, rest assured that there is a 95 percent success rate for this surgery and a very good prognosis for recovering vision after the transplant.

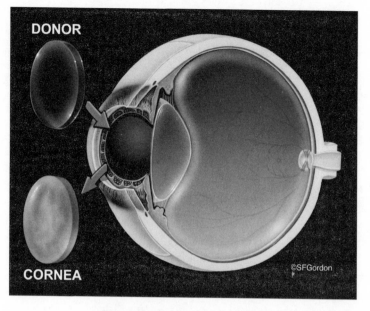

DONOR

CORNEA

©SFGordon

Figure 9. Corneal Transplant

Corneal Transplant Surgery

Replacing a clouded cornea is the only way to restore full vision after it becomes irrevocably damaged. The success rate for corneal transplant surgery, which is approximately 90 percent (and as high as 95 percent in correcting keratoconus), depends on the amount of damage the eye has sustained. It's important to remember that a cornea transplant can restore vision only if the rest of the eye is functioning properly.

Corneal transplantation is one of the most delicate and dramatic operations in all surgery. It is performed under an operating microscope. It can be done at any age, under either general or local anesthesia, and is usually performed as an outpatient procedure.

A team effort is required for cornea transplants. After the death of a donor, the family must make known their intention to donate the corneas immediately so that the corneas can be removed, ideally no more than fifteen hours after death. Technicians retrieve the tissue and rate the health of different layers of the cornea. The transplant staff is assembled, and the patient in need of a cornea is offered the opportunity for surgery. Due to improved efficiency in eye banking, surgeons are now often able to schedule the procedure (instead of needing to perform it immediately after the donor cornea is available) which alleviates much of the transplant patient's anxiety.

With corneal transplant surgery, as with all surgery, your doctors and hospital should know about all your medications before the operation. If you are having a cornea transplant as an outpatient, make sure you take someone with you to drive you home afterwards. You will probably be able to return home after resting only a few hours following your operation.

Corneal transplant surgery should be painless. You will receive either local or general anesthesia, depending upon your individual situation. Nervousness will probably be the biggest problem you encounter, so try to place yourself in as calm a state of mind as possible. Intravenous sedatives work beautifully, with very few side effects. If you're still concerned, don't be afraid to ask your physician if it's possible for you to undergo general anesthesia. If you're going to be knocked out (with general anesthesia), there is little likelihood that you will have nausea and vomiting afterwards. In fact, a scratchy throat may be the worst aftereffect you experience from undergoing a cornea transplant.

Only the central part of the cornea is used for transplantation. The surgeon uses a very sharp, circular instrument (a trephine) to outline a circular ring of tissue (called a *button*) in the donated cornea. A similar opening, depending on the condition of the cornea and the surgeon's technique, is then cut out of the donor cornea. After the donated button of cornea is placed in the patient's eye, it is sewn into place with suture material so fine it's difficult to see with the human eye (it's approximately one-fourth the thickness of a human hair). If an intraocular lens or cataract must be removed, that procedure is performed at the same time as the cornea transplant.

Postoperatively, some corneal surgeons adjust the stitches and leave them in the eye for a long time, even many years; others remove the sutures selectively after healing. When I perform this surgery, I prefer to use interrupted stitches, so that a broken or loose stitch will not be a problem and early suture removal will not jeopardize the other stitches. The surgeons performing cornea transplants are very highly trained, and no matter which technique they use, corneal transplant surgery has a great success rate.

Some physicians have the patient use steroid eyedrops for up to a year. I try to get my patients off the steroid eyedrops within six weeks if there is no inflammation or previous scarring (which carries a higher risk of postoperative rejection episodes). As I've pointed out several times, all steroid drugs have eye side effects—like accelerating cataracts—that make them very risky to use, especially over long periods of time.

Because it's usually the inner lining of the cornea that needs to be transplanted, full-thickness cornea transplants are the most common ones performed. Variations, however, exist there as well. If the injury (like a chemical burn) affects only the outer layers of the cornea, for example, only the outer layers of the donor cornea need to be transplanted into the recipient's eye.

In uncomplicated conditions, corneal transplantation is 90 percent successful. After surgery, some people have astigmatism (caused by irregular healing of a circular wound) and require a contact lens to obtain best vision. The success rate of corneal transplantation is lessened in cases in which there is perforated injury of the eye, irregular scaring, thinning or ulceration of the cornea (from recurrent herpes infections, for instance), or severe dry eye.

Dr. Abel's Tip

If you've had a cornea transplant, you may have to wear a hard contact lens for your best-corrected vision due to astigmatism.

Complications

Like any surgery, corneal transplantation has some risks, but as our techniques improve these risks are diminishing. One percent of the time the donor cornea is not a good one and will never provide good vision, so a second transplant is necessary. Fortunately, this situation is unusual because eye banks now examine the eyes thoroughly before they make them available to transplant surgeons.

The most frequent complication following corneal transplant surgery, as I mentioned above, is astigmatism. Because the cornea transplant wound does not heal exactly the same all the way around, a certain amount of astigmatism is inevitable. Astigmatism is not as great a problem as it used to be, however, because we've developed ways to reduce it with various suture techniques and wound modifications, even after healing has begun.

More serious but far less frequent complications of corneal transplant surgery include hemorrhage, infection, chronic inflammation, retinal detachment, wound rupture, cataract formation, and delayed glaucoma. While patients should always measure risk versus benefit when deciding to have a surgical procedure, in the case of corneal transplant surgery, the chances of success greatly outweigh the risk of either failure or the development of a serious complication.

Even if there are no complications, cornea transplants take three to twelve months to heal. The eye needs to be protected very carefully during that time.

Occasionally, the body rejects the donor cornea because it is a foreign tissue. This is called *corneal graft reaction*, and usually occurs within the first six months following surgery. The symptoms of graft reaction are red eyes, weeping, pain, and suddenly decreased vision. Immediately report any such symptoms to your ophthalmologist—do not wait until your next appointment to do so. If you develop symptoms of graft reaction, start using cortisone eyedrops immediately, and make sure you always have a prescription for these eyedrops on hand in case a rejection reaction occurs. The trigger events for corneal graft reactions (rejection episodes) are transfusions, immunizations (including flu shots), and injury. I advise my patients to avoid immunizations following a cornea transplant, if it's at all possible. Sometimes, no matter what precautions the patient and I take, a graft reaction occurs anyway. However, I have found that using an eyedrop like Pred Forte four times a day for five days can stop graft rejections caused by these trigger events, and save the transplanted cornea.

Dr. Abel's Tip

If you've had a cornea transplant, you must be aware that a transfusion, a flu shot, any vaccination, or an allergy could stimulate a corneal graft reaction. If you need a vaccination or transfusion, you should be on strong topical steroid eyedrops four times a day for the day of the vaccination and for four days afterwards.

Dr. Abel's Post-Corneal Transplant Instructions

You should rest quietly at home for the first twenty-four hours after your corneal transplant surgery. On the second day after surgery, you can resume most of your normal activities, if you follow these guidelines:

1. Protect your eye by wearing either the shield you're given after surgery or glasses at all times. I strongly suggest that you wear glasses (your regular glasses, sunglasses, or nonprescription glasses) to cover your eye during the day and the shield at night. When resting, always place the eye shield over the operated eye.
2. You may bathe and shower, but keep the eye protected with an eye shield or a protective covering for 1 month.
3. You may gently wash any excess secretions from your operated eye using a soft, white washcloth.
4. Moderate amounts of stooping, bending, and lifting—up to 30 pounds—are allowed.

5. Please place your medications in your operated eye regularly. You can't afford to miss even one application. There's no reason to take a chance of developing an infection or serious inflammatory reaction just because you didn't apply your medication on schedule. For the first week, your medication will be a combination antibiotic/corticosteroid, four times a day. Usually, after the first week, the antibiotic is discontinued, and a pure corticosteroid is used in decreasing amounts—for example, three times a day for one week, followed by twice a day for one week, and so on. I have always found it easiest for patients to apply the eyedrops by leaning the head back (or lying down) and placing the drops in the inner corner of the eye with the eye opened or closed. If it is closed, the patient doesn't have to look at it; he can feel the drop go in and merely has to blink for it to coat the cornea. I ask patients to keep their treated eye closed for fifteen to twenty seconds and dab the excess in the inner corner away gently with a clean tissue.

6. Vision improves slowly after corneal transplantation. Don't worry if your vision is slightly decreased immediately after your cornea transplant. The decrease in vision in the early postoperative period is due to mild inflammation and tight sutures. The sutures are usually removed after surgery (they don't dissolve by themselves), and your ophthalmologist will adjust your glasses or prescribe a semirigid contact lens (to correct astigmatism) to provide your best-corrected vision. Every eye and every cornea is unique, so your situation will be different from every other patient's.

7. Cornea transplant rejection, a known complication, may occur suddenly or slowly but the symptoms of blurred vision, tearing, and irritation should alert the patient to begin cortisone (or prednisone) eyedrops (which should always be on hand in the refrigerator), and call the eye doctor immediately. I always give my patients written instructions as a reminder of these symptoms and what to do should they occur.

8. If at any time you experience pain, increased redness, a sudden decrease in vision, or flashing lights, notify your ophthalmologist immediately. Do not wait until your next appointment!

Alternative Treatments After Corneal Transplantation

Along with the standard medications and precautions that must be taken after a cornea transplant, I recommend that my patients take these further steps:

- Supplement with essential fatty acids (500 mg twice a day with meals and a fat-soluble vitamin) to stabilize the tear film, along with artificial tears. (See Chapter 14 for more information. There are many essential fatty acid supplements available.)
- Take vitamin C, to stabilize corneal curve and aid wound healing, up to 2 grams (2000 mg) a day. (Hint: Don't immediately start taking 2 grams of vitamin C daily if you've only been taking a small dose or none at all previously, because it can give you diarrhea. Begin by taking 500 mg once or twice a day, determine your tolerance for increasing the dose, and gradually increase it to 2 grams a day.)
- Take the full complement of vitamins that you usually take.
- Control allergy conditions. Take 1000 mg of quercetin a day to avoid sneezing and itchy eyes.
- Take zinc, which is well known to improve wound healing (30 mg daily for two months).
- Be well aware of drugs that may affect healing. For instance, Israeli researchers discovered that the drug colchicine delays the healing of corneal ulceration.
- If you are going to get a vaccination (tetanus, typhoid, measles, and especially, a flu shot) after having a cornea transplant, treat that eye with cortisone drops (such as Maxidex or Pred Forte) four times a day for five days following the vaccination. The same applies to getting a blood (or blood product) transfusion, so be sure to alert your ophthalmologist if you're getting a transfusion.
- Use artificial tears to keep the surface of the cornea moist. While the corneal surface is irregular after surgery (after all the sutures are removed, the contour becomes normal), it's important to keep the surface well moisturized, since dry spots that would irritate the cornea might develop.
- Don't forget that the body is in repair at night. Have you ever noticed that your mouth ulcers or a cut finger heal during the night? All day long, you keep touching the area that's sore, but overnight, it heals. Likewise, your eyes heal at night, without movement and exposure to bright lights, so make sure you get regular sleep following corneal transplant surgery.
- A patient who has a cornea transplant is a patient for life. If you have had a cornea transplant, you need to protect your eye from trauma and be more sensitive to eye symptoms and any changes in vision you experience. You need to have a long-term relationship with your doctor. If you move, get the name of a cornea specialist in the area you're

moving to, preferably someone who has had a year of postresidency fellowship training in cornea transplant.

The Need for Cornea Donors

In the United States, thousands of people are now awaiting cornea transplants to restore their vision. The need for donors is always great.

Although potential donors don't need to have had perfect vision, the cornea must be healthy to be used for transplantation. With few exceptions, healthy donor tissue (screened for diseases like hepatitis and AIDS) is usable from people of almost any age—from 1 to 75 years old. Factors like sex, race, color of the iris, or the previous vision of the donor have no influence on the success of the procedure. No major religion bans the donation of corneas.

My home state, Delaware, has an eye bank (the Medical Eye Bank of Delaware, Inc., part of the Lion's Eye Bank of Delaware Valley) to help people from the region regain their vision. The eye bank screens all tissue carefully to insure that it is healthy and in good condition for transplantation. Your state probably has an eye bank of its own. To find out about it, ask your ophthalmologist.

Please consult your state eye bank or your ophthalmologist about becoming a cornea donor. Again, you don't need to have perfect vision to provide the gift of sight to someone else.

Corneal donation is increasing all over the world. In Italy, the donation rate was very low until a 1994 tragedy took the life of an American child named Nicholas. Nicholas's parents donated all his organs, including his corneas, for transplant to Italians needing organ transplants. The public was so touched by this gesture from the American parents that organ donation soared. The tragic loss of one child's life resulted in saving many, many lives. Don't wait for tragedy to strike to make the decision to become a cornea donor.

Tables 20 and 21 summarize my recommendations regarding diet, lifestyle, and nutritional supplementation following corneal transplant surgery.

Table 20. Alternative Treatment Following Corneal Transplant Surgery

Diet and Supplementation	Lifestyle	Water and Digestion
• Increase your Omega-3 fatty acid intake by consuming flaxseeds or flaxseed oil, and dark leafy green vegetables, fatty fish, turmeric, and other sources mentioned in text; or supplement with DHA 500 mg twice daily with meals. • Eat plenty of fresh fruits and vegetables to help you avoid dry-eye symptoms and improve your overall health. Increase use of antioxidant supplementation, especially quercetin and vitamin C. Make sure you're getting sufficient zinc. • Avoid artificial sweeteners; use Stevia or D-xylose instead. Avoid products containing sugar. • Avoid refined foods, harmful fats, and supermarket oils. • Don't eat anything you're allergic to so that you limit the possibility of sneezing or having itchy eyes. • Supplement your diet with: vitamin C (2000 mg daily) zinc (30 mg daily for two months)	• Realize that you will have a long-term relationship with your eye surgeon. • Be cautious with any exercise program after having a corneal transplant. Don't engage in boxing or other contact sports. Wear protective glasses during racquet sports. • Get plenty of sleep (the eye heals at night). Try to relax and deal positively with stress. When stress is high, cortisone levels go up and melatonin is suppressed, adversely affecting sleep. • Smoking will increase coughing, which is not good for your eye after a cornea transplant. • Be your own doctor. Pay attention to what your body is telling you. If your eye is irritated, or if you're producing tears or mucus, find out why.	• Drink eight 8-ounce glasses of water daily, but not with meals. • Eat slowly, in a relaxed setting, so you digest your meal properly. • Take digestive aids if necessary. Try supplementing with Betaine (a weak hydrochloric acid) for one month. • Increase the amount of fiber in your diet to encourage regular bowel habits.

**Table 21. Further Ways to Encourage Healing After
Corneal Transplant Surgery**

Other Diseases/Drugs	Whole Body
• If you have bad allergies, avoid having a cornea transplant during allergy season. • If you have keratoconus, make sure you don't have mitral valve prolapse, since the two conditions may coexist. • Avoid systemic steroids. Be aware of topical steroid side effects. • Always keep eyedrops on hand in your refrigerator in case you get a graft reaction.	• Be extra conscious of the condition of your eyesight. • Be vigilant with your food intake to maintain bodily health. • Keep a calendar on which you record your medication and supplement regimes so you'll know when you started taking something new. • Exercise gently to reduce stress (which produces cortisol).

CHAPTER 11

The Not-So-Odd Couple: Dry Eyes and Arthritis

Myth: Only drugs will relieve the symptoms of arthritis.
Fact: The Omega-3 essential fatty acids and the supplement glucosamine will relieve arthritic pain and dry-eye symptoms in many cases.

- *Fifty-two-year-old Lois came into my office for her regular checkup limping badly and using a cane. As she sat down, I said, "I'll bet your eyes are bothering you today, aren't they?" She said, "How did you know?" I explained that I see many patients whose arthritis—especially rheumatoid arthritis—affects their lacrimal glands so that they're unable to produce tears. Lois told me that when she gets up in the morning, her eyes are so dry that she has to put cold cloths on them immediately. She also can't read for more than ten minutes at a time before her eyes start hurting. Although Lois used to be able to get into a hot, steamy shower to make her eyes feel better, now she can't walk very well, so that remedy's out. Furthermore, she's had to take an anti-arthritis drug (Plaquenil) that's a derivative of the antimalarial chloroquine which, in high doses, can sometimes affect the retina. (Lois hasn't had any problems so far, and we check her color vision regularly to catch this type of damage early, if it develops.) Twenty years ago, Lois took gold for her arthritis, but developed an allergy to that old-time remedy. She has tried a variety of NSAIDs, which alleviated the pain but gave her gastrointestinal bleeding (a common side effect of these drugs). Lois's story is not unusual. Her next treatment step was to take prednisone, which she understood would be for the rest of her life. So I asked Lois if she'd be willing to try a variety of natural remedies, as well as an exclusion diet, before committing herself to the steroids, which can accelerate osteoporosis and even cause melting of the cornea when the dry-eye condition is severe.*

Lois agreed to try my suggestions and eliminated the nightshade plants (eggplant, peppers, and tomatoes), dairy products, and refined wheat products from her diet; started taking chondroitin and glucosamine sulfate for her arthritis; took flaxseed oil capsules twice a day (for both her dry eyes and arthritis); added supplements of vitamins E and A, as well as a B complex; and began mixing Knox gelatin with her orange juice at breakfast. (Studies have shown that consuming Knox gelatin can prevent people with severe arthritis from requiring a hip transplant.) In addition, I put plastic plugs in her tear ducts to maintain the tears that she did have (a typical therapy for severe dry eyes), and instructed her to use artificial tears during the day and ointment at night to supplement her tears. Three months after beginning this treatment regimen, Lois walked in without her cane. She didn't know which of the steps she'd taken was the most helpful, but she was willing to continue all of them to be able to shower again, drive her car, and have her eyes be more comfortable (especially when she remembers to blink). I wish more patients like Lois, and even those who have less severe and long-standing arthritis, would be willing to try the natural remedies before committing themselves to a long-term course of steroid drugs with all their potential side effects.

• I'm glad to say that my lectures to colleagues on the role of nutrition in eye health have borne some fruit. An increasing number of optometrists and, now, ophthalmologists have begun to develop their own nutritional regimens. These eye doctors start by prescribing nutritional therapies for their patients or family members and then when they see the results, try them themselves. My colleague Bob Cole, O.D., in Bridgeton, New Jersey, for instance, after seeking my advice on the subject, started suggesting that his patients who had dry eyes eat fish and take essential fatty acid supplements. One of the first patients to whom he made this recommendation found that her dry eyes improved almost immediately after she began taking an essential fatty acid supplement twice a day with her meals. A month later when she came in to pick up her new glasses, she called Dr. Cole out of his examining room to tell him, "Not only do my eyes feel much better, my arthritis is gone!" Dr. Cole was thrilled that this natural remedy for dry eyes and arthritis had helped her, and has since began recommending it to his other patients with dry eyes.

The famous diagnostician Henrik Sjögren described the triad of symptoms comprised of dry eyes, dry mouth, and arthritis now called Sjögren's syndrome. He was the first to realize that these three seemingly unrelated symptoms are connected on a deeper level.

Severely dry eyes can be caused not only by eye diseases but also by *systemic* (whole body) conditions, particularly connective tissue diseases like rheumatoid arthritis, systemic lupus, scleroderma, and polymyositis.

Each of these is an inflammatory condition in which our own antibodies attack tissue linings. These antibodies can destroy tear glands, joints, and salivary glands, producing the symptoms seen in dry eyes, arthritis, and dry mouth. It was this hidden connection that Dr. Sjögren observed in the syndrome that now bears his name.

Dr. Abel's Tip

The conjunctiva is a mucous membrane similar to many other body surfaces and joints. Therapy not only for dry eyes but also for joint diseases like arthritis lies in their lubrication through nutrition, using Omega-3 essential fatty acids, glucosamine sulfate, and water.

All elderly people can have decreased production of watery tears, but rheumatoid arthritis patients develop dry eyes especially often. According to the 1997 Eagle Vision Yankelovich Partners Survey, one out of every five Americans (nearly fifty-nine million) has dry-eye symptoms, as do 50 percent of people over age 65. Thirty-seven million Americans have arthritis, either osteoarthritis (from wear and tear) or rheumatoid arthritis (an inflammatory disease).

Let's learn a little more about these cousins, dry eyes and arthritis, and what we can do about them.

Anatomy of Dry Eyes

Tears are not just water. They have three separate components: (1) oil (from the Meibomian oil glands in the eyelids); (2) mucus (from the goblet cells deep inside the eyelids); and (3) watery tears (the "aqueous" tears from the lacrimal gland and accessory lacrimal glands located in the conjunctiva of the eyelid).

The innermost layer of tears in direct contact with the eye is the mucous layer, which is also called *mucin*. The mucin coats the surface of the cornea. The middle layer is the watery tears, which stick to the mucin and keep the eye moist. The outer tear layer is composed of oil from the Meibomian glands; it is deposited like an oil slick on the outside of the watery tears to slow their evaporation from the surface of the eye.

When the tears become more mucoid (and therefore less watery), so that you find them sticking in the corner of your eye in the morning, dry-eye symptoms may develop. People are most susceptible to this condition in the winter (when the heat is on in the bedroom) and in airplanes.

The oil in the tear film retards evaporation of the bulk of the tears (the watery component). Many people, however, have too much lipid (fat or oil) in their tear film, and studies have found that people with oily eyelids have a poor distribution of the outermost, lipid tear layer. This can lead to more rapid tear film breakup and perpetuate increased evaporation. In other words, people may have plenty of tear volume, but a poor oil slick on the top. The unprotected areas of watery tears can evaporate as a result, leading to the development of dry eyes.

Dr. Abel's Tip

The first symptom of dry eyes may be oiliness or even excessive tearing, along with burning and irritation. The tear film has three layers (watery, mucoid, and oily), and most people with dry eyes do not have enough of the watery layer. Nevertheless, the dry eye may actually seem wet, because the lacrimal gland is still stimulated to produce tears that evaporate too quickly from the eye because of a problem with another component of the tear film.

Reasons for Dry Eyes

I am surprised by how many people over age 50 have dry eyes. To me, this indicates that there are many unrecognized interactions between their food, medications, subtle medical conditions, and even imbalances throughout their bodies. In fact, I used to develop very dry eyes myself on airplane flights and during hot, dry weather.

We now understand that tear deficiencies can be associated with numerous medical conditions besides arthritis, including systemic lupus, taking multiple medications, sarcoidosis, diabetes, salivary gland disease, and gradual dehydration. For instance, older people don't drink very much water, and that's one reason they become incapacitated easily in hot climates, during water shortages, or in outbreaks of diarrheal disease. Even younger people can become dehydrated by drinking too many sodas and caffeinated beverages that stimulate the need to urinate without supplying the body with much water. That's one of the reasons I emphasize over and over that everyone must drink greater quantities of good water.

Many medications, both prescription and over-the-counter, can affect the tear film that bathes your corneas. You may not realize that the antihistamine you need to take during allergy season contributes to your eye irritation and burning. Other types of medications, including psychiatric drugs like Prozac, can cause both dry mouth and vision problems. Gastrointestinal tract medications, cold remedies, drugs for dizziness and motion sickness, and even birth control pills can contribute to dry eyes. A study examining 2520 patients at The Johns Hopkins University Hospital found that antihistamines, antidepressants, antipsychotics, diuretics, antiemetics (antinausea drugs), and certain high blood pressure medicines all increase the likelihood of developing dry-eye symptoms. The greater the number of these drugs you take, the greater your chance of developing dry eyes. I've found this to be particularly true in people over 55 who already have some decrease in their tear volume.

If you take any of these kinds of medications or your eyes seem to be drying out more than they used to, ask your doctor if the medication may be contributing to the problem. It is very difficult to read a drug's package insert and determine whether a medication causes dry eyes because it's often worded ambiguously. You can bet, however, that if a drug causes dry mouth and aches and pains, the eyes can also be irritated by it. For people who must take one or more of these medications, a reduction in their dose is sometimes helpful. Otherwise, it's important to look for an alternative medication.

Many other factors can contribute to the development of dry eyes, including:

- Drinking too much coffee
- Cigarette smoke (including secondhand smoke)
- Air conditioning or heat
- Ultraviolet light
- Staring at your computer for a long time without blinking
- Wearing contact lenses
- The dry air in airplanes

Something as simple as not blinking often enough can cause a serious dry-eye condition to develop. Conversely, having an eye problem can change the rate at which you blink, either helping to heal the problem or making it worse. Japanese researchers, for example, discovered that the rate at which we blink is controlled by the condition of the eye's surface. The surface of the eye needs to be wet; if it's not (when the surface of the eye is damaged, for instance), people blink more often, make more tears, and even squeeze the eyes to drain their accessory lacrimal (tear) glands, thereby making the eyes wetter.

In other words, the eyelids are involved in keeping the eyes moist, and the severity of dry eyes can be evaluated by measuring the rate of blinking. On the other hand, with aging or contact lens wear, our corneal sensitivity decreases. As a result, we don't feel the discomfort and may blink far too infrequently, irritating the eye. Patients with thyroid eye disease suffer chronic irritation, because their lower lids don't move during blinking, so the blinking is incomplete. Even if these patients have an adequate volume of aqueous tears, they aren't spread across the surface of the eye properly.

If people are preoccupied, as when they're staring at a computer, they blink less often. The Japanese investigators found that decreased blinking while using a computer creates a major risk of developing transient, or short-term, dry eyes. There's no long-term risk from this type of dry eyes, because people eventually stop working at the end of the day.

Diabetic patients may experience dry-eye symptoms, especially when their blood sugar levels are high. It's possible that the elevated sugar in the tears makes the tears more syrupy, causing burning and irritation. Immediate relief can be achieved by using artificial tears, but the ultimate goal should be to regulate blood sugar more tightly.

Dr. Abel's Tip

Blink regularly and completely, making sure that your eyes are really closing. If you don't blink often enough, your eyes dry out.

Symptoms of Dry Eyes

Symptoms of dry eyes include a "gritty" feeling; redness or burning; decreased quantity or quality of tears; and difficulty reading for prolonged periods because of discomfort.

People have variations in their tear film level throughout the day, so I've found that treatment intensity is often determined by patients' own sense of well-being. In other words, if a patient is just miserable, I prescribe an intensive treatment regimen for as long as it takes to make that patient feel better. Then, when the condition has stabilized, I reduce treatment intensity and work with the patient to figure out how to prevent the situation in future by adjusting his or her lifestyle and diet.

Ophthalmology residents are taught that the most common cause of corneal irritation in both eyes (called *bilateral chronic keratitis*) is—you guessed it—dry eyes. Therefore, when a patient describes a two-month or longer history of irritation symptoms (whether it's described as feeling as if there's a foreign body in the eye, or even having excessive tearing at times) and is carrying a bagful of eyedrops, the ophthalmologist is taught to think immediately of dry eyes. In this situation, more than just eyedrops will be required to keep the surface of the eyes wet for a long period of time. It may be time to plug the tear ducts, but it's certainly time to begin nutritional therapies.

Diagnosis of Dry Eyes

Diagnosis of dry eyes is generally made by a test called Shirmer tear testing. After the eye is anesthetized (with eyedrops), a strip of paper is placed on the outer one-third of the lower eyelids, and the amount of tears is measured after five minutes.

The tear film can also be examined with a slit lamp, which will reveal disturbances in the tear film layer. Other observations that can be made via the slit lamp—such as debris on the lashes or lids, "scalloping" of the lid surface, folds in the conjunctiva (the "white" of the eye), and mucus accumulation in the corner of the eye—are helpful in diagnosing dry eye.

Fluorescein dye can also be used to detect dry or dehydrated spots on the cornea. This dye colors the tear film so that it can be visualized under blue light. The time it takes the colored tears (as tinted by the dye) to break up is called the "tear film breakup time," is useful to making a diagnosis of dry eyes. The dye also shows up in the crevices between surface cells (which shouldn't be visible in a healthy eye) and can reveal ocular surface disease. Other dyes (such as rose bengal or lissamine green) stain areas on the cornea and the conjunctiva to show where the mucous tear layer is deficient.

There may be an irregular curve to the corneas. This situation can develop for many reasons. The corneas may be bulging with keratoconus. There may be dry spots at the edges of the patient's contact lenses. There may be the beginnings of a pterygium—a growth that comes from the nasal side of the eye and extends onto the cornea. Or the cornea may have developed a thinned area. People with irregularly curved corneas frequently develop dry-eye symptoms. When the eyelid, like a windshield wiper, goes over the bump, it doesn't distribute the watery tears in the little depression in front of the bump. If the patient is wearing a contact lens, the eyelid goes over the contact lens but doesn't touch the cornea on either side. Additionally, while blinking can spread tears over the damaged corneal surface to protect it, the mechanical scraping of the eyelid over a wound on the cornea can make it worse.

New diagnostic tests can evaluate how syrupy the tear film is, so that it can be adjusted. A device called the Tearscope allows the doctor to evaluate the lipid and watery components of your tear film, so you can be given exactly the right therapy. Unfortunately, this equipment is expensive, and the test is not covered by most insurance plans.

While I will mention many of the artificial tears available when I discuss conventional therapy, I will do so only to give you some information about the possibilities for treatment. Every patient is unique, and treatment must be designed individually for each person, taking into account age, career, lifestyle, and overall state of health. Keep in mind that environmental factors—like the heat drying out the air in your apartment, or your car's air conditioning vents being pointed right at your eyes—may contribute to your dry-eye symptoms. Correcting these environmental problems must be part of your treatment.

Dr. Abel's Tip

If you are diagnosed with dry eye, ask your doctor what symptoms you should be on the lookout for, as well as the result of your Shirmer tear test measurement.

Since the symptoms for many minor eye conditions are similar to those of dry eye, it's important to confirm the diagnosis. The only way to confirm the diagnosis at the present time, however, is to see if the therapy—whether conventional, alternative, or a combination of both types—is successful. Only you and your doctor can determine the right course of therapy for you.

Conventional Therapy for Dry Eyes

I will do whatever is needed to heal my patients, whether the therapy is conventional or alternative. Some of each may be necessary. I generally rely on the patient's symptoms to determine how to supplement with artificial tears.

If a patient is really miserable, we not only pursue an aggressive course of treatment, but look at the environment as well. One of my younger patients, J. T., had frequent episodes of red eyes with dry-eye symptoms. He had an unstable tear film, swollen and red conjunctiva, and excess mucus collecting both on his corneas as well as under his eyelids. We treated him with several conventional therapies, none of which was terribly effective. Though resistant to alternative treatments, he briefly tried Chinese medicine, which, as it so often does, made his symptoms worse for four or five days before any improvement was seen. J. T. was even evaluated at the National Eye Institute in Bethesda, where ophthalmologists came up with some novel treatments for him. Simultaneously, J. T. and his wife recalled that his symptoms had begun to develop when they moved into their new house. When his symptoms continued to worsen, J. T. decided to have all the air conditioning ducts in their house cleaned. As the fumes and solvents from the new house disappeared and the house's air circulated through clean ducts, treatments to remove J. T.'s excess mucus were instituted, and his eyes improved considerably within two weeks. I cannot tell you categorically that cleaning the air conditioning ducts in J. T.'s house completely solved the problem, but it certainly helped. I urge you, however, to try to leave the house for several days if you're going to have such a service performed. In that way, any health problems you may be experiencing because of dirty heating or air conditioning ducts won't be worsened by the process of cleaning them.

Dr. Abel's Tip

If you have dry eyes, be sure you don't have an eyelid infection or eyelashes that turn in and avoid steroids. Increase humidity and add an air purifier in your bedroom. Supplement with transiently preserved artificial tears, or a type of artificial tear you find comfortable. Ask your doctor about punctal plugs, which will help reduce your eyes' demands on your tear glands.

Any therapy for dry eyes should restore the tear film so that symptoms disappear. Conventional treatments for dry eyes include:

- *Using artificial tears a few times a day.* There are three types of artificial tears: preserved (with benzalkonium chloride or EDTA), transiently preserved, and nonpreserved.

  1. Preserved tears are slightly toxic and cause problems if used frequently by people with damaged corneal surfaces. For instance, patients with severe dry eyes, a recent cornea transplant, or recent refractive surgery (to correct nearsightedness) should probably use one of the other two types of tears.

  2. Transiently preserved tears contain preservatives that degrade on contact with either light or the patient's eye. They are more cost-effective and convenient than nonpreserved tears, while being minimally irritating. These products include Refresh Tears (0.5 percent carboxymethylcellulose) and Gen Teal (sodium perborate).

  3. Nonpreserved tears are meant for single-dose administration (to avoid bacterial contamination and to decrease all toxicity) and are more expensive than the other two types. Most of the lubricating ointments do not have preservatives, and I recommend using the lubricants at night because they blur vision, but support the tear cells during sleep.

I recommend trying transiently preserved tears first, because they are less toxic than the regular artificial tears and less expensive than the nonpreserved artificial tears packaged in individual doses. Remember that only you and your ophthalmologist, however, can determine the exact course of therapy that is right for you. Keep in mind, too, that you may need to adjust therapy as your eye (and body) conditions change.

To find out what type of artificial tears you're using, read the label or ask your pharmacist.

- *Preservative-free ointments, especially at night.*
- The eye pellet Lacrisert (which is made of hydroxypropyl cellulose, and is biodegradable) lasts for sixteen to eighteen hours, but it is a pellet, not an eyedrop, so it requires moderate dexterity to use. Ask your doctor if it's appropriate for you.
- *Plugging the lower lid puncta* (the opening to the tear outflow into the nose) with a temporary or more permanent silicon plug. This option produces a very satisfactory result because it enables you to maintain your own tear film. It is simpler than it sounds to manage, often brings immediate relief, and is especially helpful for anyone with a tear deficiency. If there is a lipid abnormality, however, it causes excessive tearing.
- Treating *blepharitis,* a bacterial infection that often accompanies dry eyes. Warm compresses, cleaning the eyelids with Ocusoft™, and erythromycin antibiotic ointment are the usual protocol for treating blepharitis. This treatment program is used for several weeks at a time.
- *Using a humidifier at home and/or the workplace* to keep the air from drying out in the winter.
- *Repositioning heat and air conditioning vents.* Make sure any such vents at home (or in the car) are not pointed in the direction of your face.
- *Protecting your eyes from wind and moisture* by wearing protective eyeglasses outdoors.
- *Remembering to blink,* especially while working at your computer.
- Using Cyclosporin A, an oral drug taken by organ transplant patients to prevent rejection reactions. Cyclosporin is now available as eyedrops to prevent corneal transplant rejection and eye inflammation. It is proving safe and effective for severe external ocular inflammations, as a product called Restasis™. Interestingly, a veterinarian discovered that this human antirejection drug is a marvelous treatment for dogs with dry eyes. More than sixty species of dogs have dry eyes. Many of you with dogs are probably constantly cleaning the mucus from their

eyes without realizing that this is a sign that the dog is suffering from dry eyes. Veterinarians have occasionally treated dry eyes in dogs by adding the antiglaucoma drug pilocarpine to their food to stimulate digestive enzymes and tearing. Perhaps some day we will investigate this option for humans, although too much of this type of drug can cause sweating, cramps, and increased heart rate.

Alternative Treatments for Dry Eyes (and Arthritis)

The alternative treatments for dry eye are synonymous with what I recommend for arthritis (excepting, of course, eyedrops). Some of the therapies that I've found to be helpful are:

1. Using similasan eyedrops, a homeopathic herbal preparation containing 6x dilutions of apis, euphrasia, and sabadilla. I have found them very comforting, but not much different from the minimally preserved artificial tears.

2. *Checking your medications to make sure none is contributing to drying out your eyes and affecting your joints.* If you're uncertain, consult your physician or pharmacist about the side effects and possible interactions of the medications you're taking. Make sure your ophthalmologist knows all the medications you're taking, so that he or she can determine if they are causing your dry eyes. Likewise, inform your other doctors about your dry-eye symptoms.

3. *Trying an exclusion diet just to be sure that your condition is not being exacerbated by what you're eating.* The usual culprits include the nightshade plants (eggplant, peppers, white potatoes, cucumbers, and tomatoes), milk, wheat, and other allergy-inducing foods. My preference is to remove as many of these foods as possible from your diet for one month while the other remedies are taking hold. After one month, begin adding the foods back one at a time, and you should be able to determine whether any one of them is causing your dry-eye and arthritis symptoms.

4. *Supplementing your diet with essential fatty acids* (500 mg once or twice a day) *and a fat-soluble vitamin* (like vitamin A or E). I cannot tell you how many times a week my colleagues call to tell me that flaxseed oil (or another essential fatty acid) supplements really work for their families, their patients, and themselves in relieving dry eyes as well as joint pain. In handling essential fatty acid supplements, it's important to remember to keep the oils in the dark in the refrigerator;

look for a pressing date on the label to ensure freshness; and take them with meals and a fat-soluble vitamin to protect the good fats from going rancid. More than 500 mg of essential fatty acids daily may thin the blood. If you are on any blood thinners (including regular use of aspirin or NSAIDs), you should inform your physician when you begin to supplement with essential fatty acids. You may require a prothrombin blood test to determine how fast your blood is clotting. Most people, however, have no adverse reaction to essential fatty acid supplements. I like to think of DHA (fish oil) and flaxseed oil as being nature's nonsteroidal drugs without the complications.

5. *Taking a combination of glucosamine and chondroitin sulfate, which has been shown to improve symptoms dramatically.* Louis Lippiello, Ph.D., a biochemist at Medical Professional Associates of Arizona, told the New York Times in January 1998 that he'd found in both cell cultures and dogs that, while glucosamine and chondroitin sulfate independently increase synthesis of cartilage, the two increase cartilage growth even more efficiently when used together. Glucosamine (the major component of chondroitin in sulfate and shark cartilage) has been studied extensively in double-blind studies comparing it to the NSAIDs (which only provide brief, symptomatic relief). These studies showed that, after one month, glucosamine sulfate provided as much pain relief as NSAIDs and, after two months, was better tolerated and more effective than the synthetic NSAIDs. Glucosamine sulfate not only improves symptoms but helps repair damaged joints. The sulfate portion of this compound contains sulfur, which is essential in the construction of connective tissues like cartilage, tendons, and ligaments. It also inhibits the enzymes that destroy cartilage. There are no reports of adverse reactions or adverse drug interactions. It's been suggested by Michael Murray, M.D. (author of the *Encyclopedia of Nutritional Supplements,* 1996), that higher doses are necessary if the patient is taking diuretics (diuretics increase urine output, so all nutrients are flushed from the body at a greater speed). For my patients with arthritis and/or dry eyes, I recommend 500 mg twice a day, which can be increased with no side effects. Dr. Murray's recommendation is considerably higher—500 mg three times a day, and occasionally more for individuals weighing more than 200 pounds. Again, it's interesting that what works for arthritis also works for dry eyes.

6. *Building up your antioxidant bank account.* Make sure you take the following:

• A multivitamin once or twice a day, depending on the content of the vitamin pill and the advice you're given by your doctor.

- Vitamin A, 10,000 IU twice a day for the first two weeks, and then once a day, with essential fatty acids and a meal. People who have a vitamin A deficiency are known to have dry eyes as well as dry skin and hair.
- B vitamin complex, 50–100 mg daily. If you take 50 mg, for instance, that is a small enough dose to allow for the other B vitamins in your multivitamin or in your food, but is adequate to provide these necessary nutrients.
- Zinc, 7.5 to 30 mg daily. Zinc is fundamental in healing.
- Magnesium, 500 mg daily, to dilate your blood vessels. (It's the tiny vessels that bring blood to your tear glands.)
- Calcium, 750 mg daily, at a different meal from your magnesium.

7. *Drinking lots of water.* Not only is it a way to rehydrate your body, but these glands that make the tear film are very sensitive to loss of fluids.

8. *Eating fruits and vegetables as part of a balanced diet.* It's easier to digest plant foods than high-fat meals. If your blood supply is in your gut digesting a fatty meal, it's not being pumped to the head.

9. *Avoiding transfatty acid-containing foods, like margarine.*

10. *Avoiding artificial sweeteners.* I can assure you that patients who consume a lot of artificial sweeteners (in diet sodas or foods) tell me that their eyes feel much better when they stop.

If you have dry eyes and/or arthritis, don't despair. You don't have to watch sad movies and slice onions to survive. We're continuing to find new treatments, especially natural therapies, that will affect not only your eyes but your whole body, with fewer risks than synthetic medications.

Tables 22 and 23 summarize my recommendations regarding diet, lifestyle, and nutritional supplements.

Table 22. Prevention/Alternative Treatment of Dry Eyes

Diet and Supplementation	Lifestyle	Water and Digestion
• Decrease the "bad fats" in your diet: saturated fats, hydrogenated fats, and transfats. An easy way to do this is to avoid packaged and hydrogenated foods. • Increase your Omega-3 fatty acid intake by consuming flaxseeds or flaxseed oil, dark leafy green vegetables, fatty fish, turmeric, and fish oil, or supplement with DHA 500 mg twice daily with meals. • Avoid artificial sweeteners; use Stevia or D-xylose instead. • Eat lots of fresh fruits and vegetables. • Supplement your diet with: vitamin A (20,000 IU daily for the first month, then 10,000 IU daily) vitamin A eyedrops, if they're available in your area chondroitin and glucosamine sulfate (100–500 daily) B complex vitamin (50–100 mg daily) sublingual vitamin B_{12} vitamin C (1000 mg three times daily, if tolerated) vitamin E (400–800 IU daily with a meal) calcium (750 mg daily, at a different time from magnesium) magnesium (500 mg at bedtime) zinc (30 mg daily for several months) copper (2 mg daily while taking zinc)	• Stop smoking. • Reduce your consumption of alcohol and caffeine. • Find enjoyable ways to relax. By stimulating the parasympathetic nervous system (which empties the colon), you will also be contributing to tear production. • Gradually begin an exercise program.	• Drink eight 8-ounce glasses of water daily, but not with meals. Water is extremely important to tear formation; don't be a prune! • Avoid the nightshade plants (eggplant, tomatoes, peppers), milk products, and wheat products for one month to see if they're contributing to your symptoms. • Eat slowly, in a relaxed setting, so you can digest your meal properly. • Take digestive aids if necessary. Try supplementing with Betaine HCl (a weak hydrochloric acid) for one month. Take 40 grains (260 mg equivalent) with pepsin at bedtime. Or use Progest (from Phytoformica), a mixture of Betaine (155 mg) and glutamic hydrochloride and other digestive enzymes for one month, if tolerated. This mixture is especially good for older people. Biozyme™ has less acid and other enzymes.

Table 23. Further Ways to Treat Dry Eyes and Arthritis

Other Diseases/Drugs	Whole Body
• Rule out other diseases that could be causing your symptoms, including gallbladder and Parkinson's disease, which can also produce blocked oil glands. • Be aware that caffeine, sodas (i.e., sugar), alcohol, and many kinds of drugs (antihistamines, psychiatric drugs, diuretics, antispasmodics, and others) dehydrate your tear film. • Eliminate unnecessary medications. See if you still need the medicine, or whether there's a more natural alternative. • Manage chronic diseases like high blood pressure, atherosclerosis, elevated cholesterol, osteoporosis, and indigestion.	• Take periodic breaks from computer work. Blink often, and do eye exercises that will relax your eyes. • Keep a calendar on which you record your medication and supplement regimes, so that you'll know when you started taking something new. • Gently massage upper and lower lids a couple of times a day to stimulate the tear glands. • Walk, drink water, and meditate. Meditation fosters relaxation, and relaxation increases parasympathetic nervous system action, which mediates tearing.

CHAPTER 12

Kids: Pediatric Eye Problems and Concerns During Pregnancy

Myth: Children will tell you if they have an eye or vision problem.
Fact: Hours and days often elapse with a child squinting and tearing before they complain, so be vigilant about your child's eye health.

Most adults are used to dealing with medical experiences, but they can be frightening to children. If you are sensitive about people touching your eyes, the feeling may have begun during childhood visits to your doctor's office that featured eye swabs, tongue depressors, or having your eyes held open for a look with a bright light. In order to lessen children's anxieties before an eye exam, I put the eyedrops they're going to receive in my own eyes first! I lie down on the floor and talk to the child, who's actually paying attention by then. I drop an anesthetic eyedrop into the corner of my eye with my eye closed. Still lying on the floor I explain, as I blink, that the drop will run into my eye and I'll feel a little burning sensation. I dab my eye with a tissue, look around the room, and get up smiling. I then ask the child if I may put the same drop in his or her eyes to make him or her feel better. I usually give children anesthetic eyedrops so that the dilating drops won't sting and the lights from the eye exam won't be painful. After I've administered the anesthetic drops, I explain that I need to give the child other drops (the dilating drops), so I can see the inside of the eyes. After my lying-on-the-floor performance, one of my young patients called me "Dr. Nutsy," but she also seemed to enjoy her exams over the years.

Children, perhaps even more than adults, require regular eye exams. There are not many differences between the eye exam in an adult and a child, except that children are more likely than adults to catch diseases like measles, mumps, and pink eye, and they are (hopefully) more closely observed for variations in their appearance and behavior than adults. As for eye size, you'd think that little folks would have little eyes, yes? Actually, the front of the eye is fully developed and has reached its adult size by the time a child is three years old. The back of the eye continues to grow through the teenage years.

It's important that the doctor always treat your child as the most important person in the room. Computerized images, toy dogs or other animals, or cartoons on the walls can help to keep children's attention while the doctor is looking at their pupils and eye movements.

Dr. Abel's Tip

Eye doctors—and all doctors—must always speak directly to your child. If one of your child's doctors does not treat him or her like the most important person in the room, redirect the conversation to include your child.

Children have the ability to accommodate (focus) to a much greater extent than adults. You may have noticed that infants are able to focus on objects held very close to their eyes, converging their eyes to see it with both eyes (that is, *binocularly*). This is called the *accommodation reflex*. After infancy, we begin to lose accommodation (focus power) with age.

Because of accommodation, young children always need a dilated examination to evaluate their true vision. In infants, this sometimes requires using the strongest eye medicine, atropine ointment, to dilate the pupils.

Hopefully, the child will voluntarily put his or her chin on the slit lamp, but an infant must often be held so that the doctor can see into the baby's eyes; mother or father can be very helpful during this part of the examination. Here again, it's important for the eye doctor to make sure the child is not frightened by the equipment and experiences the eye exam as an interesting encounter, not as a frightening one. (See Chapter 4 for a description of the slit lamp portion of the eye exam.)

Congenital Eye Problems

Children's eye conditions are often diagnosed earlier than a similar condition might be in an adult, either because the child is born with the problem or because adults are paying close attention to the child. In other words, an adult will often ignore his or her own problem, but pay attention to a child's.

Infants' eyes need to be observed very closely by both doctor and parent. For instance, infants' eyes are very vulnerable to infection just after birth, which is why all infants receive an antibiotic eye ointment at birth. (The antibiotic ointment replaces an older treatment, silver nitrate, which was more toxic; 5 percent povidone iodine might be an even better future choice because of its broader antimicrobial spectrum.)

Infants may also be born with shaking eyes that never focus, called *nystagmus*. This rare condition can recur in response to many stimuli, including neurologic conditions. It occurs most frequently in albino children, whose eyes appear to be pink or brown. In addition to nystagmus, these children may have a decreased potential for vision in later life.

Children who are born with persistent tearing or multiple infections may have an undeveloped opening in the tear duct that drains from the eye into the nose. If the passageway between eye and nose does not connect spontaneously by the age of one, it should be opened (probed) by a pediatric ophthalmologist. This treatment is extremely effective in opening the channel. If the condition remains untreated, persistent tearing and an infection of the lachrymal sac in the inner corner of the eye (through which the tears exit the eye) may occur, so it's important to have it attended to as soon as possible.

Infants may be born with "white pupil syndrome," in which the pupil of the eye is white instead of black. It is usually caused by a congenital cataract (one that's present at birth), which causes a profound disturbance of vision and requires immediate evaluation and early treatment. This is an emergency. If the congenital cataract isn't removed within four to six weeks, optimal vision potential will not be reached. The child won't complain, since he or she never had better sight, but may lose all potential for good sight if not treated before the age of one. The presence of a congenital cataract should be obvious to an experienced pediatrician. However, if your child's eyes don't look normal to you, ask the doctor— don't just worry about it.

White pupil syndrome can have other causes, including infection or even a tumor, like an eye tumor called a *retinoblastoma*. These still-rare tumors appear to be increasing in incidence, especially among baby boys. For reasons that aren't understood, all cancers in infants have increased since 1979, as researchers from the University of Massachusetts and the National Institutes of Health reported in April 1998. Central nervous system tumors in baby boys (including retinoblastomas) jumped from seven cases per one million infants born between 1979 and 1981, to twenty-one cases per one million infants born a decade later (1989–1991). Treatment of these and similar tumors with chemotherapy and local radiation has been able to save many eyes, but it often leaves the child with less vision than is desirable. Early detection of this disease is important, because it can spread to the liver and throughout the rest of the body—a very good reason for your child to have an eye examination early in life. Another rare tumor of the eye muscles is a rhabdomyosarcoma, which usually occurs in 2- to 8-year-old children. Its rapid progression in a bulging eyelid makes it noticeable. Immediate surgery is necessary.

Dr. Abel's Tip

Have your child's eyes examined before the age of 5—or earlier, if there are any problems that you or your pediatrician notice.

A Newborn's Retina

The *peripheral retina* (the part of the retina that supplies peripheral, or side, vision) is the last part of the eye to develop fully in an infant. If the peripheral retinal blood vessels are still growing when a premature baby is born, they are susceptible to high levels of oxygen, which can cause the growing blood vessels to spasm (that is, to go into vasospasm). The still-immature blood vessels can then begin to grow out of control, damaging the eye early in life, and even causing possible detachment of the retina.

This sensitivity to oxygen in premature infants places them at risk of developing a disease called retinopathy of prematurity (ROP). Thus their eyes need to be monitored very closely, especially when they're in incubators with high oxygen levels. While it's important for the preemie to get the oxygen—the lungs having not yet fully developed—these children must be followed closely by pediatric ophthalmology specialists (or retina specialists) to catch the first signs of any problems in the retina. If you have a premature infant—whether in an incubator or not—make sure his or her eyes are checked by a specialist before he or she is 4 weeks old—it's when most ROP is detected. Don't assume this will happen either—ask, especially if you've had your baby over a weekend or holiday, when many specialists are not routinely at the hospital.

Laser therapy may be beneficial in stopping blood vessel growth. If laser therapy doesn't work, then cryotherapy (freezing) is the treatment of choice here. Infants with ROP need long-term follow-up because of their high incidence of crossed eyes and large degrees of nearsightedness.

Strabismus (Crossed Eyes)

Children can develop misaligned or crossed eyes, a condition called *strabismus*. Strabismus can be caused by any poor coordination of the muscles that move the eye; even a fever can bring out previously unnoticed strabismus. A child usually suppresses the resulting double vision, not readily bringing it to his parents' attention. Care is required here: the child can subsequently develop *amblyopia*, or lazy eye, if the two eyes are not used equally. It is thus very important that you *pay attention* to whether or not your child's eyes move together. Although strabismus is usually corrected easily, the inability of the eyes to move together can be a sign of serious illness, signaling any number of problems, including trauma, brain tumor, stroke, or a central nervous system disease like cerebral palsy. If your child is diagnosed with strabismus, make sure these more serious conditions are ruled out.

The brain controls the six eye muscles around each eye like marionettes, so it requires a lot of work for the two eyes to move together. It's no wonder that both children and adults occasionally develop double vision in response to a fever or not using one eye for a while. (For instance, when there is a cataract in one eye, people sometimes lose the ability to look straight ahead with both eyes.)

Unilateral strabismus occurs when one eye moves independently of the other. The condition may be due to one weak muscle or a lazy eye (which we'll talk about later). Occurring more often is *bilateral strabismus*, a "cross-eyed" condition. Deviations in eye movements may be vertical (up and down), but are usually horizontal, with the eyes turning in (or out). While these unconnected eye movements may be disconcerting to other people, they are not noticed by the child.

In evaluating a child with crossed eyes, the eye doctor uses prisms to determine the amount of deviation (i.e., crossing of the eyes). This is always done for both distance and near vision (with the child looking at the eye chart across the room, then at a picture of a clown or animal up close). Before considering corrective surgery, the eye doctor needs to measure the child's eyes in many directions, since the deviation varies from different positions of gaze. Other than corrective surgery to redirect the eyes in a straight-ahead position though, patching or glasses may be sufficient.

If the problem was not completely corrected, or was overcorrected, by the first surgery, it can be repeated. Now I'm sure you don't want a repeat performance here, but sometimes it is necessary. So be sure to seek out a specialist who performs many such surgeries, and don't be afraid to ask about his or her success rate. This is your child—make sure the surgeon is experienced.

In older children and adults, strabismus surgery is performed with adjustable sutures (not usually an option for young children). The eyes are tested on the day following surgery to see if they are properly aligned. If a minor adjustment in the eyes' alignment is necessary, it can easily be done at that time, using eyedrops for anesthesia.

Pediatric ophthalmologists know they have to pay close attention to mothers' descriptions of their children's eye symptoms. If you feel that your child's doctor is not paying attention, find another doctor. The only time the mother is wrong about strabismus is when the child is very small and has an epicanthal fold in the inner corner of the eye. In this case, the eye opening is small initially—it will enlarge as the child grows—and the child does not really have a focusing problem.

Dr. Abel's Tip

Crossed eyes can be corrected. Locate the surgeon in your community who's most familiar with eye muscle surgery.

A condition that may resemble congenital esotropia to a worried parent is *accommodative esotropia*, which develops in children who are very far-sighted. They have an overactive focusing mechanism that causes the eyes to turn inward. One clue for parents is that these children's eyes tend to turn in more when they are looking at close objects than when they're looking at objects far away. Fitting the child with the right glasses will immediately straighten the eyes, solving the problem. Bifocals may be required if the distance correction is not sufficient. Surgery is not indicated unless the condition cannot be completely corrected with glasses.

Amblyopia

Amblyopia develops when the brain shuts off an unwanted image. This can happen in children with strabismus whose brains reject the image from the crossed eye (the brain can't process more than one visual image at a time and does so only for the image in focus). It can also happen in children without crossed eyes but whose eyes have very different vision (that is, one is very nearsighted and the other is not). Amblyopia is truly a case of "use it or lose it"—if the brain shuts off the eye for long enough, its vision can be severely diminished or even completely suppressed.

Two or three out of every 100 people has a condition in which one eye sees less well than the other. In half of them, it is due to a muscle imbalance so small as to go unnoticed. In the other 50 percent of cases, amblyopia develops because the affected eye is out of focus—that is, it's not being used to see effectively. Don't fail to screen your child for this common condition.

Amblyopia can be treated in most cases. Placing a patch over the good eye at any time during early life may restore vision in the affected eye by forcing it to work. The old rule of thumb was to patch the good eye for one week for each year of a child's life (in a six-year-old child, in other words, to patch for six weeks) to stimulate the amblyopic eye. We no longer follow this old rule, because such long-term patching isn't necessary. Now, a patch is worn full-time only initially, and then for just a few hours each day for several weeks. Atropine drops are another option (see page 388).

If the child's amblyopia is due to a muscle imbalance, surgical correction will improve the eye's position. However, the use of a patch is still necessary, usually before surgery. Glasses may also be needed before or after surgery.

Children who do not see well in one eye after the age of 7 may lose all the sensitivity that allows good vision in that eye. This is one of the reasons I insist every child should see an ophthalmologist by age 5.

Children and Glasses

Being able to focus (and see) well influences the development of good vision. But how does sight develop? How does vision evolve as a newborn turns into a child? We don't know. We do know, however, that if the two eyes do not grow and develop together in childhood, any number of visual problems can arise in adulthood.

Every child *must* have an eye exam before the age of 5. Parents should be even more vigilant if (1) there is a family history of eye or vision problems; (2) the child has some complaint; (3) one eye appears to turn in (or out); (4) the child has headaches; (5) the child has trouble recognizing letters with either eye; or (6) the child has multiple physical or developmental problems. It is almost always the parent who recognizes a vision problem in a child of preschool age, so trust your instinct and judgment.

The part of the eye exam in which the doctor determines how well your child sees and corrects to "best vision" with glasses is known as *refraction*. The technology used by the eye doctor to ask, "Which is better, number one or number two?" depends upon his or her training, and whether the doctor's practice is dedicated to pediatric ophthalmology. The doctor will often need to hold the lenses in front of a small child.

Some people are unable to see well at distance because of the refractive error called nearsightedness, or *myopia*. Other people (usually adults) don't see well close up, which is called farsightedness, or *hyperopia*. Farsightedness is less likely to be detected in children because they have a lot of accommodation. But both these conditions can begin in childhood, and each can be corrected by glasses that make light focus at the proper place on the retina.

Nearsightedness (seeing better close up than at distance) develops when the eye is longer than normal (23 mm), or because the cornea is more curved than normal, which causes light coming from distant images to focus in front of the retina instead of on it. Only by bringing the object closer does the image come into focus on the retina.

Farsightedness (seeing better at distance than close up) is less easily detected in children who can still see well at both distance and near, because they still have accommodation reserve. A farsighted individual has a short eye or flat cornea, and doesn't refract, or bend, light enough. This produces a blurred image that can be focused on the retina only by viewing an object far away or by using the muscles in the eye to accommodate or focus.

Astigmatism is another type of refractive error that can develop in children and can be corrected by glasses. Remember that your child's eyes are different from every other child's eyes. The cornea, unlike the dome of a church, may not have the same curve in all directions, and an uneven corneal curve is usually responsible for astigmatism. While most people have a small amount of astigmatism, it has no effect on their vision because the tear film neutralizes it. If your child is astigmatic, however, it should be corrected by his or her glasses prescription.

It's important to realize that the eye exam performed in a pediatrician's office often screens for visual acuity in each eye separately. The ophthalmologist, optometrist, or pediatric ophthalmologist will take the exam one step further and look for refractive error in both eyes at the same time. Are the eyes working together? Is there appropriate depth perception? There is also an important distinction between visual acuity and perception. In other words, the child may see the fine print, but may not be interpreting it meaningfully. Multiple learning disabilities also exist in which visual acuity may be normal, but reading, perception, calculations, and writing may not follow.

Sight is a physiological trait, but vision is learned. When the eye doctor talks about *sight*, he or she is usually referring to visual acuity. This means that the child doesn't have significant amounts of near- or farsightedness or astigmatism, that his or her eyes focus (accommodate) properly, and that both eyes work together.

Vision, however, is a learned skill that implies a proper interpretation of what is seen. Researchers have learned that there are numerous aspects of vision that affect learning, including:

- Eye-hand coordination
- Visual imagery (being able to picture something in the mind)
- Eye-movement coordination (the ability to move the focus of the eyes from place to place)
- 20/20 acuity (i.e., the ability to read a blackboard at a normal classroom distance)
- Eye teaming (moving the eyes together)
- Focus (accommodation, or being able to focus close up and far away)
- Visual perception (the ability to tell the difference between letters, for instance).

If your child is lacking in any of these particular areas of vision development, he or she may have learning difficulties. Signs of vision difficulties in a child include:

- Losing his place frequently or skipping a line while reading
- Skipping small words or altering the beginning or ends of words while reading
- Moving the head instead of the eyes while reading
- Needing a finger to keep the place while reading after the age of 7
- Being labeled as having an attention problem when reading

If you have concerns about your child's vision and performance in school, consult a pediatric ophthalmologist.

Colorblindness is a problem your child will probably not be able to describe to you, so the pediatric ophthalmologist (or your family ophthalmologist) should test your child's color vision. One out of eight Caucasian boys has some form of colorblindness, while only one in thirty girls is colorblind.

It's hard for children to describe not seeing well, so parents should pay close attention to any complaints a child makes about vision. If a child is having headaches, it might be from straining to see, in which case he or she probably needs glasses. (If the child is having headaches and they are not the result of a vision problem, he or she needs to be taken back to the pediatrician, who may refer the child to another specialist.)

Dr. Abel's Tip

If eyedrops are prescribed for your child, it's important to get them into your child's eye. Try to make it into a game, so that your child is not frightened by the eyedrops and isn't caused any extra pain or discomfort. If you pretend to put drops in your own eye, make sure you're using just artificial tears, not an actual medication!

One child in four has a vision problem that may cause delayed progress or behavioral difficulties in school. Squinting, rubbing the eyes, closing an eye, having one eye turn in (or out), tilting the head, placing the head close to reading material, having a short attention span, avoiding reading or other close work, or experiencing headaches and dizziness can all be signs of a vision problem.

If your child has both a vision problem and hearing loss, the combination can make school very difficult. Hearing loss, for instance, can contribute to problems while a child is learning to read. Nearly 15 percent of children ages 6–15 suffer from some level of hearing loss. Most of these children have loss of high-frequency hearing, which makes it difficult for them to distinguish consonants; loss of low frequency hearing makes it difficult to distinguish vowels. If your child is not hearing (as opposed to not listening), he or she may be suffering unnecessary difficulties in school that could be corrected with hearing aids. A device that can detect hearing loss in newborns is now available, but universal screening is currently required in only a few states. This situation must change. It has been reported that hearing loss in infants is twenty times more common than either sickle-cell anemia or hypothyroidism, two conditions for which infants are routinely tested.

A new concern for parents is software firms that market computer programs for infants who are 9 months to 2 years old. Dubbed *lapware*— because the child has to sit on a parent's lap to reach the computer— the programs are under attack from numerous child development experts. Many children possess neither the motor nor cognitive skills required for computer games at 9 months of age, and child psychologists worry that these games may produce anxiety that will interfere with later learning. Some experts are also concerned that infants' eyes may be damaged by focusing on a computer screen at such a young age.

I strongly urge, as I've said before, that all children have an eye exam before going to school. Make sure your child is getting the proper nutrition so that his or her eyes (and the rest of the body) get off to the right start. (I'll discuss nutrition more later in this chapter.)

Do your best to get glasses for your child that he or she really likes. Let your child participate in the selection of the glasses' frame, even if it costs a little more money—if the child hates the glasses, he or she won't wear them. Even though a child may balk at wearing glasses, do your best to make sure he or she complies, with the goal of maintaining healthy eyes in a healthy child.

Dyslexia

Dyslexia is a learning disability most frequently characterized by difficulty in learning to read (although other learning disabilities are frequently present and may interact with dyslexia). It's important to examine the eyes of children with learning disabilities because one or both eyes may be focusing incorrectly, contributing to problems with schooling. Although eyes that are out-of-focus are not the usual cause of learning difficulty (which may promote hyperactivity in children), it does happen. This possibility should be eliminated first, because none of the educational tests or systems designed to deal with learning disabilities will detect it.

Yale University School of Medicine researcher Sally E. Shaywitz, M.D., and her colleagues recently provided the first evidence that dyslexia is a disease of the brain. According to Dr. Shaywitz and her team, dyslexia is an inability to look at the visual representation of sounds—i.e., the printed letters on the page—and turn them into words. Using the latest brain imaging techniques, Dr. Shaywitz and her colleagues showed that the area of the brain that processes the written word just doesn't work properly in dyslexic individuals. Hopefully this finding will result in the development of therapies for dyslexia that attack its cause instead of its symptoms.

Other researchers at the Center for Molecular and Behavioral Neuroscience at Rutgers University, in Newark, New Jersey, announced in May 1998 that they'd found an organic problem in the portion of the brain that processes rapid auditory information (spoken language) in dyslexic children. Paula Tallal, Ph.D., and her colleagues published a paper in the May 7 issue of the *Proceedings of the National Academy of Sciences* reporting that dyslexic children's brains contain very few of the specific type of brain cells that process rapidly heard sound. The resulting inability to decode ordinary language in infancy contributes to the development of dyslexia in childhood, Dr. Tallal and her colleagues concluded.

Children with dyslexia and other learning disabilities need to be put on structured diets that eliminate artificial sweeteners, nonfruit sugars, and caffeine before they are given drugs like Ritalin and amphetamines. (A good book to read about these overprescribed drugs is *No More Ritalin* by Mary Ann Block, M.D.)

Some children, particularly boys, just aren't ready to read at age 4 or 5. If your child is having trouble learning to read because of dyslexia, please realize that he or she is not incapable of learning, but may just need a little extra help. A learning disability does not reflect upon your child's intelligence, and should not be an insurmountable barrier to achievement. I am dyslexic, and it did not stop me from becoming not only a physician, but a surgeon and a specialist. I believe it is crucial to make reading—and all types of learning—fun and interesting for all children, no matter what their age or level of achievement. If your child has a learning disability, it's even more important to make learning fun, not a chore.

Vision therapy can play a role in selected cases of dyslexia (which cases can only be determined by trial and error), because its exercises are designed to keep the eyes working together. (See Eye Aerobics in Appendix F for more information about vision therapy.) To read quickly, the eyes must see clearly and function together. (A one-eyed person, however, can read just as quickly as a person with two eyes.) Although vision therapy has been reported to help children with learning disabilities, it's not for everyone, because not all learning disabilities have the same causes.

Dr. Abel's Tip

There have been some exciting developments in the field of vision therapy. New techniques are being created for treating stress and learning disabilities as well as for enhancing vision. Keep in mind, however, that vision therapy does not help everyone and that undertaking it requires practice by your child and support from you.

Being dyslexic myself, as I said, I can tell you how hard it is to catch up in reading and writing skills when the class moves ahead of you. This is especially true if your dyslexia is not recognized and you are thought to have a behavior problem, not a learning problem. It wasn't until I became an ophthalmologist that I recognized my own dyslexia. The sooner you can obtain help for your child, the happier he or she will be. Identify learning disabilities early and be aware that nutritional factors may aggravate or improve these conditions. Be a medical detective for your child.

If your child is not performing well in school or is slow learning to read, ask your pediatrician to test him or her for attention deficit disorder (ADD). While ADD and attention deficit hyperactivity disorder (ADHD) are usually treated by psychologists and education specialists, your pediatrician should be able to help you find a specialist.

Dealing with a Child's Vision Loss

If your child or the child of someone you love has an eye problem that limits his or her potential vision, it's important to remember this: A child knows only what he or she has already seen and experienced. A child does not miss vision that he or she has never had; for example, a child with vision in only one eye appears to live normally. Remember that it's us, the adults, who feel sad and traumatized by the fact our child doesn't see well from one or both eyes. Don't let this distress lessen your ability to deal with the situation. A child will utilize the vision he or she possesses much better than any adult whose vision becomes impaired. Furthermore, there are many resources in our educational system and many optical devices to maximize children's vision and life potential.

Nutrition for a Healthy Child

Our mothers all told us to eat our vegetables when we were kids, and now that we're parents, we're discovering that Mom was more right than she knew. Research shows that fruits and vegetables contain numerous substances called *phytonutrients* that are crucial to maintaining our health. While we can obtain some of these substances by taking single supplements, whole foods contain numerous phytonutrients—some of which we haven't even identified yet—that work together much more effectively than they do when taken in supplement form. Because children are children, however, we still need to add a supplement to make sure they consume all the required vitamins and minerals. Make sure you give your child a good children's multivitamin—and not one that's loaded with sugar.

One-fourth of American children are now overweight, and it's likely that bad childhood habits (like snacking on junk food) will continue into adulthood. Studies indicate that a lean diet in childhood may cut risks of cancer and heart disease in adults. This is not to say that children should be on fat-free diets, because the correct amount of the "good fats" is required for eye and brain development. Nevertheless, it's now known that the cholesterol plaques that clog our arteries start to develop in our teens. Keep fresh fruit and vegetables (like cut carrots and celery sticks) around for the kids to munch on instead of chips and other junk food. If you're short on time (and who isn't?), when you do cook, make enough for two meals so there's something good to eat later in the week—or later that evening, if you have teenagers!

You, the parent, must set an example for your children. If you eat and enjoy healthful food, your children are more likely to eat and enjoy healthful food. Clear the pantry of white bread, candy, cookies, and other processed foods that contain empty calories, lots of sugar, and unhealthful transfats. Serve fresh fruit and green leafy vegetables, fish, organic meat and poultry (in small quantitites), nuts, peanut butter (the nonhydrogenated variety you can buy at the health food store), freshly squeezed juices, and lots of good water. A diet that is cardioprotective for you will also protect your children's health.

Throughout *The Eye Care Revolution*, I've urged you and your family members to build up your antioxidant bank accounts by consuming adequate amounts of vitamins, minerals, and phytonutrients. Your child needs a full antioxidant bank account, too. Children burn up huge amounts of energy, which means they are generating lots of cellular waste for their antioxidants to clear away. As most children spend a great deal of time outdoors, they particularly need to be protected from sunlight's damaging free radicals. While this can be done from the outside—with sunscreen, sunglasses (nonscratch, nonbreakable ones are best), and appropriate clothing—you need to protect your child on the inside, too, through proper nutrition. And, as I'm sure you remember, childhood can be a very stressful time. Stress also generates free radicals that need to be neutralized by antioxidants.

Here are a few pointers to help you make sure your child is being adequately nourished and building up a healthy antioxidant bank account (for more complete information on nutrition and supplementation, refer to Chapters 14 and 15—but check with your pediatrician before giving your child supplements meant for adults).

Carbohydrates

Carbohydrates are a major source of fuel for the body. The simple carbohydrates—found in milk, white sugar, molasses, fruit and fruit juices—are also called simple sugars, and are used just like sugar by our bodies. The burst of energy provided by these foods is short-lived and can contribute to weight gain. Complex carbohydrates, which are used more slowly by our bodies and provide more sustained energy, are obtained from vegetables, grains, and fruits. Foods that are rich in complex carbohydrates also provide fiber.

Fats

We—and our children—need a certain amount of the right kinds of fats and even cholesterol for good health. Fats are major sources of energy; they lubricate our joints; they are required for the fat-soluble vitamins (A, D, E, and K) to be absorbed; and they contribute to soft skin, shiny hair and, yes, *healthy eyes*. All our cell membranes are made of fats, and some fats are essential to the proper functioning of the immune system. An extremely low-fat diet has been linked to numerous problems in children, including impaired vision, stunted growth, and limited mental development.

Fats are classified as *saturated* (found in animal products like meat); *monounsaturated* (found in olive and canola oils, the best fats to use for cooking); *polyunsaturated* (in flaxseed and DHA); and transfats (in hydrogenated products like margarine). We are just discovering how damaging transfats are to human health. Transfats block the functioning of the fats we require most, the essential fatty acids. Unfortunately, transfats are often found in the foods kids like the most; the packaged foods that line supermarket shelves, such as cookies, crackers, and potato chips.

The essential fatty acids are found in monounsaturated and polyunsaturated fats. They are required for proper brain functioning (50 percent of the fat in the brain is the Omega-3 essential fatty acid DHA), good vision, and healthy cell membranes. The two major groups of essential fatty acids are the Omega-3 and Omega-6 fats. The standard American diet is high in Omega-6 fats and extremely depleted in Omega-3 fats, creating an imbalance between Omega-6 and Omega-3 essential fatty acids that appears to contribute to the development of numerous chronic illnesses, including allergies; hyperactivity; some vision problems; autoimmune diseases; and arthritis.

Dr. Abel's Tip

Avoid empty calories. Serve your family green and yellow vegetables, the "good fats," and plenty of fiber. Eliminate packaged foods, simple sugars, and refined flour. Substitute healthful food ingredients where possible (there are many excellent cookbooks that explain how to substitute healthful ingredients for unhealthful ones). Start early on good nutrition for your children to reduce their risk of obesity, cancer, and heart disease later in life.

The vegetable sources of Omega-3 fats include: walnuts and walnut oil; flaxseeds and flaxseed oil; canola oil; and green leafy vegetables. The photonutrient content of green vegetables is one of the reasons that nutritionists advise us to eat five to nine servings of fruits and vegetables every day.

Protein

Protein is an important source of energy but it should be consumed in moderation. Eating a diet that is too high in protein may cause many health problems, including obesity (from the saturated fat in meat and cheese), even in children.

Fiber

Fiber helps to cleanse our intestines, which even kids need. There are two types of fiber. The first, soluble fiber, dissolves in water. It is found in peas, lentils, beans, oats, barley, fruits, and vegetables. Soluble fiber helps to digest food, burn calories, and control blood sugar in diabetes. The second, insoluble fiber, does not dissolve in water. It can be obtained from grains, vegetables, and fruits; it helps prevent numerous intestinal problems by causing food to move through the bowel more quickly. Most fiber-rich foods contain a mixture of soluble and insoluble fiber, which is why it's better to get fiber from food than from laxatives. High-fiber foods include: acorn squash, lentils, kidney, navy, and pinto beans, broccoli, Brussels sprouts, cabbage, kale, peas, radishes, spinach, winter squash, yams, apples, blackberries, blueberries, pears, raspberries, and whole grains (brown rice, oatmeal, and whole wheat).

Vitamins

Vitamins are crucial for the development of a growing child. Every reaction in every cell in the body requires enzymes, and vitamins are cofactors that help these reactions to proceed properly. Vitamins are either fat-soluble or water-soluble.

Vitamin A is essential for vision (its deficiency can cause blindness and can be fatal) because it's part of the visual pigment and contributes to the functioning of both the cornea and tear film. Vitamin A–rich foods include broccoli, cantaloupe, carrots, cherries, dandelion greens, sweet potatoes, and tomatoes.

Foods that are rich in vitamin A generally contain one or more of the other carotenes. Beta-carotene, vitamin A's precursor, is probably the best-known carotene; it is found in the same foods as vitamin A. Lutein, another carotene, is especially important for eye health and maintaining good sight. Lutein is the yellow pigment found in the macula (the center of the retina). It is second only to vitamin E in inhibiting the buildup of fats in the macula and lens and therefore is very important in protecting against macular degeneration and cataracts. Food sources of lutein include algae, green leafy vegetables (especially spinach), corn, eggs, and fruit (apricots, apples, cranberries, citrus rinds, and plums).

The food sources for the carotenes (there are more than 600), which occur together, include: apricots, broccoli, cantaloupe, carrots, collard greens, dandelion greens, kale, kumquats, mustard greens, papaya, pumpkin, red peppers, sea vegetables (seaweed), spinach, sweet potatoes, Swiss chard, tomatoes, and winter squash.

The B vitamins are water soluble, and their primary function is to assist nerve functioning. The B vitamins include thiamine (B_1), riboflavin (B_2), B_6 (pyridoxine), B_{12}, niacin, pantothenic acid, biotin, and folic acid. Three major studies in different countries have shown that folic acid prevents neural tube birth defects (like anencephaly, being born with only a partial brain and no skull, a rapidly fatal condition). Folic acid also helps prevent heart disease, but all the B vitamins are crucial to our health.

Vitamin C is also water-soluble. It helps lower cholesterol, is present in every cell, and recharges vitamin E and other antioxidants. Vitamin C helps make collagen, which helps strengthen capillaries (small blood vessels). Vitamin C is the second-most important antioxidant in the lens, after glutathione, which is manufactured by the liver.

Vitamin D is the only vitamin that acts like a hormone. We manufacture vitamin D in our own skin after exposure to sunlight—unless we aren't exposed to sunlight or live in a northern climate, in which case a vitamin D deficiency develops. Vitamin D is available in very small amounts from a few foods, including cold-water fish, liver, butter, and egg yolks. It should be included in any good multivitamin.

Vitamin E blocks the breakdown of fats. Fats become rancid as a result of oxidation, which vitamin E prevents. It may, therefore, play a role in preventing blood cell agglutination, heart disease, and neuropathy (pain).

Vitamin K is essential to the production of several blood-clotting factors. We synthesize most of the vitamin K we require in the intestines. If food isn't being absorbed properly in the gut, however, a deficiency can develop, the major symptom of which is easy bruising. Vitamin K is widely distributed in vegetables, and it's very easy to overdose with supplements. Simply eat lots of vegetables, and you'll have plenty of vitamin K.

Phytochemicals

Phytochemicals are the nutrients found in plants. They give fruits and vegetables their brilliant colors and taste, as well as protecting them from ultraviolet light. Phytochemicals fight free radicals and have anti-inflammatory properties. Bioflavonoids are a large subcategory of phytochemicals. They appear to have powerful antioxidant and anticancer properties, as well as generally increasing immunity, protecting the liver, and facilitating blood flow (including blood flow to the brain and retina). Quercetin is perhaps the most potent antioxidant and antihistamine. It's found in red onions, red grapes, and garlic; it helps prevent fluid accumulation in the middle ear and sinuses, as well as blood vessel leakage in diabetics.

Bilberry has a well-known positive effect on night vision. Known commonly as the English blueberry, bilberry is actually a member of the grape family. Just some of the other foods rich in bioflavonoids are: apples, asparagus, lima beans, garbanzo beans, soy beans, beets, berries, broccoli, Brussels sprouts, cabbage, carrots, eggplant, garlic, grapes, onions (many different types), peppers, radishes, sweet potatoes, and tomatoes. The spices ginger, parsley, rosemary, sage, thyme, and turmeric are also rich in flavonoids.

Minerals

Magnesium is the natural calcium channel blocker. It lowers blood pressure by dilating and relaxing blood vessels, stopping vasospasm (which is a cause of sudden death), and helping control the tendency to develop high blood pressure. Magnesium also contributes to the production of neurotransmitters like serotonin (low serotonin levels have been linked to depression and other ills). Calcium is needed for bone growth, along with vitamin D.

Refined Sugar and Artificial Sweeteners

Avoid refined sugar for your child. It rots the teeth, contributes to obesity, and is suspected as a cause of behavioral difficulties in children. If your child develops the habit of eating fresh fruits and vegetables, that good habit will automatically cut down on sugar and junk in his or her diet.

Avoid artificial sweeteners (such as aspartame). Like monosodium glutamate, the chemicals in artificial sweeteners can weaken nerve cells, including the nerve cells in the brain and the eye. Our bodies don't know how to detoxify these chemicals. If your child is diabetic or has hypoglycemia, use stevia or D-xylose as a sweetener.

Eggs and Milk

Don't completely avoid eggs. The most recent research shows that consuming up to six eggs a week does not contribute to high cholesterol levels. Eggs are very close to being the perfect food, providing very high levels of protein, lecithin, and vitamins. Eggs high in Omega-3 essential fatty acids (from organically fed chickens) are now available.

Although milk is important for growth, you (and your child) can obtain all of the nutrients in milk from other sources without worrying about what else is concentrated in milk (like antibiotics, hormones, pesticides, and other chemicals). The move toward organic foods will hopefully make wholesome milk a good idea for a growing child in the near future.

Pesticides and Other Toxins

Avoid as many pesticides and other toxins in food as you can. Buy organic produce when possible; always wash fruits and vegetables well, and peel them, when possible, to remove pesticides. Children are more sensitive to pesticides and other chemicals than are adults—children's cells divide rapidly as they grow, so they are especially susceptible to cancer-causing chemicals. Children's nervous systems are also actively developing, so any neurotoxins they consume can do a great deal of damage. Primarily, however, children are more sensitive than adults because they are smaller: The skin of one apple is a much larger percentage of a child's daily food intake, for instance, than it is of an adult's. If the apple skin has pesticide on it, it's a bigger dose of poison for a child than for an adult. Children can also have strange eating habits, often insisting on eating only one food for several days at a time. Therefore, they will ingest a large amount of any chemical in or on that food. As well as being high in animal fat, meat, poultry, and dairy products can be sources of growth hormones, antibiotics, and other chemicals and can be contaminated with bacteria, viruses, and parasites. This is not meant to scare you or your children, but is just a word to the wise. If you are unable to buy all-natural meat, poultry, and dairy, try to shop at a store where you trust the freshness of the meat and dairy foods. Some dairies now state that their cows are not given growth hormones, so read the label. A new source of hormone- and antibiotic-free meat is buffalo, which is available in many stores and restaurants.

Baby Food

If you have an infant or toddler, consider making your own baby food. If you're unable to do that, try to find a source of organic baby food, which many companies now sell. In February 1998, the Environmental Working Group (an activist group in Washington, D.C.), revealed results of a study showing that more than one million children under 1 year old are exposed to excessive amounts of pesticides in their baby food. These organophosphate pesticides may cause brain and nervous system damage in infants. They are also present in mother's milk.

Food Allergens

Identify your child's food allergies and/or sensitivities. Zoltan P. Rona, M.D., suggests in *Childhood Illness and the Allergy Connection* that middle ear infections, asthma, and hyperactivity can be prevented and treated by using complementary options like nutritional therapy. Dr. Rona also points out that identifying and treating food allergies early may save you and your child a lot of worry.

Dr. Abel's Tip

If your child has allergies, recurrent middle ear infections, or is excessively irritable, try dietary substitution and alternative therapies before routinely relying on antihistamines, antibiotics, or psychoactive drugs. If your child has an active infection, however, it must be treated with antibiotics before turning to natural methods.

Eye Injuries and Emergencies

Eye emergencies are geniune emergencies. Be prepared! Permanent vision loss—partial or total—can result from ignoring signs of an eye emergency, especially in children. Even if there's no pain, seek medical care immediately if your child develops any of the symptoms of an eye emergency. Keep in mind that your child may have trouble describing some symptoms of eye injury or other emergency, so pay attention when he or she mentions any problem related to the eyes. Remember, children may not tell you if they were hit or who hit them. Battered children often do not reveal injuries out of fear, or to protect the batterer.

Symptoms of eye trauma or emergency can include:

- New onset of crossed eyes
- Change in the color of any part of the child's eye, especially the development of a white pupil
- Persistant tearing or redness
- Swelling of the lid
- Double vision
- Aversion to light (photosensitivity)
- Sudden development of "floaters" (a child may have particular trouble describing this)
- Sudden development of flashes of light
- Sudden development of clouded, blurred, or wavy vision
- Pain
- Partial loss of vision
- Sudden blindness (however fleeting). If your child experiences a loss of sight, but it returns within five minutes or even an hour, the child has still experienced blindness. *This is an emergency!* Consider any loss of sight an emergency until proved otherwise, and seek medical care immediately.

Being hit in the eye is no joke. Kids need to understand that hitting someone in the eye in real life is much more horrible than the way it's shown on TV or in films. The consequences can be severe, causing grief to patients and families, and too often resulting in loss of ability to read, watch television or movies, or drive a car. It can affect the injured person's entire life.

Dr. Abel's Tip

Select nonviolent toys for your children. Guide their cultural experiences, including television watching, away from the gratuitously violent, and watch TV and movies with them. It's important for you to do as you want them to do.

Fists and thrown rocks are the major causes of eye trauma in children, particularly in boys. Other causes of eye trauma include: sports injuries, airbags, fireworks, toys, motor vehicle accidents (car, motorcycle, bicycle), and lawn mower injuries. An injury can occasionally mean perforation of the eye. Kids tend to injure their lids and tearducts more frequently than adults do. Corneal abrasion can result from being scratched by a fingernail, dog or cat claw, baby, plant, or a piece of paper. You may wish to buy unbreakable polycarbonate safety glasses for your child to wear when engaging in contact sports.

Trauma to the eye can result in bleeding inside the eye; broken bones around the outside (orbit) of the eye; double vision; a corneal injury that can lead to scarring and vision loss; retinal detachment; cataract; and infections that can threaten vision, among other serious consequences.

Prevention of Eye Trauma

To protect your child against eye trauma as much as possible, I recommend taking the following steps:

1. Have your child wear polycarbonate eyeglasses during sports or any kind of activity that could result in glasses being broken or eyes being hurt.
2. Educate your children about eye trauma.
3. Select sports activities carefully.
4. Avoid ballistic toys (like those that shoot missiles) and real guns.

Treatment for Trauma

Eye injuries are usually treated with antibiotic ointment, patching, and pain relief (usually with NSAIDs). A bandage or a medicated contact lens may sometimes be required to shield a corneal abrasion from being scraped by the eyelid during blinking.

If your child gets a foreign body in his or her eye, have him or her blink rapidly to encourage the tears to wash it away. Don't let the child rub the eye, which can further irritate it and possibly scratch the cornea! If blinking does not cause the tears to wash the object out of the eye, grasp the upper eyelid gently and pull it out (away from the eyeball) and down over the lower lid. Hold the upper lid in this position for a few seconds. This should cause even more tears to run out of the eye, and hopefully wash the foreign body out.

If neither of these techniques works and you can see the foreign object in the eye (an eyelash, for instance, or a piece of dirt), hold the eyelids apart and, with a Q-tip, try gently to brush the particle out. (You may want to ask someone else to help you do this.)

If your child gets a piece of metal or glass in his or her eye, seek emergency care immediately. If you are unable to coax any other type of foreign body out of the eye with tears or a tissue, call your eye doctor or go to a hospital emergency room where there is an ophthalmologist on call right away. If you think that you removed a foreign body from your child's eye but the pain or redness in the eye increases, call your eye doctor or go to a hospital emergency room immediately. Don't wait and hope it will just go away—a foreign object in your child's eye won't go away by itself. A piece of dirt, wood, or metal can scratch the cornea, potentially leading to scarring, infection, and vision loss.

I must repeat a final word of caution: If your child suffers an eye trauma, even having a piece of dirt in the eye that you're unable to dislodge, *seek medical help immediately.*

Guarding Your Child's Eyes

Look at and into your child's eyes—there is much you can do to determine whether he or she has a vision problem. If one eye doesn't seem to be working properly, cover the opposite eye with the palm of your hand (or have the child cover his or her eye with his or her hand) and make sure he or she can see well from each eye. Look at the pupils, and make sure they constrict together in response to bright light. You might even notice the first signs of an eye problem in a photograph, if the light reflex (in the pupil of the eye) doesn't look right.

Watch your child's eyes focus—is there squinting or frowning? Look for signs of allergy, like red eyes, a rash around the eyes, or even dilated pupils. Remember that children are more sensitive to chemicals like bug sprays.

If your child appears to have any eye problem, call your pediatrician immediately. Have your child's eyes examined by an eye doctor by the age of 5, or younger, if the child was premature or has any specific eye-related health problems. Give your child a head start on the road to good health through proper nutrition. Protect your child from eye injury by avoiding violent games, sharp objects, and toy weapons.

When should you rush a child to the eye doctor or hospital? Here's a brief guide:

Code White

If your child has any of the following symptoms, take him or her to see the pediatrician and ask if the problem could be related to the eyes.

- Is slow to read
- Does poorly in school
- Turns or tilts head to see or hear
- Can't see or read road signs while playing car games

- Shows tendency for one or both eyes to turn in or out when tired
- Has frequent headaches
- Is hyperactive
- Experiences excessive tearing (Make sure you get a referral to a pediatric ophthalmologist.)
- Holds reading material unusually close, squints or is very sensitive to light

Code Yellow

Have your pediatrician obtain an early referral to an ophthalmologist if your child has any of these symptoms or conditions. (A premature infant should be examined by a pediatric ophthalmologist.)

- Swelling of eyelid
- Discharge from the eye
- Red conjunctiva (i.e., the white of the eye is red)
- White instead of dark pupil
- Droopy lid
- Crossed eyes
- Black or bruised eye
- Shaking, unfocused eyes
- One eye seems smaller than the other
- Persistent rubbing of the eye (or eyes) by child

Code Red

Seek medical care immediately if your child displays any of these problems. Go to an emergency room, and make sure the ophthalmologist on call is summoned to examine your child.

- There is any injury to the eye.
- The child says he or she cannot see.
- The child closes his or her eyes (won't or can't keep them open).
- The child won't stop touching or rubbing the eye.
- There is blood on the lid or in the white of the eye.
- There is blood in the eye so that you can't see the pupil of the child's eye.
- The eye seems enlarged or the cornea cloudy.

Look at your children's eyes. If you notice or suspect any problem, ask your pediatrician who usually tests children's eyes. Report all eye symptoms and signs of allergies to your pediatrician.

Advice to Pregnant and Lactating Mothers

The best advice I can give pregnant or lactating mothers is to *plan ahead*:

1. Take a multivitamin daily.

2. Don't smoke and try to avoid secondhand smoke.

3. Pay particular attention to the B vitamins. We know that 400 micrograms of folic acid daily will help prevent spinal cord defects (such as anencephaly and spina bifida) in infants. The B vitamins are important for all nerve functions.

4. Likewise, the essential fatty acids insulate all nerves and retinal cells. Fifty percent of the fat in the brain is comprised of the essential fatty acid DHA (from algae or fish oil), which also makes up the majority of fat in the retina. Furthermore, since the mother contributes to the child's physical and neurological development, she can easily become depleted of essential fatty acids herself. Without adequate replenishment of these good fats, postpartum depression and memory loss can occur over the short term, and it's possible that diseases like multiple sclerosis can develop in the long term. Make sure you are consuming a proper amount of Omega-3 essential fatty acids. There is some evidence that pregnant women who have diets very low in the essential fatty acids have an increased risk of having low-birth-weight infants; higher rates of mental retardation have also been linked to very low essential fatty acid consumption during pregnancy.

5. Avoid most medications, including antibiotics and steroids. Remember that eyedrops are concentrated medications that enter your system and therefore your baby's system. Avoid them unless they are essential for your health. Avoid nonorganic deodorants, shampoos, hair sprays and other inhalants, if possible, or use them in well-ventilated areas. What you put on your skin enters your bloodstream, so try to use natural cosmetics during pregnancy, too.

6. Avoid refined sugar, white flour, and heavy meals in general.

7. Minimize or eliminate your alcohol consumption. One glass of wine a day is cautiously recommended, but it's important to seek and follow your physician's advice.

8. Consume lots of glutathione-boosting compounds like avocado, egg, and garlic.

9. If you are breast feeding, don't do so immediately after exercise. Researchers at the University of Indiana have found that vigorous exercise reduces the levels of certain immunoglobulins in breast milk for

an hour. Since mother's milk is the major defense against infection for a child under six months, this is important to note.

10. There is some hint that infants who are breast fed have lower rates of learning disabilities. Breast feeding may also neutralize your child's hereditary tendency to develop allergies.

Dr. Abel's Tip

Breast milk is of the greatest value to an infant, followed by soy milk. Cow milk may be the least healthy, since it contains nonnatural additives.

11. Avoid foods to which you are sensitive or allergic while pregnant or breast feeding, because your child may develop the same sensitivity.

12. Pregnant women should avoid contact with cats, raw meat, and nonpasteurized milk, all of which are potentially contaminated with toxoplasmosis. This parasitic organism can cross the placental barrier into the child and has an affinity for the eyes and brain, where it can cause serious disease.

13. Avoid the following herbs, which may increase the risk of miscarriage: balsam pear, barberry root bark, cascara, chervil, Chinese angelica, feverfew, hernandia, hyptis, juniper bean, may apple, mountain mint, mungwort, pennyroyal, pokeroot, rue, senna, southernwood, tansy, thinja, and wormwood. Consult a top-notch alternative physician before you take *any* herbs during pregnancy.

14. Get plenty of rest—you'll need it!

15. It's always important to have the support of the baby's father, whether in maintaining a clean environment and a healthful diet, or in deciding who gets up and takes the dog out.

16. Relax and enjoy your pregnancy and new child.

CHAPTER 13

Other Eye Diseases

One morning at my office, I saw seven-year-old Karen, who'd had a red, sensitive eye for two days. The slit lamp examination of Karen's eye revealed the typical curlicue-shaped ulcer caused by a herpes simplex viral infection. As I was telling Karen's mother, Ann, about the infection, I noticed a fever blister on Ann's lip, and I realized that Karen's mother had accidentally passed on the infection to her child. Herpes infections are very easily transmitted—a kiss can do it. I explained that the herpes virus that causes fever blisters and this kind of eye infection (ocular herpes, which is not related to what we call genital herpes) is contagious in individuals who've never had it before, much like its cousin, the virus that causes chicken pox. I recommended that Ann treat her lip, avoid recurrences (by using zinc oxide to protect her lips in the sun and not eating chocolate), and not kiss anyone else while she has an active fever blister on her lip. My advice was very serious: ocular herpes can produce a dangerous infection of the eye.

Infectious agents other than the herpes virus—both viruses and bacteria—also cause eye infections, some of which can be very serious. I'll discuss some of the commonest, and how to prevent and treat them, in this chapter. I'll also describe some uncommon, noncontagious eye conditions, like retinitis pigmentosa, to give you an idea of what these unfamiliar names mean. Remember, every person and every eye is unique. If you or someone you love has one of the eye conditions I describe in this chapter (or elsewhere), work with your ophthalmologist to determine the best course of treatment for the individual involved.

Herpes Infection

Anatomy

Herpes virus infection is the leading cause of corneal damage and blindness in developed countries. *Ocular herpes*—*Herpes simplex* Type 1 virus—can cause eye, oral, and genital lesions and is very widespread: 90 percent of people have antibodies indicating they've had contact with the herpes simplex virus. A healthy immune system generally controls this virus, and most of us will not experience a serious herpes outbreak.

Genital herpes—*Herpes simplex* Type 2—will not be discussed here, since it is extremely rare for genital herpes to infect the eyes.

We develop an active infection, often a cold sore, the first time we encounter the *Herpes simplex* Type 1 virus. However, as most of us know from painful experience, having cold sores once does not protect us from having them again and again. Herpes virus outbreaks (like cold sores) may recur in numerous, complex ways for two reasons:

1. Unlike the antibodies we make in response to most other infectious agents (bacteria and viruses), herpes virus antibodies do not provide immunity. In other words, they do not protect us from future infections (as the antibodies we make in response to a polio immunization do, for instance).

2. The herpes virus is not eliminated from the body after an outbreak heals. Instead, it persists in almost a perfect symbiotic relationship with our bodies, hiding in nerve fibers, nerve cells *ganglia*, or the *myelin sheaths* covering nerve fibers. Generally, the immune system keeps the herpes virus under control and it lives peacefully inside us. However, if the immune system is disrupted or immunity is suppressed for some reason, the dormant herpes virus can grow out of control, causing lesions on the skin, in the mouth, or in the eye. Once you have had a herpes infection in the eye, it can reemerge in response to sunlight hitting the eyelid, to an injury, or to stress, all of which suppress immunity to varying degrees. Herpes eye infections recur in at least 25 percent of cases.

Herpes simplex is not the only virus that can infect the eye. Infections of the lids, conjunctiva, and cornea are caused by other viruses, including *Herpes zoster* (which causes chicken pox and shingles), Epstein-Barr virus (which causes mononucleosis), cytomegalovirus (CMV, which can cause severe, often blinding, eye disease in AIDS patients and other immuno-compromised individuals), and *Mollusca contagiosum* (a virus that infects the skin). *Herpes simplex* Type 1 virus is by far the commonest of these, however. In the eye, it produces blisters, conjunctivitis, and inflammation of the cornea. For the sake of simplicity, throughout this discussion I will refer to *Herpes simplex* Type 1 virus as the herpes virus.

Herpes infection creates particular patterns of disease on the surface of the cornea, visualized as either a branching, tree-shaped pattern called a *dendrite*, or a broader, lake-shaped pattern known as a *geographical corneal ulcer*. As soon as I (or any ophthalmologist) sees either of these patterns of infection, it's clear that the patient has a herpes eye infection.

The herpes virus can also cause inflammation called *herpetic keratitis* in the cornea, which can provoke an allergic reaction or cell death (*necrosis*). A sympathetic inflammation, known as *uveitis*, can develop inside the eye.

Symptoms of Ocular Herpes Infections

1. Red eye
2. Tears
3. Light sensitivity
4. Irritation (severe discomfort)
5. Some vision loss, as the lesion gets closer to the center of the eye, or as inflammation inside the eye (uveitis) develops and scar tissue forms.

Because of the danger that herpes presents in the eye, if any of these symptoms arise, you should see your eye doctor immediately. Ophthalmologists call ocular herpes "the great masquerader" because it can resemble any number of eye conditions. Herpes infection is so potentially threatening to sight, however, that most ophthalmologists treat people who have symptoms of ocular herpes as if they have the infection until it's proved that they don't.

Conventional Therapy of Herpes Infections

Fortunately, early therapy will control ocular herpes infections, and we have a number of conventional drugs, both eyedrops and pills, that are very effective against them. (See Table 24.)

To treat viral infections, we must stop the virus from growing. Viruses are made up of genetic material similar to that found in people (although the genetic material is arranged differently in viruses from that in people). This is one reason why viruses are so hard to treat. Medications that stop viruses from growing by interfering with their enzymes can also affect

Table 24. Antiviral Drugs Used to Treat Viral Eye Infections

Drug Type	Form	Used For
Eye Drops/Ointments		
Acyclovir	3% ointment	Herpes simplex keratitis
Trifluridine	1% eyedrop	Herpes simplex keratitis
Systemic Drugs		
Acyclovir	IV injection	Herpes zoster infection
Valtrex	Oral capsules/tablets	Herpes simplex and Herpes zoster infections
Famvir		
Foscarnet	IV injection	CMV retinitis (in AIDS)
Ganciclovir	IV injection or injection in eye	CMV retinitis (in AIDS)

Every patient is different, so your ophthalmologist may prescribe any of these drugs for a viral infection.

human enzymes negatively. As a result, people frequently have allergic (and other) reactions to antiviral medications, even when they are applied topically (through eyedrops or ointment, or even via a skin cream).

Therapy for ocular herpes is quite individual. In some cases, the herpes infection has been brought on by using another medication; steroid eyedrops after a mild injury can lead to the development of a herpes lesion several days later, for instance. Although it sounds contradictory under other conditions, it may be necessary to use steroids to treat herpes eye infections, either to quell the accompanying uveitis or to treat an inflammatory lesion in the center of the vision. Herpes infections in the eye must always be treated aggressively enough to stop them as soon as possible, because untreated herpes infections often scar the cornea and result in some vision loss.

Oral and intravenous antiviral medications (like acyclovir) are also available for treating viral eye infections, but are generally used only to treat severe, debilitating eye disease with potential for spread. Since they are toxic, these drugs should be used sparingly. The usual regimen for treating viral eye infections, in the order in which they are generally used, is:

1. Topical Viroptic (eyedrops), five times daily.
2. Topical acyclovir ointment, if available, as backup.
3. Oral acyclovir, if the eyedrop medications aren't effective.
4. Topical 5 percent iodine (povidone), which is an antiseptic. Potassium iodide (a form of iodine) was used to treat herpes infections 150 years ago, before specific antiviral drugs existed. In those days, iodine eyedrops were combined with scraping the ulcer off the surface of the

eye. We now know that iodine, which is still placed in the eye prior to eye surgery, can also eradicate the herpes virus.

5. Intravenous anti-herpes medications such as acyclovir, foscarnet, or ganciclovir. Although these drugs could be made into eyedrops, the FDA has yet to grant approval for this route of administration. Each of these drugs is very effective in treating herpes infections, and there's reason to believe they'd be very helpful in treating ocular herpes, as well.

Prevention of and Natural Therapy for Herpes Infections

1. Avoid nuts, and chocolate. These foods are high in arginine, which stimulates the growth of herpes viruses.

2. Supplement with L-lysine (500 milligrams daily). Lysine helps counteract the herpes virus's stimulants.

3. Treat dry eyes and other causes of conjunctivitis involving the cornea, so the herpes virus does not have a fertile ground in which to grow. (This is another reason why essential fatty acids and other natural methods of treating dry eyes are so important.)

4. Avoid topical steroids wherever possible, because their suppression of immunity can allow the herpes virus to grow out of control and establish an infection in the eye.

5. Identify the triggering event(s) for recurrences. These are different for different people, and can include trauma, exposure to strong sunlight, fever, stress or psychiatric disturbance, and even menstruation.

6. Attend to eye trauma early. Use appropriate patching, foreign body removal, antibiotic ointment, eye-moisturizing drops, or a bandage contact lens to heal the eye surface quickly and avoid infection.

7. If you have ocular herpes, start using antiviral eyedrops as soon as you suspect that an outbreak is beginning and always keep a prescription on hand.

8. Make sure you're consuming enough selenium (garlic and onions are two natural sources, and selenium is available as a supplement).

9. A natural treatment for herpes virus infections is Juglans rogia, which is made from immature English walnuts and contains the antioxidant quercetin. In an alcohol preparation applied to fever blisters on the lips, it immediately kills the herpes virus.

10. Olive leaf extract is also reported to be an effective antiviral and antibacterial agent.

A British researcher has patented the use of Earl Grey tea bags as a treatment for ocular herpes infections of the lip or genitals. To use this remedy, dip the tea bag in hot water for two to three minutes and then allow it to cool for two to three minutes before applying to lip or genital lesions. I don't know if the Earl Grey treatment works. My personal recommendation for treating herpes infections is antiviral eyedrops or 5 percent iodine, which kills the organism after one minute's contact.

Most episodes (about three-quarters) of ocular herpes do not recur. Nevertheless, everyone should be aware that they may recur and must be able to identify their symptoms.

Although I have limited my discussion here to *Herpes simplex* Type 1, *Herpes simplex* Type 2, which causes genital herpes, is on the rise. The Centers for Disease Control and Prevention (CDC) reported in October 1997, that, unlike other sexually transmitted diseases, genital herpes is soaring in young Caucasians. According to the CDC, as many as one in five Americans over the age of 12 is infected with *Herpes simplex* Type 2, reinforcing the perception that herpes feasts on our society. If we don't keep our immune systems sound, viruses will soon be above us on the food chain.

Another type of herpes virus, the *Herpes zoster* virus that causes chicken pox and shingles, usually causes a systemic infection but can also affect the eye. *Herpes zoster* infections can reappear as shingles (also called *varicella*) twenty years after a person has had chicken pox, when the immune system becomes depressed for any reason or after taking high levels of steroids. Shingles may produce a great deal of pain around the eye, a condition that is called postherpetic neuralgia. It has a characteristic appearance on the face and around the eye, and requires systemic (oral or intravenous) antiviral therapy to stop its spread—eyedrops won't stop this infection. However, although it can be very painful and take a while to disappear, a *Herpes zoster* reactivation (i.e., shingles following chicken pox by many years) generally resolves with no negative aftereffects.

Alternative treatments for shingles include capsicum cream applied to the facial skin (but definitely not to the eye), which helps take some of the pain and tingling away, and 5 percent iodine drops directly to the lesion on the skin.

Pinkeye (Epidemic Keratoconjunctivitis)

Epidemic conjunctivitis, or pinkeye, is a well-known, contagious viral disease that spreads through communities in the fall, spring, and winter. It usually results in red, irritated eyes and disappears in three days to two weeks. In serious cases, vision can become impaired if the condition is not attended to as soon as possible by an eye doctor.

Pinkeye is usually caused by a virus named *adenovirus*, and it spreads in many ways, including through close contact with people who have colds or even swimming in contaminated water. (You should be aware that chlorine does not kill everything in the water in a crowded pool.) If your child has pinkeye, don't let him or her go into the pool. It is important to note that adenovirus has many different varieties (serotypes) which have a five- to twelve-day incubation period before they cause disease.

We're learning that, in addition to adenovirus, pinkeye can also be caused by other viruses that infect the human respiratory tract and eye. These viruses often cause colds or other respiratory infections (which means that a cold caused by one of these viruses can result in pinkeye). They include: rhinovirus, respiratory-syncitial virus, influenza virus, coxsackie virus, and certain enteroviruses (which usually affect the gastrointestinal tract).

Symptoms of Pinkeye

Pinkeye is characterized by a rapid onset of redness and irritation in one or both eyes. The eyelids will frequently be "glued" together in the morning from a discharge that's secreted overnight. The eyes are light-sensitive, and feel itchy and gritty. The eyelids are generally swollen, and occasionally the lymph nodes in front of the ears and down the neck are also swollen.

After the acute conjunctivitis phase passes (in three to five days), the infection gradually resolves and symptoms slowly disappear over the next ten days to two weeks. If the infection doesn't subside in this period of time, however, the virus may infect the cornea, creating little clouded areas (opacities) in the cornea. If these cloudy areas are in the center of the cornea, they can result in vision disturbance and light sensitivity. Because of the corneal involvement, adenovirus outbreaks that occur as sudden epidemics of pinkeye are called *epidemic keratoconjunctivitis* (EKC), meaning an outbreak of infectious conjunctivitis affecting the cornea. If your child's symptoms linger, make sure to take him or her to the eye doctor. Kids who have pinkeye often have it more than once, and parents often just use leftover ointment instead of returning to the doctor.

Conventional Treatment of Pinkeye

We know much about adenovirus (and, for that matter, the other respiratory system viruses and enteroviruses), but we don't know much about how to treat these infections. All of our therapeutic efforts have been failures—but then, neither have we cured the common cold. Although we are making progress, viral infections (like colds and flu) are difficult to treat.

In the past, nothing could be done to treat the viral infection, but antibiotics (like the sulfa drugs) were often prescribed anyway. Since antibiotics attack bacteria, not viruses, they were rarely effective (unless a bacterial infection was also present). Unfortunately, medicine hasn't really made much progress in combatting viruses, even today.

I have found that 1 percent silver nitrate or 5 percent povidone/iodine will help eliminate the virus-infected cells by exfoliating the surface of the eye, as well as killing the virus itself. Both of these preparations have been used for decades. Silver nitrate is the old-time prophylaxis put in newborn babies' eyes to prevent eye infections, and 5 percent iodine is used in modern eye surgery to neutralize all bacterial contamination prior to the surgical procedure. These may be effective therapies against pinkeye, but they are not commonly known, so you may want to remind your eye doctor about these "new" old remedies.

Artificial tears, over-the-counter painkillers (usually NSAIDs), and cold packs applied to the eyes help to relieve discomfort. In rare, severe cases, topical steroids need to be prescribed to control the inflammation.

Prevention and Alternative Treatment of Pinkeye

Prevention of pinkeye involves stopping its spread from person to person. Avoid touching the infected eye, wash your hands frequently with antibacterial soap, use paper towels and facial tissues instead of cloth, avoid eye makeup and contact lens wear until the infection has healed, and stay home from work (or keep your child home from school) as directed by your eye doctor. If cloth towels are used by the person with pinkeye, place them in an area where no one else will use them, and wash all towels and linens (like pillowcases) in hot water.

Homeopathic eyedrops, placed in even just one eye, appear to be effective in treating pinkeye in both eyes, according to a 1995 study. Some homeopathic remedies used commonly for pinkeye include:

- Apis (for itching and burning eyes and hot tears)
- Belladonna (for eyes with burning pain, dilated pupils, and light sensitivity)
- Euphrasia (for allergic pinkeye);
- Ferrum phosphate (if pinkeye is diagnosed very early)
- Hepar sulfate (when eyes and eyelids are very sensitive to touch, cold, and light)

• Mercurius (for a several-day-old infection in eyes that have a profuse, burning discharge)
• Pulsatilla (for eyes that burn, itch, and have a thick discharge at night that glues the eyelids shut)

The basis of homeopathy is the axiom "Like treats like." Homeopathic remedies are extremely dilute preparations. It should be remembered that a remedy like belladonna is used in a very weak preparation when treating a red eye. For example, I have found a 5 percent iodine solution to be the most effective treatment for this common problem.

Styes

Anatomy

A stye is an infection of the eyelid usually caused by staph bacteria. It can result in swelling on the inside or outside of the eyelid, or a general eyelid inflammation. If the external portion of the eyelid is swollen, the stye involves inflammation of a hair follicle and its associated glands; swelling on the underside of the eyelid involves the oil glands (meibomiam glands). The swelling increases for a week or so and then generally begins to subside, sometimes rupturing. (The fluid or pus that seeps out of a ruptured stye can be gently blotted away with a clean, white cloth, and is nothing to worry about.) People with very oily eyelids or blepharitis (oily eyelids that become infected) can have recurring styes.

Conventional Treatment of Styes

The first-line treatment for styes is hot compresses and antibiotic eyedrops or ointments to attack the staph infection. Styes are generally self-limiting; if the swelling and inflammation do not respond to this treatment, it may not be a stye. Since you need a prescription for antibiotic eyedrops to treat a stye, be sure to let your eye doctor know if the stye does not go away within the amount of time he or she tells you it should.

Easily mistaken for a stye is a chronic inflammation (a bump) on the eyelid called a *chalazion*. It is larger than a stye, and is inside the eyelid itself. A chalazion points either toward the outside of the lid, or toward the inside (toward the eye). Oral antibiotics (such as erythromycin, 250 mg twice a day between meals for three days), steroid eyedrops, and warm compresses may speed its resolution. A chalazion must be surgically removed, however, if it disturbs vision or looks so unsightly that it disturbs the patient. This surgery generally takes ten minutes to perform under local anesthesia, and produces great results.

Prevention and Alternative Treatment of Styes

People who are prone to developing styes can help prevent their recurrence by washing their eyelids carefully with a very gentle soap and warm water several times a day. This keeps the excess oil secreted by the hair follicle glands from providing fertile ground for the growth of staph bacteria.

If a stye begins to develop, however, a number of herbal treatments have proved to be helpful in healing it:

- Chamomile has been recommended as an herbal treatment for styes for centuries. Make some chamomile tea, let it cool a bit, soak compresses (made from white cloth, and use a clean one each time) in the tea, and apply them to the affected eyelid several times a day.
- Echinacea is an herb that has well-known antibiotic and immune-stimulating properties. Echinacea can be taken orally as a tea, an extract, or in capsules.
- Garlic has potent antibiotic properties. When you have a stye, either consume more garlic in your food or take a garlic supplement (up to 2000 mg daily).
- Goldenseal is considered to be both an antibiotic and an immune system booster. Warm compresses can be soaked in goldenseal tea and applied to the eyelid several times a day. You can also wipe your lids with Ocusoft™.

I also suggest that you take a multivitamin once or twice daily, as an extra insurance policy.

Ocular Surface Disease

Ocular surface disease is a combination of three clinical conditions: *seborrhea* (oiliness); *staph* (bacterial infection); and *sicca* (dry eyes).

Seborrhea is oiliness of the skin of the eyelids. It can result in dry, flaky eyelashes and redness and itching of the eyelids. A change in tear film complexion, when it becomes oilier than usual, can accompany eyelid seborrhea. You can treat the condition by watering down the tear film with eyedrops.

Why does the tear film become oilier? In part, it's because of the toxins produced by the staph bacteria growing on the lid. These staph bacteria also create toxic substances that break down the long chain of fatty acids (the good fats) into small molecules that irritate the conjunctiva and cornea, giving rise, in turn, to scales, redness, itching, and opacities (cloudy areas) in the peripheral cornea. Meanwhile, the dry-eye condition stimulates the Meibomian glands to make more oil, creating the seborrhea (oily) component. This increased oil is a good medium for growing staphylococcus and other bacteria; and the growth of bacteria creates chronic blepharitis (infection and eyelid inflammation), which may have acute flare-ups.

The best way to manage ocular surface disease is to attack the bacterial component first, by using antibiotic ointment nightly (if not more often, as directed by your doctor) in conjunction with using warm compresses and moisturizing drops throughout the day.

When people have significant eyelid seborrhea, in association with seborrheic dermatitis, it's often called *acne rosacea* or *adult acne*. This condition does not occur by itself, as we've discussed. Poor digestion is often a culprit in rosacea, and digestive enzymes (containing hydrochloric acid, pancreatin, bile, and pepsin, taken with meals) can be helpful in healing it, as can lactobacillus/acidophilus. Try a health food store that has regular deliveries of active-culture yogurt; the plain flavor, without sugar, is best. Taking a good multi-B vitamin complex daily, along with an additional 50–100 mg of vitamin B_2 (riboflavin), can also be helpful in healing and preventing rosacea.

Some people have a tendency to have scales on their eyelids and grow their own staphylococcus. These are the same scales that can be found on hair shafts on the leg, on the back of the neck, or in the nose, and mild irritation stimulate the bacteria, causing redness and inflammation. Our own bacteria, however, generally tend to keep more militant organisms at bay. When the balance of these organisms is thrown out of whack, an aggressive microbe can overgrow our more benign, friendly organisms, similar to what can happen in the gut (when antibiotics destroy the bacteria that keep candida in check, for instance).

Trachoma and Inclusion Conjunctivitis

Trachoma and inclusion conjunctivitis are both caused by chlamydia, a very small bacterium that also causes other serious illnesses, including pneumonia. Chlamydia, like *herpes simplex*, can have a genital, as well as an ocular component. People with unexplained eye infections should always look for associated genital symptoms occurring in the same time period as the eye infection to assist the doctor in making a diagnosis. Parents should be aware that chlamydia can also cause conjunctivitis in newborns if it is passed from mother to child during childbirth.

Trachoma, an infection of the upper eyelid conjunctiva (the lining of the upper eyelid), is rarely seen in the Western world because rapid antibiotic therapy eradicates its cause (i.e., chlamydia). In the developing world, however, blindness from trachoma is caused by lid scarring, loss of tears, and secondary bacterial infection of the cornea. When people in these regions suffer from vitamin A deficiency, corneal blindness often occurs. It's amazing to me that a small amount of something so simple as vitamin A could save the sight of so many children around the world, yet they continue to suffer. If it were up to me, 5 percent iodine would become the treatment of choice around the world for trachoma because of its effectiveness, safety, and affordability.

Inclusion conjunctivitis, which affects the lower eyelid conjunctiva (the lining of the lower lid), is more common in the West than trachoma and may actually be spread by close contact. Inclusion conjunctivitis is often carried and spread by pigeons and other birds who carry chlamydia. Treatment of these disorders, which affect the whole body, is oral or injected antibiotics.

Chlamydia infections need to be treated promptly, because they can lead to scarring of the cornea. One study found that an herbal treatment was better than a placebo, but no one in his right mind would use a placebo in treating an infection that can scar the cornea. This is a situation in which Western medicine can cure a potentially blinding condition. The cornea is usually scarred from a secondary, superinfection with other bacteria, which can develop if the chlamydia infection is not treated promptly. Corneal transplantation is required in many such cases. Don't forget that corneal scarring is the fourth-leading cause of blindness throughout the world after cataracts, glaucoma, and diabetes.

Noninfectious Eye Conditions

Retinitis Pigmentosa

There are several forms of retinitis pigmentosa, a slowly progressing deterioration of the retina that results in diminished vision over time. It is often a hereditary disease. Excessive amounts of cortisol produced in response to extreme stress may also contribute to the development of retinitis pigmentosa.

Immunologist Alfred Sapse, M.D., announced at a medical conference in March 1998 that not only do elevated levels of cortisol contribute to the development of retinitis pigmentosa; treating people with anticortisol drugs improves their condition. Dr. Sapse, who left the University of California Los Angeles to start his own company, Steroidogenesis Inhibitors Inc., is developing anticortisol drugs. Reducing stress, Dr. Sapse points out, also lowers dangerously high cortisol levels. He argues that retinitis has two separate components, one of which is hereditary and the other autoimmune. The autoimmune component is stimulated by cortisol, and the anticortisol drugs like those Dr. Sapse is developing will attack that part of the disease.

The retinal damage caused by retinitis pigmentosa can be detected as early as 10 years of age. The rods that govern peripheral vision are affected most severely first, and peripheral vision gradually diminishes as the condition worsens. The pigment of the retina degenerates in a way that indicates retinitis pigmentosa. Eventually, the optic nerve disc takes on a waxy appearance; cataract may develop, and central vision is affected.

There is no conventional treatment for retinitis pigmentosa, except in the case of a hereditary type of the condition, in which large doses of vitamin A may be helpful. Your ophthalmologist can tell you which kind of retinitis pigmentosa you have.

Alternative treatment of retinitis pigmentosa also employs vitamin A (up to 30,000 IU/day). Other suggestions for alternative treatment of this difficult condition include:

- Supplement with DHA (fish oil or microalgae-derived)
- Take B vitamins (especially B_{12})
- Improve digestion with enzymes
- Decrease stress
- Avoid UV light by wearing sunglasses outdoors
- Improve liver function with silymarin
- Supplement with lutein (10–20 mg)

Optic Neuritis

Optic neuritis occurs when the optic nerve becomes inflamed in conditions like multiple sclerosis, in which nerve demyelination (destruction of the protective myelin sheath around the nerve fibers) takes place. Optic neuritis can also be caused by any one of several other conditions, including lack of blood flow to the retina and optic nerve, diabetes, syphilis, trauma, chemical poisoning and, rarely, even tumor.

Optic neuritis produces a sudden loss of visual acuity and pain with movement of the eye. The eye doctor can diagnose optic neuritis by examining the retina, which is usually swollen. Blood vessels around the optic nerve head can appear engorged, and there are sometimes small hemorrhages visible near the optic nerve.

Currently, there is no effective conventional treatment for optic neuritis. Ophthalmologists occasionally attempt to treat optic neuritis with high doses of oral steroids, but these are minimally effective and have numerous side effects.

I have had four patients with optic neuritis treated successfully by a local Chinese traditional medical practitioner with whom I often work. Chinese traditional physicians believe that optic neuritis (sudden loss of vision) is related to a stagnant or congested liver, as well as a weak heart. In cases of ischemic optic neuritis, we used antioxidants (multivitamin, B complex, vitamin E, and alpha lipoic acid) to decrease inflammation and Chinese herbs (a ten-herb combination called Salvia sho wu) to move the blood, as is used for ischemic heart disease. Other heart-strengthening supplements that can be used in appropriate cases are CoQ10, astragalus, ginseng, and hawthorne. (Don't use these herbs, however, without the advice of an accomplished herbalist and the approval of your physician.)

Transient Ischemic Attack (TIA)

A transient ischemic attack (TIA) is a small stroke. Its symptoms are an irregular heartbeat and low pulse. A doctor can easily detect a blocked carotid artery in the neck, a very common cause of strokes (which can also be caused by blood vessels leaking or breaking in the brain). Because the optic nerve fans out into both sides of the brain, and a stroke in any number of areas can affect one of the optic nerve's branches, these small strokes can cause vision disturbance or loss.

People usually recover fully from TIAs without much treatment. Beta-blocking eyedrops can be implicated in decreasing heart rate or blood pressure. Identifying the cause of the TIA so that preventive measures can be taken to prevent its recurrence is essential. Taking aspirin on a daily basis to thin the blood can also be useful to prevent recurrence.

Grave's Disease

Grave's disease is a thyroid disorder. It can result from hyperthyroidism (the production of too much thyroid hormone), from hypothyroidism (the production of too little thyroid hormone), or from an autoimmune-like condition. We see low-thyroid Grave's disease more often in the elderly. It is sometimes difficult to detect.

You can determine whether your thyroid is potentially underactive by taking your basal temperature. Place a thermometer under your arm in the morning before you get out of bed, and leave it there for at least ten minutes. A temperature below 97.0, is a low reading. If this is the case on succcessive days, it's a good indication that your thyroid is underactive. You can ask your doctor to test your thyroid function.

As we've discussed elsewhere, conditions throughout the body can and do cause eye symptoms and diseases. Grave's disease is a perfect example of a disease in a remote part of the body (the thyroid gland) resulting in eye symptoms. In fact, all the visible symptoms of Grave's disease occur in the eye, and include prominent eyes (because the eyelid retracts), bulging of the eye, and dry eyes (which can result in corneal abrasion). The muscles that control the eyes are sometimes also involved, which causes double vision. Very rarely, is the optic nerve involved, which can cause total loss of vision.

Treatment of Grave's disease involves reducing the excess thyroid hormone (the most common cause) by using radioactive iodine to inactivate the thyroid gland. Once the thyroid gland is essentially destroyed, the treated person must take artificial thyroid hormone for the rest of his or her life—which is really not so bad. It's easier to take thyroid pills than to risk blindness. For bulging eyes (perhaps the most telling symptom of the disease) there are other treatments: prednisone treatment, radiation, or surgical decompression to remove parts of the eye's orbit.

Remember: If you have any symptoms of Grave's disease, see your doctor immediately.

Bell's Palsy

Bell's palsy affects one side of the face, right or left, with temporary paralysis. The larger nerve that controls the facial muscles become inflamed at the point where it leaves the skull. It's not known why the nerve swells, or why only one of the nerves is affected. The condition generally develops quite suddenly, usually overnight, and can be painful on the affected side of the face or in the ear on that side of the head. In fact, Lyme disease can sometimes trigger Bell's palsy. It affects men and women without regard to age. It recurs in fewer than 10 percent of individuals; in only 1 percent of cases are both sides of the face affected.

The major concern in Bell's palsy is damage to the eye, which usually does not close properly. Open to dust and pollution, the eye may dry out, leading to the development of corneal ulcers. It's important to wear a patch to protect the eye and use moisturizing eyedrops to keep it from becoming very dry. Temporary lid suturing may be required.

Another concern is the affected individual's response to suddenly having a face that can't be controlled. Just imagine how frightening this can be: a person who was perfectly healthy yesterday, wakes up with a partially paralyzed face. Sometimes a patient with Bell's palsy may require psychological counseling during recovery, and a caring physician should be alert to that possible need and ready to provide a referral.

There is no completely effective treatment for Bell's palsy, although surgery to relieve the pressure on the affected nerve may be suggested. Steroids or corticotropin (a hormone produced by the pituitary gland) are sometimes administered for a short period of time (two weeks or less) to help speed natural recovery. Recovery usually begins within two days, with significant recovery usually occurring in two or three weeks. Eighty-six percent of patients recover completely. If no improvement is seen after two months or more have passed, however, the patient will probably not recover completely. People who have high blood pressure, complete facial weakness, pain other than in the ear, changes in tearing, and are older than 55 may not recover totally.

Tumors

The first sign of a brain tumor may be an eye symptom like uncontrolled tearing or decreased peripheral vision (or other vision loss). An eye/brain symptom, like increasingly severe headaches, might be the first sign. If these or any other symptom sends the patient to the eye doctor, the doctor may uncover other clues suggesting the presence of a brain tumor. An examination of the inside of the eye may reveal optic nerve swelling (blurred cup margins or disc swelling), the appearance of "cotton wool" spots, retinal hemorrhage, or blood vessel abnormalities.

If a brain tumor is suspected, the eye doctor will refer the patient to a neurologist or neurosurgeon for further evaluation. In many cases, the suspicious symptoms are caused by other problems and do not signal the presence of a brain tumor. Even if a brain tumor is diagnosed, don't panic. Neurosurgery has become so sophisticated that the prognosis is good for most patients.

PART V

DIET AND NUTRITION

CHAPTER 14

Food for Sight: Don't Stop Thinking About Tomorrow . . .

No Kaffir [a pejorative name for indigenous people] cuts his beard or hair, nevertheless there are very few with long beards, as their hair grows but little, and it does not turn white until they are of a great age. It is common among these Kaffirs to live to ninety and a hundred years of age.

—*From the diary of a Portuguese explorer who visited Mozambique in 1609, recorded by official historiographer George McCall Theal (Records of South-Eastern Africa, Vol. VII, Printed for the Government of the Cape Colony in 1901).*

In 1609, the average Portuguese man didn't expect to live past the age of 50. The unnamed seventeenth-century explorer later quoted by George McCall Theal, the official historian of the South African Cape Government in 1901, was quite impressed when he encountered people native to South Africa's tropical paradise who lived twice as long as he and his fellow "civilized" Northern Europeans. Perhaps he did not make the connection between quality of life, diet, and the South Africans' longevity. We certainly understand this correlation today.

My nutritional education began in earnest while I was a young medical student, but I didn't acquire it in medical school. Unfortunately, my instructors who were so learned in anatomy and biology didn't understand that nutrition is the foundation of good health. I attended medical school during the magic age of medicine: We learned to diagnose, prescribe the appropriate drug, and wait for the symptom to go away. Who needed nutrition? We had drugs that cured everything.

I remember asking one of my professors about the fundamentals of a good diet. He waved me off with the abrupt comment, "Just eat whatever you like. Nutrition is vastly overrated. No one needs to take vitamins."

My mother Ruth was a "health nut" who monitored my diet closely during childhood (she always caught me sneaking bacon into the shopping cart, and promptly removed it) and advocated balanced meals. "No dessert unless you eat your salad and vegetables" was her daily refrain.

My mother deplored the lack of nutritional education in medical school. She thought that Linus Pauling and Albert Szent-Georgi, advocates of taking vitamin supplements, must be right about us needing greater quantities of vitamins than we could obtain either in food or by manufacturing them in our own bodies. She was pleased when I began to study nutrition seriously and especially happy when I married a woman who cleared the pantry of packaged and refined foods. In nearly everything she taught me about diet and nutrition, Mother was right.

Early on in my career, I began to notice that those patients who were really sick—not just with eye diseases, but also with an assortment of problems including diabetes, heart disease, and high blood pressure—shared something important. They all had terrible diets. They ate meat every day, lots of fried and processed foods, and hardly any fresh vegetables or fruits. At that time, I began to explore the link between nutrition and health with the same level of seriousness I'd given to my medical studies. And I continue to keep up with the latest nutritional research, just as I keep up with new techniques in ophthalmology.

If you are satisfied with the state of your health—if you feel good all the time, you seldom catch colds or the flu, have no stomach problems or allergies—then you're probably on the right track. If you're like most people, however, and suspect you could feel better when you wake up every morning, or you have recurrent health problems (herpes or yeast infections, frequent colds, sinus problems, or chronic fatigue), the information in this chapter is vitally important for you. Best of all, it's simple to learn. The hard part about making dietary changes—if you're like me—is deciding to do it and then following through.

Antioxidants and Free Radicals

It doesn't matter if you are currently healthy or sick, young or not-so-young, you can have a positive effect on your health *starting today* by changing your diet. By consuming adequate quantities of antioxidants, you will be protecting your eyes and body against the many ravages of modern life.

On the other hand, if you're consuming nutrient-poor foods, you're probably also *not* eating nutrient-rich foods. (A person can consume only so much food in a day.) The most important role played by an antioxidant-rich diet is to protect against damaging free radicals, which contribute to many degenerative diseases like cataracts, arthritis, diabetes, and perhaps even some effects of aging itself.

A free radical is an incomplete molecule, which is why it's so unstable. Free radicals lack one negative charge (one electron) to balance the molecule's positive charges and stabilize it. If, for example, a balanced molecule is a table with four legs—two positive and two negative charges balancing each other—then a free radical is a three-legged table, missing an electron and always off-balance. To achieve balance, the free radical is always looking for an electron to complete its structure. Free radicals obtain those electrons by attacking other molecules and stealing an electron, damaging the second molecule in the process.

Free radicals are formed when molecules are metabolized; that is, when they interact with oxygen (which is why the process that creates free radicals is called *oxidation*).

Oxygen is required to sustain human life, but it can also produce tissue damage. Metabolism is literally a fire inside that consumes nutrients through their interactions with oxygen. This process, which energizes our bodies, also generates free radicals and other damaging waste products.

We also produce free radicals in response to outside environmental factors, including excessive sunlight, tobacco smoke, preservatives, pesticides, industrial chemicals, air pollution, and stress.

Free radicals attack the retina, muscles, joints, cell membranes, the lining of the coronary arteries, and DNA (the genetic material). Free radicals cause the general wear and tear on our bodies associated with aging, as well as contributing to the development of cataracts, cancer, arthritis, and heart disease. They are only stopped from wreaking this havoc on the body's tissues when they are neutralized by antioxidants.

Since we gain most antioxidants from the food we eat, we must make intelligent decisions about our diets. Think about your antioxidant bank account: you're constantly withdrawing from it, but are you making enough deposits? Your diet directly influences your immune system and its ability to combat illness; a poor diet, for instance, encourages the growth of disease-causing viruses.

Our eyes depend upon antioxidants for protection from disease. Clinical studies show that the risk of developing cataracts can be decreased by more than half by eating fruits and vegetables rich in vitamin C, as well as the antioxidants vitamin A, E, selenium, and glutathione. The risk of developing glaucoma can be lowered by consuming high levels of vitamins C and B_{12}. The risk of developing macular degeneration is reduced by maintaining high levels of vitamins E, A, the carotenoids (beta-carotene and lutein), and the amino acid taurine (found in egg whites). Diabetic retinopathy can be delayed (or prevented) by consuming vitamin C along with alpha lipoic acid, bilberry, and other bioflavonoids.

The Road to Good Health and Better Vision

- Stay fully involved in maintaining your health through good nutrition and supplementation.
- Employ alternative and Eastern medicine therapies to prevent illness and maintain health.
- Use Western medicine prudently when required.

We already know that eating properly can replace certain medications for many people. A good diet is far less toxic and certainly less expensive. In 1996, the U.S. public spent $88 billion on drugs—a figure that does not even include all the over-the-counter drugs purchased.

Recognizing that food can replace medicine, pharmaceutical companies and food manufacturers have begun to create products containing food-derived nutrients. According to *Food Processing Magazine* publisher Bob Messenger, 55 percent of food companies and 36 percent of pharmaceutical companies are developing "nutraceutical foods" in response to public demand.

Until now, food manufacturers have primarily emphasized creating foods that stay fresh on the grocery shelf for a long time. But foods with long shelf lives often contain poisonous transfats, which interfere with normal body processes. That innocent-looking cracker that you slather with peanut butter or cheese is, most likely, poisoning you. On June 8, 1998, the *New York Times* reported that, according to USDA researchers, the following foods contain high percentages of dangerous transfats: crackers (40 percent), chocolate chip cookies (36 percent), margarine (32 percent), and potato chips (30 percent). (These percentages obviously vary from one brand to another.)

Unlike such food components as fat, salt, and calories, the transfat content of packaged foods doesn't have to be listed on their labels. The Washington-based food-safety watchdog group Center for Science in the Public Interest has been lobbying the FDA since 1994 to require manufacturers to include transfat content on food labels. Although the FDA has not yet done so, the public is increasingly refusing to buy transfat-filled packaged foods, and manufacturers are responding.

I know it's difficult to avoid packaged foods entirely. But if you and your family limit them as much as possible, you will have taken a major step toward avoiding illness.

Four Easy Steps Toward Achieving Longevity, Good Health, and a Lifetime of Good Vision

1. Eat a salad every day. The darker the greens, the better.

2. Replace candy dishes with bowls of fruit; keep sliced vegetables (like celery and carrots) available in the refrigerator.

3. Don't eat red meat every day. Substitute other forms of protein, like turkey, chicken, eggs, beans, and my favorite, fish (which I eat about three times a week). Eating red meat once a week, in small quantities, probably won't hurt healthy people who really like it. Try and buy natural beef that does not have added hormones and antibiotics. Another excellent source of red meat is buffalo meat, which is raised on wild grasses.

4. Start replacing the sodas, other packaged drinks, and even the commercial fruit juices in your refrigerator with good bottled or filtered water or freshly made juices. Buy a good juicer. Experiment with different combinations. This can be great fun for the entire family. You'll find your kids will drink more juice and less soda after they become involved.

Dr. Abel's Food Pyramid

The food pyramid shows how to balance the different kinds of foods we should eat each day. Those foods that should be eaten sparingly, if at all, are in the top portion of the pyramid, and those foods that should be most plentiful in the diet are at the base of the pyramid. Different nutritional philosophies result in very different food pyramids. In one, carbohydrates may be at the very top of the pyramid, with a caution to eat them sparingly, while in another, carbohydrates are the diet's staple food. As theories of nutrition come and go, so do food pyramids.

Most people concerned about nutrition agree that consuming at least five fruits and vegetables a day is ideal (hard-liners say ten, and Japanese nutritionists recommend consuming twenty different fruits and vegetables daily). I suspect, however, that fewer than 5 percent of Americans actually consume five servings of fruits and vegetables every day.

I recommend avoiding large amounts of dairy because of the hormones and antibiotics fed to the animals. In fact, the growth hormone commonly given to cows may increase breast and prostate tumors, since glands tend to store these fat-soluble substances.

The U.S. Department of Agriculture's food pyramid suggests consuming fats, oils, and sweets only sparingly; two to three servings of dairy daily;

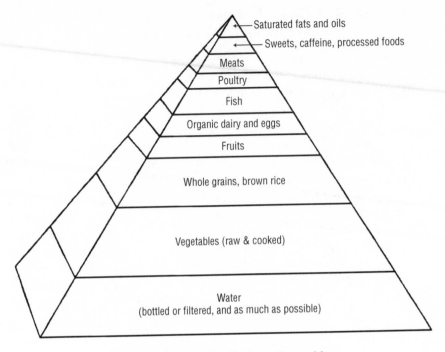

Figure 10. Dr. Abel's Food Pyramid

two to three servings of protein (meat, poultry, fish, dry beans, eggs, and nuts) daily; three to five servings of vegetables and two to four servings of fruit daily; and six to eleven servings of carbohydrates (bread, cereal, rice, and pasta) each day.

As you will see from my food pyramid, I think a healthful diet should consist primarily of vegetables (raw and cooked), whole grains, Omega-3-rich fats, and fruits, along with judicious amounts of protein (from beans, nuts, organic dairy, natural poultry, natural meat, and fish). Sweets, caffeine, processed foods (including pasta and bread), and saturated fats should be consumed in very small quantities, if at all. My food pyramid is built upon a base of water, our most important and most neglected nutrient. (See Figure 10.)

A Most Important Element: Water

Everyone should drink six to eight glasses of water (8 ounces each) every day. It's very important to keep our bodies properly hydrated, because dehydration affects every organ in the body. Severe dehydration can result in death—it's not the diarrhea that kills people during cholera outbreaks, it's the resulting dehydration. Older people are extremely vulnerable to dehydration. Even well-cared-for and affluent elderly people can easily become severely dehydrated, which can lead to mental confusion and kidney dysfunction, among other serious problems.

Water transports all the nutrients throughout our bodies and helps us to maintain a constant internal temperature. It helps create the fluid in our eyes, the blood that brings nourishment to them, and the lymph fluid that carries away waste products. Water also carries waste out of the rest of the body, primarily through urine and sweat. This is why regular exercise speeds our metabolism and contributes to health (and weight loss) by allowing us to sweat toxins out through the skin. To keep this cycle of nutrition and waste removal flowing, it's important to replace the fluids and antioxidants we lose by sweating.

The Importance of Good Digestion

What's good for the digestion is good for the macula. Remember, it takes only twenty minutes for the nutrients—and the toxins—you eat to reach your eyes. Certain eye diseases correlate with specific dietary deficiencies. Macular degeneration, for example, is a disease of poor digestion. Glaucoma is a disease of stress, which disturbs digestion. Cataracts are caused by an antioxidant deficiency that allows free radicals to damage the lens of the eye (adding to age-related damage to the lens). Dry and red eyes result from poor diet and digestion. All good health, including eye health, begins in the bowels.

Having low stomach acid doesn't help digestion, so stop taking your antacids unless your doctor prescribed them. There are plenty of natural substances that aid digestion, including:

- Plant-derived digestive enzymes (amylases, cellulases, lipases, and proteases).
- Animal-derived digestive enzymes (elastases).
- Microbe-derived digestive enzymes (from acidophilus or lactobacillus cultures, which can be obtained from sauerkraut, yogurt, and supplements). Take probiotics on an empty stomach.
- Fiber, both soluble and insoluble.
- Natural betaine and other forms of hydrochloric acid (to make up for deficient stomach acid). Many elderly people make decreased amounts of stomach acid and bile and so cannot absorb vitamins B_{12}, C, or the fat-soluble vitamins.

- Inulin from onions and Jerusalem artichokes, which promotes healing of colon surface cells.
- Aloe vera, apple cider bitters, cayenne pepper, comfrey root, fennel, ginger, garlic, and licorice root, which all have anti-inflammatory effects.

Make sure you're eating an adequate amount of fiber-rich foods, which naturally contain both soluble and insoluble fiber. Soluble fiber promotes normal bowel function, while insoluble fiber decreases toxicity in the colon.

Be good to your gastric mucosa. A healthy intestinal lining protects against the development of *leaky gut syndrome*, which can cause inflammatory bowel disease and other autoimmune disorders. It's crucial to provide a high level of the substances that maintain normal intestinal permeability by using supplements if necessary (see Chapter 15). It's also important to block the overgrowth of fungus, which causes a breakdown in food digestion and absorption.

Food Sensitivities/Allergies

Hidden food allergies may cause much of the ill health people endure on a day-to-day basis. There are two types of food sensitivities: (1) food "intolerance," which generally implies that the enzyme needed to break down the suspect food is missing; and (2) true food allergies, in which an allergic attack is mounted by the immune system whenever certain foods are eaten.

Food sensitivities may play a role in causing various chronic conditions, including arthritis. Some researchers claim that even rheumatoid arthritis can be significantly improved by identifying foods to which one is sensitive and removing them from the diet. It's strongly suspected that the nightshade plant foods contribute to osteoarthritis in aging individuals. The nightshade plants produce a number of poisons—the "deadly nightshade" belladonna is one—and it's thought that the same chemicals are present in smaller quantities in the edible members of the family (green peppers, eggplant, tomatoes, and white potatoes).

Migraine headaches can be triggered by foods in sensitive people. According to a study published in the *British Medical Journal*, the foods most often linked to migraines are: alcohol, bananas, cheese, chocolate, eggs, milk, preserved meats, tomatoes, yeast, yogurt, and foods containing nitrites or monosodium glutamate.

Sensitivities can be provoked by growth hormones, antibiotics, and other chemicals routinely added to animal feed. Milk cows are given so much penicillin (to prevent infections in their udders from the milking machines) that federal standards have been established to regulate how much penicillin milk can contain before it has to be (literally) dumped.

One of the commonest intolerances is to lactose, the sugar in milk. The symptoms of lactose intolerance include gas, diarrhea, and abdominal pain.

Fewer people have a true milk allergy, which causes nasal congestion, hives, headache, urinary frequency, and loss of protein in the urine. Unlike food intolerance, which causes symptoms only in the area where the food is not processed properly (the intestines), a food allergy can cause symptoms all over the body. Dr. J. C. Breneman, M.D., author of *Basics of Food Allergy*, points out that "Food allergy can do anything to any part of the body."

The most allergy-provoking foods are eggs, milk, the nightshade plants, shellfish, and wheat.

Some physicians and alternative practitioners believe that gallbladder disease results from food allergy, and that elimination diets can be very helpful in managing it.

We don't understand the mechanisms of all food sensitivities/allergies, but that doesn't mean we should ignore them. As doctors and patients, we need to act on what we observe and, if it leads to an improvement in health and well-being, to figure out its underlying scientific mechanism later.

We require energy to fuel the basal metabolism that allows us to go on living. The energy we gain from carbohydrates, proteins, and fats (which provide twice as much energy as either carbohydrates or proteins), is stored in various forms, including fat, in the body. While sugar is also a source of energy, its contribution is fleeting—it is broken down immediately and either used right away or stored as fat.

While fat provides energy, too much of the wrong kind of fat contributes to obesity, clogged arteries (atherosclerosis), heart disease, stroke, and other degenerative conditions. People with a lot of body fat may actually be poisoning themselves by accumulating toxins in their own fat. And eating a diet high in animal fat means you may be ingesting dangerous amounts of the antibiotics or pesticides consumed by the animal and stored in its fat.

Fats are classified as *saturated*, found in animal products like meat; *monounsaturated*, found in olive and canola oils, the best fats to use for cooking (I personally prefer to use olive oil); *polyunsaturated*, found in flaxseed, algae, and fatty fish; and *transfats* (found in hydrogenated products like margarine).

Saturated fats are generally solid at room temperature, and are found in pork, beef, dairy products, coconut, and chocolate. Hydrogenated products (cocoa butter, vegetable shortening, and margarine) contain high levels of saturated fats as well as transfats.

Monounsaturated fats are generally liquid at room temperature. Olive oil has the highest percentage of monounsaturated fats of any generally available vegetable oil. It has long been associated with the low rate of heart disease and cancer in people who eat a Mediterranean-style diet, which is high in fat from olives and olive oil. A study performed by an international team of researchers, including Walter Willett, Ph.D., an epidemiologist at the Harvard School of Public Health, suggested in early 1998 that women who consume monounsaturated fat (like that found in olive oil) have a lower risk of developing both breast cancer and heart disease than women who consume mostly polyunsaturated fats (highest in corn, sunflower, and safflower oil). Interestingly, the *amount* of saturated fat in the diet appeared to have no impact on the women's chances of developing heart disease or breast cancer, although the researchers stressed that their findings are preliminary. (They cautioned, however, that limiting calories and controlling weight certainly lowered women's risk of developing both diseases.)

My review of the literature has led me to believe that DHA, the twenty-two-carbon molecule with six double bonds, is the key ingredient for our health. DHA is a basic component of every cell membrane in our body when it is connected to an Omega-6 fatty acid and phosphatidyl choline. This fat sandwich keeps the necessary ingredients in and selects only certain products outside of the cell.

In the brain and retina there are two DHAs with a phosphatidyl choline in every cell membrane because this fatty acid conducts nerve transmissions faster than any other molecule. Therefore, DHA is a must for sending light impulses through the eye to the brain.

The essential fatty acids are required for healthy cell membranes (to keep blood vessels from leaking, for instance), proper immune system functioning, and visual acuity. They transport and help metabolize cholesterol, regulate stomach secretions and smooth muscle contraction, and are important for growth, particularly in infants. I've discovered that some patients' eye problems, particularly dry eyes, are helped by adding Omega-3 essential fatty acid supplements to their diets. The essential fatty acids must be acquired from food.

The two major groups of essential fatty acids are the Omega-3 *(alpha-linolenic acid)* and Omega-6 *(linoleic acid)* fats. The essential fatty acids are very fragile, and must be handled with care. If you buy oils rich in essential fatty acids (like flaxseed oil), make sure that they are cold pressed (without using heat), have the date of the pressing marked on the bottle (to ensure freshness), and are bottled in dark containers (to protect against damage from light). You should never cook with oils high in essential fatty acids.

Omega-3 essential fatty acids are found in flaxseeds and flaxseed oil, walnuts and walnut oil, fat-rich fish (like salmon and mackerel), and dark green leafy vegetables. Flaxseed oil is very fragile, and should never be heated. (It can be sprinkled on salad, for instance, or on cooked vegetables, without being heated.)

The Omega-3 essential fatty acid that we consume from green vegetables, is poorly converted in our bodies (with the help of vitamins C and B$_6$, zinc, and other coenzymes) into docosahexaenoic acid (DHA) and eicosapentaenoic acid (EPA). It is better to take DHA directly.

DHA can also be acquired by eating fish, which is why it is commonly called "fish oil." DHA *makes up about 30 percent of the fat in the brain, retina, and adrenal glands.* In addition to contributing to brain and eye health, DHA protects against heart disease. British researchers have found that diets containing a lot of fish cut deaths among heart patients by as much as 35 percent, and American investigators have found that male physicians who eat fish at least once a week halve their risk of sudden death (presumably from heart disease). The best food sources of DHA are the cold-water fatty fish: salmon, tuna, mackerel, cod, herring, sardines, trout, and eel.

For people who don't like to eat fish, DHA is now available in a supplement made from microalgae, which does not go rancid as easily as fish oil capsules.

The vegetable sources of Omega-3 fats include: walnuts and walnut oil; flaxseeds and flaxseed oil; canola oil; and green leafy vegetables. The high Omega-3 content of green vegetables is one reason that nutritionists advise us to eat at least five servings of vegetables every day. Omega-3 fatty acids can also be found in legumes, eggs (particularly from free-range chickens), and herbs and spices (including mustard, fennel, cumin, and fenugreek).

Flaxseeds and flaxseed oil are probably the best plant sources of Omega-3 fats. Omega-3 essential fatty acids from flaxseeds or their oil have been shown to reduce high triglyceride levels, one of the major risk factors for developing cardiovascular disease.

The Omega-6 essential fatty acid is converted in our bodies into *gamma-linoleic acid*, or GLA. Omega-6 fatty acids are found in such vegetable oils as borage, canola, evening primrose, safflower, and sunflower oil.

While it was initially thought that we should consume equal amounts of each group, research has shown that the standard American diet is high in Omega-6 fats but extremely depleted in Omega-3 fats. This imbalance between Omega-6 and Omega-3 essential fatty acids appears to contribute to the development of numerous chronic illnesses, including allergies, arthritis, some vision problems, autoimmune diseases, some types of dementia, and hyperactivity in children.

In *The Omega Plan*, Artemis Simopoulos, M.D., points out that the American diet is fourteen to twenty times higher in Omega-6 fats than in Omega-3's, a ratio that is badly out of balance. Dr. Simopoulos compared the diet eaten on the Greek island of Crete to seven other regional diets, including those of the Greek mainland and Japan. She found that the Crete diet is more healthful than the Japanese diet, even though it contains 40 percent more fat, because of its high Omega-3 essential fatty acid content. Dr. Simopoulos also compared a modified version of the Crete diet to the American Heart Association diet (a very-low-fat diet). Among people who'd had a previous heart attack, the Crete diet provided a better chance of survival from a second heart attack and reversal of heart disease.

By itself, no single nutrient can guarantee good health, and the essential fatty acids are no exception. They require vitamins E, A, C, B_3, and B_6, as well as the minerals zinc, selenium, and manganese, for proper absorption.

Hydrogenated fats and oils are produced by a manufacturing process that chemically adds hydrogen to the oils to give them a longer shelf life and make them solid at room temperature. Margarine is made from cottonseed oil, to which bubbled hydrogen (which makes it "hydrogenated") and nickel are added to make it solid; other additives give it color and make it taste like butter. Crackers, chips, many kinds of dips, and vegetable shortenings contain hydrogenated fats as well as transfats.

We are just discovering how damaging transfats are to human health. Found in processed supermarket oils, margarine, and artificial "cheese foods," transfats block our use of the fats we require most (i.e., the essential fatty acids) and do all kinds of mischief in our bodies. Hydrogenation takes a harmless, unsaturated fat and turns it into a harmful transfat.

Technology has provided yet a new worry—the "fake fats" like Olean (Olestra) and Simpless. Fake fats block the production of cholesterol in the liver; therefore, they also block the liver's other functions, including the production and release of glutathione, which is vital to eye health.

These fake fats leach nutrients out of the body, as well as causing cramps and diarrhea in some individuals.

Remember that *fat-free* does not mean "calorie-free." Many fat-free foods (including those made with fake fats) have just as many calories as similar foods not marketed as fat-free. In addition, fat-free foods are generally unsatisfying, causing us to eat more because we're still hungry after consuming whole packages of fat-free chips—an important consideration if you are trying to lose weight.

Phytochemicals and Bioflavonoids

Phytochemicals are the nutrients found in plants. Vitamins, for instance, are phytochemicals. Other phytochemicals are called "bioflavonoids," or just "flavonoids." Phytochemicals are often found at highest concentration in the skin of fruits and vegetables, where they give vegetable foods their color and taste and protect plants from the damaging effects of ultraviolet light. In humans, they appear to have powerful antioxidant and anticancer properties, as well as generally increasing immunity, protecting the liver, and facilitating blood flow throughout the body including the brain and retina).

Just some of the foods rich in flavonoids include asparagus, beets, broccoli, Brussels sprouts, cabbage, carrots, cocoa, eggplant, garlic, onions, peppers, radishes, sweet potatoes, tomatoes, lima beans, garbanzo beans, and soy beans, black and green teas, apples, berries, citrus fruits, grapes, and red wine. The spices ginger, parsley, rosemary, sage, thyme, and turmeric are also rich in flavonoids.

More than eight hundred flavonoids have been identified, including: anthocyanidins (from grape skins, cranberries, strawberries, blueberries, and blackberries); proanthocyanidins (OPCs, from pine bark, grape seeds, and *ginkgo biloba*); flavonones (from citrus peel); isoflavones (genistein and diadzein, from soy); catechins (from green tea, grape seeds, and pine bark); lignans (in flaxseeds); and rutin (from citrus rind, grapes, and wine).

Sugar

In the past four hundred years, the diets of almost all the people on earth have changed because of refined sugar. We worship sugar in its roles as a sweetener, preservative, decoration, medicine, and ceremonial substance. Consider the role of sweets in all major holidays; think about rewarding Johnny for going to the eye doctor with an ice cream cone. Without realizing it, we have become addicted to sugar. When our blood sugar declines, we *have* to have more.

The destructive qualities of sugar were demonstrated by the studies of Weston Price, a dentist who traveled among many indigenous peoples in the mid-1930s. Although his primary interest was in teeth and dental decay, Dr. Price learned that there was almost no tuberculosis, arthritis, or cancer among indigenous peoples in Alaska, the Outer Hebrides, or New Zealand, where—at that time, the indigenous people used no refined sugar or other refined foods.

Sugar, white flour, canned food, and processed vegetable oils all cause the emergence of cavities, narrowed dental arch, and decreased immunological resistance. As our resistance weakens, we develop bacterial and viral infections that can be fatal. Sugar eventually destroys the body; besides contributing to diabetes, it destroys the pancreas (where insulin is produced) and acts as a medium for yeast growth. Increased refined sugar consumption has also led to greater body fat and the ills that accompany obesity, like heart disease. The dawn of the heart attack era, 1895–1910, corresponds to the beginning of increased sugar consumption in the United States. By 1970, as much as 9 percent of the American diet was composed of simple sugars.

In nature, only honey and maple syrup are as sweet as refined sugar, and neither of them possesses refined sugar's destructive qualities. In addition, honey possesses healing properties. The Romans used honey to kill infections on the skin after burns, because no bacteria can live in it. Honey is also useful as an ulcer treatment, when taken in large quantities for short periods of time.

Sugar is hidden in prepared foods like ketchup, cheese dips, salad dressings, sauces, crackers, frozen vegetables, and many others. Fruit-on-the-bottom yogurt can contain as much as nine teaspoons of sugar per cup of yogurt. Please read the labels on the foods you buy!

Toxins

Our food contains many more contaminants than we really care to know about—as we discover with each new outbreak or outrage. Bacteria, viruses, parasites, antibiotics, growth hormones, caffeine, nicotine, and all kinds of chemicals are on and in the food we eat, animal and vegetable, unless we grow it ourselves. Since most of us don't raise our own food, we must find ways to protect ourselves and our families from these toxins.

Livestock, for instance, are routinely fed antibiotics. While we're consuming their meat or milk, we're also consuming the antibiotics they've been fed. The increased prevalence of antibiotic-resistant organisms in recent years has been linked by some scientists to this passive consumption of antibiotics. A study performed in the Netherlands and Denmark showed that resistant strains of bacteria were transferred from chickens who'd been fed antibiotics to the humans who later ate them, as well as to the factory workers who processed the birds.

Some pesticides and plastics act so much like hormones that researchers call them *environmental estrogens*. They have been linked to an increased incidence of hormone-sensitive cancers, including those affecting the breast, uterus, and prostate. Nearly all commercially available vegetables and fruits are sprayed with pesticides, so scrub your vegetables well, and if possible, skin them before eating.

Preservatives can also damage health. A chemical used to preserve shrimp, sodium metabisulfite, can cause reactions ranging from rash to death by suffocation. It's suspected that sodium metabisulfite may actually be causing some reactions identified as shrimp allergies. (Shellfish allergies can be life-threatening, so consult a physician if you have a bad reaction to shrimp or any other seafood.)

An elimination diet can help you determine if toxins in a particular food are causing skin conditions, chronic sinusitis, or even asthma.

Nature's Superfoods for the Eyes: Soy and Wine

Soy: The Extraordinary Legume

Soybeans have a higher protein content than any plant; they also contain vitamins, essential fatty acids, and coenzyme Q10. Soy also contains some of the most potent phytochemicals of any plant food, including daidzein and genistein, which appear to have a positive influence on hormone levels. Since high estrogen levels have been linked to the development of hormone-sensitive cancers of the breast, uterus, and prostate, soy may have cancer-preventive activities. It is also thought to reduce the incidence of colon polyps, which can precede colon cancer.

Soy has also been shown to increase bone mineral content, thereby decreasing bone fragility and helping to prevent osteoporosis. It decreases total cholesterol by balancing LDL and HDL cholesterol (which may help prevent heart disease); it dilates coronary arteries (which also prevents heart attack); and it improves kidney function in diabetic men. Soy also helps to block the growth of new blood vessels which, in the eye, can cause blindness in people with diabetic retinopathy.

Soy foods include tofu, tempeh, soy sauce, tamari, miso, natto, and "second-generation" soy foods like soy sausages and burgers.

Wine: To Your Health

One of my patients, an older woman who had always enjoyed French food—cream soups and rich sauces—told me one day that she was suffering terribly with her arthritis. I advised her to stop consuming dairy products and to substitute a glass or two of red wine for her usual dinnertime martinis. Not long afterwards, she told me that not only was her arthritis improved, but she thought her vision was better, too.

Wine is produced by using microorganisms to ferment grapes, creating alcohol. It has many health benefits, including protecting against some eye diseases. Wine contains, in a dilute state, many things necessary for health: amino acids, anthocyanidins, flavones, phenols (like resveratrol, which has antioxidant and anti-estrogen activities), tannins, small amounts of vitamin C, high levels of rutin, some B vitamins, including thiamine (which seems to be helpful in treating Alzheimer's disease), and alcohol (which, in low doses, is beneficial to circulation and the retina).

Researchers at Kaiser Permanente (in Oakland, California), found that one glass of wine (or beer) a day reduced the incidence of heart disease by 20 percent. Countries in which more red wine is consumed have the lowest mortality rates, and countries in which the least red wine is drunk have the highest. Red wine (one or two glasses a day) has been shown to decrease the risk of developing macular degeneration, possibly because of its high MSM (methanylsulfonyl-methane) content. MSM is a high-sulfur compound that is also a glutathione and lipoic acid-booster.

Both red and white wine protect against the organisms that cause food poisoning. The only difference between red and white wine is that the grapes' skins are discarded before the fermentation process begins in making white wine. The skins are left in red wine for several weeks as it ferments, not only giving the red wine its color but dissolving the bioflavonoids out of grapes' skin.

In the early 1990s, American nutritional researchers began studying the so-called "French Paradox": why the French have a relatively low rate of heart disease despite a very high fat diet. They found that the red wine the French consume along with all that filet mignon smothered under Béarnaise sauce thins the blood, lowers blood pressure, and decreases platelet stickiness, thereby decreasing the incidence of heart attack and stroke.

If you don't drink alcohol, you can obtain the same benefits from grape juice. Grape juice and grape seed extracts contain high levels of proanthocyanidins (OPCs), some of the most protective phenols in red wine.

Sulfites used as preservatives in wine may cause headaches in sensitive individuals. The FDA is considering listing the sulfite content of all foods, hopefully including wine, on their labels. If you are sensitive to sulfites but like to drink red wine, look for organic wine with no sulfites added. There is more iron in European wines than in American wines, so if iron is a problem for you, you may want to have your physician check your blood level periodically.

Other Superfoods

Remember that the egg is designed to allow a highly vulnerable, developing animal to survive. It contains nine amino acids, vitamins A, D, E, and almost all the B vitamins. It also contains magnesium, calcium, and small amounts of iron, zinc, iodine, and manganese. Because of the lecithin in egg yolk, you can eat as many as six eggs a week without affecting your cholesterol, Dean Ornish, M.D., who has redefined treatment of heart disease, still recommends egg whites on his reasonably restricted diet.

Algae, bean sprouts, broccoli sprouts, and wheat germ also contain many essential nutrients, including the Omega-3 fatty acids. I'm sure research will continue to identify many other "superfoods" for eyes and body.

Read the Label

Be aware of what you are eating. Practice defensive shopping. For example, what's in that "organic" tomato sauce? Perhaps the tomatoes were grown organically, but how much salt is in the sauce? Does it have MSG in it? Were chemical preservatives added after the organically grown tomatoes were made into a sauce?

Read the label so you can eliminate ingredients to which you are sensitive. If MSG gives you a headache, don't buy any type of prepared, canned, or frozen food containing MSG. If you don't pay attention to what's in the food you're buying, who will?

Dr. Abel's Recommendations

• Eat some protein in the morning. Eggs contain the amino acids taurine and tyrosine, which help to wake you up.

• Consume some carbohydrate at dinner. Carbohydrate helps to slow you down and put you to sleep. (If weight is a problem, you may have to limit your total carbohydrate intake.)

• Eliminate refined sugar and flour. Avoid processed grains; substitute whole grains, which contain fiber and phytic acid.

• Eat a salad every day—it's a great way to consume raw vegetables.

• Obtain your calcium from green leafy vegetables, not dairy foods.

• Shop at a market or store where you trust the freshness and quality of the food. You can't get good nutrients from bad food.

• Remember that *fat-free* does not mean "calorie free." "Low fat" foods are often high in carbohydrates, which can cause weight gain.

• Control your weight if it's a problem. Obesity is a major risk factor in worsening diabetes, heart disease, and other life-threatening conditions.

• Avoid artificial sweeteners like Nutrasweet (aspartame), which are neurotoxins. They can damage the optic nerve as well as other nervous tissues in your body. I have heard that Canadian pilots are advised not to drink too many diet sodas to avoid the possibility of seizures during flight.

• Drink plenty of water. We all need water to flush toxins from our bodies and hydrate our cells. Limit your exposure to chlorinated water by using a filter at home.

• Avoid the "fake fats" (like Simpless and Olean). They only make you hungrier (since they're unsatisfying), provide unnecessary chemicals, and serve as a source of empty calories.

• Avoid as many toxins as possible in your food, water, and air. While air pollution is hard to avoid, you can use common sense to limit your exposure. Don't go jogging alongside a busy highway, for instance, and try to avoid secondhand smoke. Handle raw poultry and meat carefully, and cook it thoroughly enough to kill bacteria, viruses, and parasites.

• Buy organic produce when you can to avoid consuming pesticides. If you're unable to buy organic greens and vegetables, scrub your produce well (it also doesn't hurt to scrub organic produce carefully—it grows in dirt, too). Even "prewashed" salad greens and cut vegetables should be washed before you eat them. Combining lemon juice and table salt creates a weak solution of hydrochloric acid that's very effective for scrubbing fruit, killing any stray organisms that may lurk on your produce.

- If it's right for you, have one glass of wine daily, but don't overdo it, or you won't receive wine's benefits.
- Relax. Create your own stress-reduction plan. Learn yoga, meditate, or just sit quietly for five minutes at the same time every day.
- Get enough sleep. Your eyes—and your body—heal themselves at night, in the dark, while you sleep.

Summary

I'm convinced that the long-term treatment and prevention of disease must utilize food, which is nature's pharmacy. While food will always be more nutritious than pills, there are oceans of evidence that we can neutralize eye and other diseases through nutrition and supplementation. Remember that the eyes are an extension of the whole body, and that anything you put into your body, good or bad, you're also putting into your eyes.

Visit the fields and the gardens in your search for better health, which starts with good nutrition. Be aware of the culprits that rob us of our nutrients: smoking, dehydration, drinking coffee, excessive alcohol consumption, poor digestion, certain diseases, certain medications, and stress.

People must have desire and discipline to manage their diets. Unfortunately, we often need to become ill before realizing we need to make new choices. As patients and doctors, we must recognize that disease prevention and management are one. Small changes can have great impact over time. Each day, examine the little changes you've already made and those you can continue to make and, day by day, you will be more in charge of improving your health and preserving your vision.

In the fifth century B.C., Hippocrates said, "Let food be your medicine; let medicine be your food." Try to follow his advice in designing your own nutritional program to protect your eyes and body. I want you to shine when you take your next eye exam.

CHAPTER 15

Supplement Your Vision

An elderly woman from Pittsburgh called me because she had seen me discuss how I manage macular degeneration, using nutrition and supplements on the television show The 700 Club. *She has the dry form of macular degeneration, with vision of 20/100 in her good right eye and 20/400 in her bad left eye. Her eye doctor, after studying extensive diagnostic photographs of her eyes, had regretfully told her that nothing could be done for her. After seeing me on television, however, she decided to ask if I thought anything could be done to keep her from losing more of her eyesight. I recommended a nutritional program (see Chapter 8) and asked that she contact me again in three months to let me know how she was doing. Three months later, she wrote to tell me that her vision had improved by five lines on the eye chart in her good right eye and by two lines in her bad left eye. Needless to say, she was very happy that her vision had improved instead of continuing to degenerate. She added that her retina specialist told her, "Whatever you're doing, by all means, keep it up."*

I agree with most nutritionists that the best way to obtain a broad spectrum of nutrients is to eat a carefully balanced diet. I also live in the real world, and know that isn't always possible. We skip meals, lead stressful lives, and eat on the run, none of which is helpful to either digestion or the absorption of nutrients. It's also very difficult to acquire from diet alone the large quantities of specific vitamins and nutrients needed to stop cataracts, glaucoma, macular degeneration, and diabetic retinopathy. Therefore, in my opinion, it's often necessary to supplement the diet with vitamins, minerals, and other nutritional substances in an intelligently designed program.

We're deficient in minerals partly because our fruits and vegetables are grown in mineral-depleted soil. As of 1964, American soil was deficient in fifty or sixty essential minerals, and the soil quality hasn't improved in recent years. Modern farming and harvesting methods, which have turned farming into factory work, are partly to blame for the poor quality of our soil. On the one hand, these farming methods have resulted in the United States having the least-expensive food supply in the world. On the other hand, we get what we pay for.

If you don't eat a primarily plant-based diet, consuming at least five different fruits and vegetables each day, you'll probably want to build up your antioxidant bank account with supplements. New phytochemicals are being discovered every day. We'll examine some of the major antioxidants that help protect us from free radicals.

Antioxidants, which abound in plant foods and can be taken as supplements (like vitamin C, antioxidant enzymes, and flavonoids like quercitin) fight free-radical damage. Cataract, macular degeneration, glaucoma, diabetic retinopathy, and dry eye are all caused in part by free-radical damage. All can be helped to various degrees by antioxidants like vitamin C, the carotenoids (especially lutein and zeaxanthin), vitamin E, glutathione, and the B vitamins.

So much research has now accumulated about the way various vitamins, bioflavonoids, enzymes, and minerals help to prevent (and, in some cases, reverse) eye diseases that it is very difficult to argue against selective supplementation.

Vitamins

Your eyes, like every other tissue in your body, are vulnerable to attack by free radicals, which are neutralized by antioxidants. Although many powerful antioxidants can be obtained from food (see Chapter 14), preventing or reversing eye diseases requires ingesting additional amounts of antioxidant vitamins.

Vitamins are classified as either fat- or water-soluble. The fat-soluble vitamins are A (and beta-carotene, its precursor, as well as the other carotenes), D, E, and K. The fat-soluble vitamins are stored in the body. The B and C vitamins are water-soluble, which means you flush them from your body and need to replace them daily.

Fat-Soluble Vitamins

The history of *vitamin A*, the first vitamin to be recognized in modern times, dates back to the ancient Egyptian *Ebers Papyrus* (1500 B.C.). When isolated, it is a yellow crystal called *retinol*—which should clear up any mystery about its relationship with the retina. Vitamin A nourishes night vision (via the rods), while a carotene related to vitamin A named *lutein* feeds the center of the retina (the *macula*), nourishing color vision (via the cones). It is also necessary to form tears to lubricate the eye, and avoid dehydration of the cornea and conjunctiva. Therefore, it is important to supplement these nutrients, especially before enduring an insult like laser treatment. Vitamin A is also essential for immunity and cell growth. Vitamin A is found at high levels in liver and other meat products, in vegetables high in carotenes (like spinach and carrots), and in fruits (especially apricots, papaya, and melons). Butter, cheese, cod liver oil, and egg yolks are also high in vitamin A, but many of these foods contain high levels of saturated fats. Foods rich in vitamin A also tend to contain one or more of the other carotenes (such as beta-carotene, zeaxanthin, lycopene, or lutein), many of which work together.

Vitamin A deficiency can not only cause blindness, it can be fatal. It manifests primarily as vision and eye problems, including poor night vision, cataracts, and ulceration of the cornea (which can result in vision loss). Too much Vitamin A, on the other hand, can produce birth defects, miscarriage, headache, vomiting, other general signs of toxicity (like rash or hair loss), and liver damage. You would have to take more than 17,000 IU vitamin A daily for at least one year to accumulate a toxic dose, however.

The *carotenoids (carotenes)* are related to vitamin A. More than six hundred carotenoids have been discovered, but only six are found in a typical American diet (alpha-carotene, beta-carotene, cryptoxanthin, lutein, lycopene, and zeaxanthin). Fourteen carotenes are found in blood, however, demonstrating that they are being manufactured by the liver. Only a couple of the known carotenes, primarily beta-carotene, are metabolized into vitamin A. Research is demonstrating that dietary carotenoids, in addition to being potent antioxidants, play a protective role in age-related macular degeneration. All the carotenes have specific functions in the retina, the lens, or cell membranes, so all are important in preserving sight. Consuming large amounts of the carotenes (and vitamin A) causes yellowing of the skin, which goes away when you lower your consumption.

The best way to ensure getting a variety of carotenes in your diet is to eat plenty of carotene-rich foods, which include: algae, arugula, bok choy, broccoli, broccoli rabe, carrots, collard greens, corn, dandelion greens, kale, mustard greens, red peppers, sea vegetables (seaweed), spinach, sweet potatoes, Swiss chard, tomatoes, turnip greens, watercress, winter squash, apples, apricots, cantaloupe, cherries, kumquats, papaya, and pumpkin.

- **Beta-carotene,** vitamin A's precursor, is probably the best-known carotene, but foods rich in beta-carotene also contain other carotenes. For beta-carotene to be metabolized into vitamin A, you must have sufficient protein as well as thyroid hormone, vitamin C, and zinc. It's impossible to overdose on beta-carotene, because the body knows when we have enough vitamin A, and stops converting beta-carotene into the vitamin. Like vitamin A, beta-carotene is crucial to preserving sight.
- **Lutein** (a carotene) is especially important to the health of the eye and maintenance of good sight. Lutein is the yellow pigment found in the macula (the center of the retina). It is a crucial protector against macular degeneration and cataracts, because it counteracts damage from ultraviolet and blue light.
- **Lycopene** (another carotene) is a very powerful antioxidant (twice as strong an antioxidant as beta-carotene) that is reported to have antitumor properties. It is most concentrated in tomatoes and tomato products (juice, paste, and sauce), and is also found in dried apricots, pink grapefruit, and watermelon.
- **Zeaxanthin,** together with lutein, forms the yellow pigment that protects the macula from light-induced damage. It's also found in small amounts in the lens (as is lutein) and may play a role in preventing cataracts.

Vitamin D is the only vitamin that acts like a hormone. It's required to maintain bone strength, muscle functioning, and mineral absorption. We manufacture vitamin D after exposure to sunlight. Without sunlight, vitamin D deficiency develops, usually manifest as deformed bones (rickets). Researchers recommend that most people under the age of 70 consume 400 IU of vitamin D daily (an amount typically contained in a multivitamin), and that people age 70 and older take 600 IU of vitamin D daily.

Vitamin E is an important antioxidant that blocks the breakdown of essential fats in cell membranes. Vitamin E is found in the retina and lens. People who consume a high enough level of vitamin E (even 60 IU, although 400 IU is a healthier level) have a reduced rate of cataract formation, according to several studies. Vitamin E works with selenium and glutathione to help protect cell membranes, and may also support immunity as well as delay aging. Vitamin E deficiency results in muscular dystrophy, neurological difficulties, and reproductive problems. Along with low bioflavonoid levels, low vitamin E allows capillary walls to weaken (including the capillaries that nourish the eyes), drusen to form in the retina (a sign of macular degeneration), and the pigment concentration in the retina to be lost (which decreases visual acuity). The signs of toxicity are muscle weakness, rash, and upset stomach. Food sources of vitamin E include asparagus, avocado, broccoli, spinach, peaches, dried prunes, beef, turkey, whole milk, soy, and cold-pressed safflower, sunflower, and wheat germ oils.

Vitamin K, which is essential to the production of several blood-clotting factors, got its name from the German word *koagulation.* It is found in many foods.

Water-Soluble Vitamins

The primary function of the *B vitamins* is to facilitate nerve impulses. B vitamins include thiamine (B_1), riboflavin (B_2), niacin (B_3); folic acid (B_4), pantothenic acid (B_5), pyridoxine (B_6), B_{12}, and biotin. Inositol and choline are unofficial members of the B vitamin family, and are often included in B vitamin complexes. (Choline is an important component of the neurotransmitter acetylcholine, and appears to help preserve memory; it is deficient in people with Huntington's disease and Alzheimer's disease.) All the B vitamins perform vital neurologic functions and many work together, so it's important to take a good B vitamin complex to maintain their balance. Diuretics, excessive sweating, alcohol, and caffeine can cause depletion of B vitamins.

Vitamin C is the second-most important antioxidant in the lens of the eye (glutathione is the first). It is present in every cell of the body, recharges vitamin E and other antioxidants, and helps lower cholesterol by binding it in the intestines. Vitamin C helps make collagen (which strengthens capillaries, including those that nourish the retina), and helps prevent cataracts by guarding the lens against free radical damage. A 1998 study performed at Tufts University in Boston found that long-term consumption of vitamin C (400–800 mg daily) can reduce the incidence of cataracts in women by 77 percent. It has also been found to lower elevated eye pressure (a risk factor for glaucoma), and is used to treat experimental corneal burns. The cornea can actually be rebuilt using vitamin C, and many cornea specialists recommend that patients with chemical burns take as much as two grams (2000 mg) of vitamin C daily. We are beginning to work with vitamin C as an eyedrop. Taken orally, it is most effective when consumed in conjunction with bioflavonoids. Vitamin C deficiency, called scurvy, weakens collagen in the body, resulting in bleeding from capillaries. Too much vitamin C can cause diarrhea, a response that varies widely among individuals. If you have this reaction, reduce your dose. (Your body will accept more vitamin C, however, when you have a cold or the flu.)

A study published in April 1998 suggested that more than 500 mg a day of vitamin C could cause genetic damage (a change in one DNA base was found in volunteers who took 500 mg of vitamin C daily for six weeks), but that short study has not been duplicated. In addition, it was performed in a very polluted city in Great Britain (pollution can also damage DNA). This result has never been seen before, even though millions of people have taken vitamin C in doses exceeding 500 mg daily for years, with no bad effects. I've definitely had fewer colds after taking two grams of vitamin C every day. I think that, pending further studies, the evidence is overwhelming that vitamin C is good news.

Enzymes

Enzymes, the major antioxidants in the body, are significant free-radical fighters. Raw vegetables are loaded with enzymes. The critically important enzymes are glutathione peroxidase, glutamine, reductase, superoxide dismutase (SOD), and catalase.

Glutathione, a pre-enzyme, is a very important antioxidant and detoxifier. Glutathione is the major antioxidant in the crystalline lens of the eye. It is found in large quantities in a healthy eye but is deficient when cataracts form. It's found in every cell, and has fourteen times the power of catalase and two hundred times the power of SOD. Glutathione is composed of three amino acids—cysteine, glutamine, and glycine—each of which has its own actions in the body. Astronauts took large amounts of cysteine each day, for instance, because NASA scientists knew it's the most effective radiation neutralizer. Glycine helps to reduce toxicity of food preservatives and other toxins. Glutamine, small quantities of which are necessary for brain and eye function, protects against macular degeneration and is important in healing the gastrointestinal tract.

Glutathione has been called the "anti-aging molecule of the future." A 1994 study of a group of thirty-three elderly individuals found that higher glutathione levels were associated with lower cholesterol, lower blood pressure, lower body weight, fewer reported illnesses, and higher self-reported health status. In contrast, elderly individuals with arthritis, diabetes, or heart disease were found to have lower levels of glutathione. A 1992 study that found glutathione levels decrease with age, and concluded that glutathione status, physical health, and longevity are closely intertwined.

Table 25. Recommended Daily Allowances of Vitamins and Minerals

Vitamin/Mineral	RDA (Women)		RDA (Men)		Toxic Level	
Vitamin A	1000	mcg	1000	mcg	50,000	IU
Vitamin D	200	IU	200	IU	1800	IU
Vitamin E	12–15	IU	15	IU	1600	IU
Vitamin K	65	mcg	80	mcg	500	mcg
B_1 (Thiamin)	1.1	mg	1.2–1.5	mg	not	established
B_2 (Riboflavin)	1.3	mg	1.7	mg	not	established
B_3 (Niacin)	13–20	mg	15–20	mg	1000	mg (variable)
B_5 (Pantothenic acid)	4–7	mg	4–5	mg	not	established
B_6 (Pyridoxine)	1.6	mg	2	mg	not	established
B_{12}	2	mg	2	mg	2	g
Folic acid	180	mcg	200	mcg	not	established
Vitamin C	60	mcg	60	mcg	not	established
Biotin	30–300	mg	30–300	mg	not	established
Calcium	1200	mg	1200	mg	not	established
Manganese	2.5–5	mg	2.5–5	mg	not	established
Magnesium	300	mg	400	mg	not	established
Iron	15	mg	10	mg	not	established
Zinc	12	mg	15	mg	150	mcg
Iodine	150	mcg	150	mcg	not	established
Selenium	55	mcg	70	mcg	200	mcg

RDA listings were designed to give the public the minimum requirements to avoid deficiency and malnutrition conditions. These minimums are constantly being raised for many of the vitamins and minerals to conform with new research as it becomes available. In the opinion of the author and many complementary physicians, many of these minimums are far too low.

Recommended daily allowances (RDAs) of vitamins and minerals are established by the National Research Council, operating under the auspices of the charter granted to the National Academy of Sciences by the Congress of the United States (last revised in 1989).

The term *recommended daily allowance* is abbreviated as *RDA; International unit* is abbreviated as *IU; microgram* is abbreviated as *mcg; milligram* is abbreviated as mg; *gram* is abbreviated as *g.* Remember that levels of fat-soluble vitamins are cumulative, so if you are using them for more than a month, be sure to stay well under the toxic dose in your daily regimen. (See appendices G and H for latest recommendations.)

Don't take glutathione supplements; instead, consume nutrients that contribute to glutathione production, such as alpha lipoic acid, N-acetyl cysteine (NAC), selenium, and vitamin B_2. Vitamin C, grape seed, Pycnogenol™, turmeric, and milk thistle also contribute to the production of glutathione.

Food sources of glutathione include asparagus, avocado, broccoli, cauliflower, garlic, onions, parsley, potatoes, purslane, spinach, squash, tomatoes, apples, pears, watermelon, walnuts, and eggs. Glutathione production is boosted by cysteine-containing foods, including beans, eggs, and whole grains. Sulfur-containing foods are also glutathione-boosters, including chives, garlic, leeks, onions, scallions, and shallots. High-sulfer foods are best consumed raw, since they're damaged by heat.

Glutathione helps produce two major detoxification enzymes, glutathione peroxidase and glutathione reductase, which prevent breakdown of cell membranes and decrease toxins like radiation, pollution, smoke, and drugs.

Glutathione peroxidase protects against eye disease (particularly cataracts), heart disease, cancer, AIDS, and numerous chronic conditions. Its deficiency is thought to contribute to growth retardation as well as to the development of anemia, disorders of the kidney, pancreas, and liver, muscle disease, and reproductive failure.

Bioflavonoids

Bioflavonoids (or flavonoids) comprise a subcategory of phytochemicals (plant chemicals). Flavonoids, along with chlorophyll and the carotenoids, give fruits, vegetables, and leaves their brilliant colors, while protecting them from the effects of ultraviolet light. In people, flavonoids appear to have powerful antioxidant, anti-inflammatory, and anticancer properties, as well as generally increasing immunity, protecting the liver, and facilitating blood flow and are often combined with vitamin C supplements. Flavonoids also prevent collagen breakdown, improving the integrity of capillaries (including those in the back of the eye). More than eight hundred flavonoids have been identified. Neither RDAs nor toxic levels have been established for the bioflavonoids, since they are only now coming under intensive scrutiny. Many researchers in the field, however, feel these compounds hold great promise as the medicines of tomorrow.

Anthocyanidins help improve circulation to the retina and other parts of the eye and slow the development of macular degeneration and cataracts. They can be obtained from bilberry, grape extract, and cranberry supplements.

Proanthocyanidins (OPCs) are powerful antioxidants extracted from maritime pine bark, grape seeds, and *Ginkgo biloba*. They are helpful in treating macular degeneration and other circulatory disorders. They appear to increase intracellular vitamin C levels, inhibit collagen destruction, and decrease capillary fragility (which may be how they help prevent macular degeneration).

Quercetin is perhaps the most potent natural antihistamine. It is useful in alleviating allergies and sinusitis, as well as countering diabetic retinopathy. It helps prevent leakage in the middle ear and sinuses, and prevents blood vessels from leaking in diabetics.

Resveratrol appears to protect against heart disease. Red wine is the usual source cited for resveratrol, but USDA researchers found that peanuts (which are technically legumes) are very high in resveratrol. A study of Seventh Day Adventists (who are mostly vegetarian) showed that those who consumed nuts (almonds and walnuts, as well as peanuts) more than four times a week reduced their heart attack risk by 50 percent.

Rutin is an anticancer substance extracted from the rinds of citrus fruits, grapes, and berries. This common bioflavonoid is often combined with vitamin C in supplements. (It is also found in wine.)

Silymarin is a bioflavonoid extracted from milk thistle that increases the glutathione content of the liver.

Minerals

Minerals are not manufactured by any kind of living creature—they are inorganic substances—but we need them to perform numerous metabolic processes. Minerals regulate the flow of fluids in and out of cells. They also mediate electrical impulses among nerve cells, thus controlling heartbeat, brain function, and vision.

Boron modulates inflammatory and immune processes, and helps to prevent bone loss.

Calcium is necessary to strengthen bones and prevent osteoporosis. The recommended 1000 mg daily can be obtained from 1.5 pints of milk, three ounces of cheddar cheese, or two cups of spinach. Supplementing is probably important for those who don't consume 1000 mg from food. Nondairy sources of calcium include almonds, broccoli, mustard greens, pinto beans, spinach, and tofu.

Chromium is an essential trace mineral that is beneficial in sugar metabolism and is said to help control both diabetes and lactose intolerance.

Copper is required for oxygen to be carried successfully in red blood cells. It also helps produce collagen, melanin (pigment in skin and hair), and the enzyme superoxide dismutase (SOD).

Iron works with copper to bind oxygen to red blood cells; its deficiency results in anemia, muscle weakness, and susceptibility to infections.

Magnesium appears to be crucial in maintaining eye health. Diabetic patients with high blood levels of magnesium are less likely to develop diabetic retinopathy than those with low levels, and it improves vision in glaucoma patients. It is the natural calcium channel-blocker, lowering blood pressure by dilating and relaxing blood vessels (high blood pressure can lead to high internal eye pressure) and stopping vasospasm (a cause of sudden death). It contributes to production of neurotransmitters like serotonin. (Low serotonin levels have been linked to depression and other ills.) Food sources include many kinds of beans and whole grains, almonds, brazil nuts, cashews, kale, mustard and other greens, spinach, bananas, blackberries, dates, dried figs, mangoes, watermelon, shrimp, and tuna.

Molybdenum is required for DNA and RNA metabolism, and contributes to creating a number of enzymes.

Potassium, along with magnesium is one of the two major minerals inside cells. It is essential in maintaining heartbeat, muscle contraction, conduction of nerve impulses, and protein synthesis. Severe potassium deficiency can be fatal (causing heart attack), but almost never occurs in healthy people. Its usual symptoms include weakness and muscle pains. People on diuretics must be especially careful to maintain adequate potassium levels, and those with kidney failure must be certain not to accumulate toxic potassium levels. Food sources of potassium include dandelion greens, Swiss chard, watercress, and meat.

Selenium stimulates immunity and speeds wound healing; its deficiency promotes cataract formation. It is an essential precursor to glutathione peroxidase, which protects not only against cataracts but also against macular degeneration, heart disease, cancer, AIDS, and other chronic conditions. Selenium toxicity produces black or fragile fingernails, a metallic taste in the mouth, garlic breath odor, nausea, and dizziness.

Zinc is a critical cofactor in several enzyme-governed functions, including immune responsiveness, protein synthesis, and gene expression. It appears to stabilize macular degeneration. Zinc deficiency causes vision disturbances, poor wound healing, mental sluggishness, and increased susceptibility to infections. Consuming too much zinc can cause copper deficiency. Signs of toxicity include nausea, vomiting, and diarrhea.

Amino Acids/Proteins

Amino acids are the building blocks of protein. Although we make most of the amino acids we need in our own bodies, the essential amino acids must be acquired from the diet or through supplementation.

NAC, or *N-acetyl-cysteine,* is a sulfur-containing amino acid that boosts glutathione production. Cysteine is one of the semi-essential amino acids, and may be one we need to supplement regularly.

Taurine is found at high concentrations in the retina, which it nourishes and defends against damage from UV light (thereby protecting against macular degeneration). Taurine is depleted in diabetics, which raises the question of whether its deficiency contributes to the development of diabetic retinopathy as well as to other complications of diabetes. It is suspected, but not proved, that taurine deficiency may contribute to the development of age-related macular degeneration and that supplementing with taurine may protect against it. Unlike the other amino acids, taurine is not incorporated into proteins, but exists independently in tissue, most abundantly in the retina, platelets, muscles, and the nervous system. It is not considered an essential amino acid because it can be metabolized in the body from cysteine. Taurine makes up 50 percent of the free amino acid in the heart and is thought to strengthen it.

Metallothionein is a protein that binds copper, cadmium, and zinc in the body. It's thought to protect the body against toxic heavy metals.

Digestive Aids

As we age, our levels of stomach acid naturally decrease—which means we shouldn't take antacids for our digestive woes. Some older people are unable to absorb nutrients from their food because of age-related changes in the intestinal environment. Don't assume you can fix every digestive tract ailment you experience, especially in older age. Be sure to ask your doctor about diagnostic tests if you experience persistent digestive difficulties. If your troubles are due to not having adequate digestive enzymes or stomach acid, there are several types of supplements that can relieve symptoms of poor digestion (bloating, gas) and increase nutrient absorption.

Other Helpful Supplements

Alpha-lipoic acid protects all cells and, unlike most substances, freely enters the brain. It is the only antioxidant that is both fat- and water-soluble; therefore, it enters and nourishes all parts of the body. People with normal metabolism and no complaints do not need alpha-lipoic acid supplementation, since it is produced in the body. However, studies have shown that patients with glaucoma experience both enhancement in color vision and generalized visual sensitivity while taking 150 mg of alpha-lipoic acid daily. It's been found to reduce diabetic cataract formation and helps burn sugar by increasing insulin's efficiency, suggesting that it may be helpful to diabetics in other ways. It also enhances the antioxidant activities of glutathione, vitamin E, and vitamin C and may possibly even substitute for them. Any eye condition that is improved by the presence of glutathione—including cataract, glaucoma, macular degeneration, and diabetic retinopathy—can benefit from alpha-lipoic acid supplementation.

Blue-green algae is perhaps the lowest link in the food chain. It contains all the essential amino acids, as well as protein, Omega-3 essential fatty acids, chlorophyll, vitamins (including beta-carotene and vitamin B_{12}), and trace minerals. It is said to increase energy, relieve stress and depression, and improve digestion, memory, and mental clarity.

Coenzyme Q10 (acetyl coenzyme A) helps cells break down food into energy. It is required for the synthesis of ATP, the cell's basic energy molecule. After about age 35, our production of CoQ10 begins to decrease, and deficiency of CoQ10 can contribute to gum disease, breakdown in the immune system, and heart failure. More CoQ10 is found in the heart, in fact, than in any other tissue in the body. CoQ10 is also known as *ubiquinone*, because it's in all plant and animal cells. The best preparation of CoQ10 comes in soft gelatin capsules with a base of soybean oil.

Collagen type II is one of the fourteen types of collagen and is the most effective in relieving symptoms of arthritis. Generally derived from chicken collagen, it contains glucosamine sulfate (which helps rebuild cartilage), chondroitin sulfate A (an anti-inflammatory substance), and the newly discovered antioxidant cartilage matrix glycoprotein, among other substances.

Pyruvate is a form of sugar (glucose) that actually may help dieters lose weight. In studies of people supplementing a low-fat diet with pyruvate, more weight and total body fat was lost compared to people on a low-fat diet alone. Gas, bloating, or diarrhea are occasional side effects of pyruvate. Pyruvate appears to protect against cataracts in lab experiments.

Phytates, also known as phytic acid (inositol hexaphosphate), is incorporated into cell membranes as phosphotidylinositol (PI). One of the components of PI, inositol, was found in one study to relieve depression and anxiety in previously unresponsive individuals. Phytates are found in high fiber foods like cereals, legumes, and vegetables.

IP₆ (Inositol Hexaphosphate): Research done at the University of Maryland School of Medicine by AbulKalam Shamsuddin, M.D., Ph.D., and colleagues conclusively shows that IP₆ is a new major anti-cancer agent.

Rain Forest Remedies for Eyes

The modern ophthalmologist's office is so filled with technological wonders that it's no surprise we forget that the first eye medicines came from plants. Acknowledging the botanical heritage of the powerful Western drugs (as well as modern Chinese herbal formulas) that we use today will help us discover the treatments we'll use tomorrow. For example, we've known how to dilate the pupil of the eyes for centuries using atropine, which can be derived from any one of several solanaceous plants, including deadly nightshade, henbane, jimson weed, and/or mandrake. The first written record of the use of atropine (or its close relative scopolamine, found in the same plants) is in the *Ebers Papyrus*, written about 1500 B.C., but it was undoubtedly used long before recorded history. Today we synthesize atropine in the laboratory, where we also search for compounds that act more efficiently with fewer side effects, since both atropine and scopolamine (whether obtained from plants or the laboratory) affect not only the eyes but also the cardiovascular, gastrointestinal, respiratory, thermoregulatory, and urinary systems.

The search for new drugs is proceeding at fever pitch because of the rapid destruction of the rain forests. The oceans, deserts, and temperate climates are also being explored for new drugs. For instance, Amylior Pharmaceuticals, Inc., is developing a blood sugar-lowering compound derived from gila monster saliva. Scientists at VIMRX Pharmaceuticals, Inc., discovered an anti-inflammatory agent for arthritis by studying the colorful sea whip. These are just two of the potential therapeutics in nature's apothecary.

A renewed interest in the plants growing in our endangered rain forests has been generated by the work of several ethnobotanists—scientists who study how primitive people used plants—and by the publication of books like *Rainforest Remedies*. Michael J. Balick, Ph.D., of the New York Botanical Garden, published a scientific report in 1995 estimating that more than three hundred drugs, worth nearly $147 billion, await discovery in tropical rain forests. Dr. Balick and his colleague in Belize, Dr. Rosita Arvigo, gave me the opportunity to visit an old Mayan Indian shaman named Ponti (nicknamed "El Santo," the saint), who had been treating people in the area for more than sixty years. In addition to maintaining some of Ponti's herbal resources, Dr. Balick and his colleagues have convinced the government to subsidize farmers who grow herbs instead of marijuana.

Furthermore, scientists like Mark Plotkin, Ph.D., an ethnobotanist associated with Conservation International, has established a program that gives economic aid to young people in South American indigenous communities so they can study and preserve traditional medicine. And researchers from Shaman Pharmaceuticals, Inc., of San Francisco, actively search rain forests in Africa, Asia, and South America for pharmaceutically useful plants. Even the National Cancer Institute maintains about 20,000 samples of plants—an amazing number—to test for antitumor and antimicrobial compounds.

I believe ophthalmologists should use both modern drugs and natural remedies whenever possible. Herbal preparations can provide safe and effective relief from many disorders without the side effects that prescription or even over-the-counter drugs often produce.

Many herbs are powerful substances—that's why they work—and they should be used with caution. If you decide to try an herbal preparation for any medical condition, research the risks and benefits, as you should with any medication. And be sure to tell your physicians, including your eye doctor.

An herb is a flowering plant lacking a woody stem that is valued for its medicinal properties, flavor, or scent. The common vernacular expands the definition to include any medicinal plant (woody or nonwoody), including spices, bark, roots, flowers, berries, or even mushrooms.

Herbal preparations are called *standardized* when they've been processed to guarantee a minimum level of the major ingredients. An effective preparation of *Ginkgo biloba*, for instance, should contain 24 percent ginkgosides (its active ingredient). Standardization provides some quality assurance and compensates for the variability of bulk herbs (herbs bought by the ounce rather than in pill form). The label should indicate if the herbal product is standardized, so *read the label*—be responsible for what you buy and put into your body. I advise all my patients and colleagues to use standardized herbs. While it may be a little more expensive, doing so will guarantee that you get the same strength in every dose.

Herbal preparations (and, in fact, all food supplements) are not regulated by the FDA, so buy herbs and supplements from well-established companies and suppliers in whom you have confidence. Most supplement manufacturers have a toll-free telephone number, so don't be afraid to call and inquire about standardization, manufacturing practices, interactions with other drugs, or side effects.

If you are pregnant or nursing, you should not take any herbal preparation without the explicit consent of your physician.

Asia's Wisdom

A Short History of Medicine

A patient tells a doctor, "I have an earache." The doctor replies:

2000 B.C.	"Here, eat this root."
1000 A.D.	"That root is heathen. Here, say this prayer."
1850 A.D.	"That prayer is superstition. Here, drink this potion."
1940 A.D.	"That potion is snake oil. Here, swallow this pill."
1985 A.D.	"That pill is ineffective. Here, take this antibiotic."
2000 A.D.	"That antibiotic is artificial. Here, eat this root."

I'm certain that twenty-first century medicine will rely on ancient healing methods utilizing herbs, for instance, in conjunction with modern medical techniques. We sometimes forget that the causes of many diseases are still just assumed, not known, and that our modern treatments are actually based on trial and error. We physicians must also encourage greater participation by patients in managing their own health—an area where Western practitioners could learn a great deal from our Eastern colleagues.

Chinese herbs, for instance, are useful in treating many eye conditions. I've had more than a dozen patients with chronic red eyes and conjunctivitis who've improved so much after a course of Chinese herbal therapy that they don't have to rely on artificial drugs constantly. In addition, many other health problems (eczema, asthma, and even indigestion) disappeared simultaneously. I've had ten patients with chronic iritis (inflammation inside the eye) who were able to decrease their high-dose cortisone eyedrops, which can accelerate cataracts and may increase intraocular pressure over time, possibly resulting in glaucoma. Two of these patients, after ten years of depending upon very strong eyedrops, discontinued them completely.

If I knew how these Chinese herbs worked physiologically, I'd be delighted to share the knowledge with you, but I don't. All I really know is that the Chinese system of using herbs to resolve disharmonies in the body does work.

Chinese traditional medicine (CTM) and Ayurvedic (Indian or Buddhist) medicine have both been used with success for millennia but remained largely unknown in the West. As the twentieth century drew to a close, however, the Western world become more aware of these two ancient Eastern health care systems. Each is so complex that it would be difficult to capture its essence in a whole book dedicated to that subject alone. That being said, I will introduce you to the fundamentals of each.

One of the biggest stumbling blocks to Westerners' understanding of Chinese traditional medicine is the unfamiliar and seemingly exotic language used to describe both illness and health. Ancient Chinese physicians developed medical concepts by observing nature and translated those observations to the human body. For instance, they often represented the kidneys by water and the brain by air. Even today, Chinese practitioners don't use Western words like fever, pneumonia, or cancer to describe illness. Instead, they use words that reflect nature, like heat, dampness, and dryness.

As a sophisticated system involving complex methods of diagnosis and treatment, Chinese traditional medicine has a track record of centuries of positive results: communism, democracy, and even monarchy have not lasted as long. Acupuncture is only one of hundreds of Chinese techniques available to us if we choose to use them and learn from them.

In learning about Chinese traditional medicine, it's important to remember that the ancient concepts underlying its methods are just as scientific as those supporting modern medicine—we just use different words to describe them. The concepts used by Chinese traditional medicine can be applied quite accurately to conditions Western doctors describe in scientific detail.

It's not necessary to be an expert in Chinese traditional medicine to benefit from its concepts either. It is, however, helpful to understand some of the important terms used, like *yin* and *yang*. Chinese texts describe yin and yang as being like the two sides of a mountain. As the sun rises and falls, one side of the mountain is illuminated, and the other is in darkness. When the sun shines on one side of the mountain, it is light, or yang; the other side is dark, or yin. As the sun passes over the top of the mountain, the dark side becomes light—yang and yin exchange.

Philosophically, yin and yang are not the same as good and bad; a more appropriate analogy is strong and weak. We need both strength and weakness. If we used the same amount of force to lift a glass of water as to open a heavy door, we'd throw the glass across the room. In Chinese theory, if someone approaches you with force, you step out of the way and meet it with lightness or weakness.

I think of yin and yang as up and down, two directions that exist together and are necessary to balance each other. Think about your diaphragm as you breathe. It moves downward as you breathe in, and upward as you breathe out. Think of that motion as a circular movement, blending one action into the other. When viewed as two parts of one motion, harmony between the two actions (breathing in and out) is achieved.

Chi is another term integral to understanding Chinese traditional medicine. Chi is energy, the driving force that circulates blood through the body. If we become excited or nervous, for example, we pump more blood, which has more energy—more chi—causing it to move.

When the body is relaxed, chi can flow freely, creating a tingling and warmth felt during meditation or Tai Chi. When chi's flow becomes imbalanced or stagnant, health declines. The body is under constant bombardment from both internal and external forces that affect the circulation of both blood and chi. The aim of Chinese traditional medicine is to use herbs, acupuncture, acupressure, diet, and exercise to encourage harmony and the flow of chi—essential energy—throughout the body to maintain health.

I had a patient who, following back surgery, became progressively depressed and noticed his vision failing. The combination of tightened back muscles and lack of chi flow up the spine blocked his thinking, clouded his outlook, and dimmed his vision. After massage and exercises, he regained his normal vision and cheerful attitude, and returned to work. Since this experience, I've seen many more examples of chi stagnation in the back associated with poor vision. When I see a patient walk slowly into the office, I always consider the consequences of a back problem for his eyes. I can see people's weak chi when I look at their eyes and observe a pale conjunctiva, droopy lid, and languishing look.

In ancient India, religious sages known as *yogis* were also doctors. Not only did these holy men have the time to study medicine, they were keen to study it because illness was viewed as an impediment to spiritual development and enlightenment. About 2500 years ago, they recorded their oral knowledge in a famous volume, the *Charaka Samhita*, one of the first compilations of medical knowledge. The medical system described in this and other texts nearly three millennia ago is called Ayurvedic medicine.

Ayurvedic medicine is based on five elements: earth, water, fire, wind, and ether (i.e., space). Additionally, Ayurveda recognizes three fundamental natural forces (known as *doshas*) that underlie everything: creation (*kapha*), destruction (*pitta*), and regulation (*vata*). The doshas act together in the human body, and when they go out of harmony, according to Ayurveda, illness results.

I believe that there is no one true church, but beliefs in many areas, and that the healing arts are no different. We are the sum of what we know, practice, have experienced, and our dreams and goals. Our experiences in health are only as great as the number of adventures we've had. I believe we must venture out from Western medicine to Asian medical systems before concluding that no answer can be found for any specific health problem. Modern Western doctors should incorporate these long-standing tools in their practices to give patients more options for healing.

Table 26. Chinese Herbs for Eye Conditions

I have used these Chinese herbs to treat various eye conditions in consultation with practitioners of Chinese traditional medicine. I do not recommend that anyone attempt to treat him- or herself using these herbs. If you have an eye problem, consult an appropriate specialist. If you need to find an acupuncturist or qualified Chinese herbal physician near you, call the National Certification Commission for Acupuncture and Oriental Medicine (703-548-0994).

Chinese Name	English Name	Action
Jú hua	chrysanthemum flower	Clears the liver and the eyes, and is used for red, painful, dry eyes, or excessive tearing. Also helps to clear floaters, blurry vision, and control dizziness.
Qing xiang zi	celosia seeds	Improves the vision, drains liver "fire." Used for red, painful, swollen eyes, and cataracts.
San qi	pseudoginseng root	Stops eye bleeding. San qi must come from the Yunan Province of China to be genuine.
Chán tuì	cicada moulting	Clears the eyes; used to treat blurry vision and red, painful, swollen eyes.
Mì meng hua	buddleia flower bud	Treats sensitivity to light, excessive tearing, red, swollen, and painful eyes.
Jou qi zi	Chinese wolfberry fruit or lycium fruit	Brightens the eyes (acts on liver and kidney deficiency), and corrects blurred vision, diminished visual acuity, and dizziness.
Huai hua mi	pagoda tree flower	Cools the liver; used to treat red eyes and dizziness due to liver heat.

Table 27. Chinese Herbal Combination Supplements for Eye Conditions
(Available from the Institute for Traditional Medicine. See Resource Guide.)

Supplement Name	Contents	Uses/Indications
Celosia 10	Celosia Rehmannia (raw) Salvia Red peony Eclipta San qi Sophora flower Chrysanthemum Lycium fruit Tang-kuei	Used to treat retinitis and other retinal diseases, as well as hemorrhage or bleeding in the eye.
Chien-Li Tablets	Chien-li-huang Cordycep/Cicada Buddleia Princepia Lycium fruit Chrysanthemum Eriocaulon Tribulus Rehmannia Celosia seed Vitex Cornus Cnidium Cassia seed Cuscuta	Aids in the treatment of cataract or any clouding of the vision due to other sources (such as trauma or infection).
Salvia Shou Wu (a five-herb combination)	Salvia Cnidium Carthamus Tang-kuei vessels Red peony	Used to move the blood and strengthen the heart as well as in treating eye disease in which there is not enough blood flow to the eyes.

PART VI

COMPLEMENTARY OPTIONS

CHAPTER 16

Exercise for Eye Health

Those who think they have not time for bodily exercise will sooner or later have to find time for illness.

—*Edward Stanley, Earl of Derby, 1873*

Scientists continue to discover new ways in which exercise is crucial to maintaining good health, including eye health. Among its many benefits, exercise:

- Lowers intraocular pressure
- Helps children avoid obesity, which can lead to diabetes
- Increases longevity
- Improves agility, mobility, and sight
- May even help prevent the development of cataracts and macular degeneration

Marvin, a 48-year-old patient of mine, was fifty pounds overweight and had a sedentary lifestyle. In addition to high blood pressure, he suffered from elevated eye pressure, which can lead to glaucoma. I told Marvin that he should begin an exercise regimen, eat only salads for lunch, and avoid desserts for the foreseeable future. To my surprise, he took my advice about limiting his calories, began a walking and treadmill exercise regimen, and lost sixty pounds. To his medical doctor's surprise, Marvin's blood pressure returned to normal, allowing him to give up his medication. I now see Marvin only once a year, because his eye pressure is normal and his eyes are otherwise healthy.

This is not unusual. My patients often ask why an ophthalmologist encourages them to begin an exercise program, to which I reply that exercise strengthens not only their bodies, but also their eyes.

If you think about it, you'll realize that exercise is crucial to maintaining eye health. Exercise helps you lose weight or maintain your optimal weight. Since being overweight is an important risk factor for developing diabetes, and all diabetics are at risk for diabetic eye disease, this concerns me. Exercise also helps to lower high blood pressure, a risk factor for developing increased internal eye pressure and possible glaucoma (see Chapter 7). The eyes are connected to the rest of the body and as exercise, strengthens the body, so does exercise help strengthen the eyes.

Aerobic exercise, using as many muscles as possible (to burn fat) is best for weight loss, according to Barbara deLateur, M.D., who chairs the Department of Rehabilitative Medicine at Johns Hopkins University. "To reduce fat, the appropriate type of exercise is prolonged, aerobic exercise using as many muscles as possible in a reciprocal, rhythmic, low-force fashion," Dr. deLateur reports. "Examples of this include walking, jogging, cycling, and rowing."

That doesn't mean that you don't have to watch what you eat if you're trying to lose weight. Research also shows that people not restricting their diets but walking thirty minutes a day did not have substantial change in weight. It's necessary to walk one hour a day, seven days a week, to lose weight if not dieting simultaneously. Cycling without reducing calories burns more fat, but it also requires cycling sixty minutes a day, seven days a week. Swimmers actually experience no weight loss at all if they do not restrict their caloric intake.

Getting Started

If you didn't previously have a motivation to exercise because of your heart or a weight problem, now you know that exercise is also crucial to maintaining eye health. So start now, following these general guidelines:

- Know your body's limits, and take your overall health situation into consideration. Get your doctor's approval and advice before starting an exercise program, particularly if you've been sedentary for a number of years. And while you're at it, find out what your pulse and blood pressure are. If you're over 40, ask your doctor if you should have an EKG to make sure your heart is healthy.
- Treat yourself to good exercise shoes, whether sneakers or high-tech running shoes.
- Always stretch before exercising. If you have knots or sore points in your muscles, see a chiropractor or get a massage, which also contributes to relaxation.

- Begin in incremental steps, whether you're doing calisthenics, playing tennis, jogging, or even just walking. Don't try to overcome an exercise deficit of several years in one weekend, or you'll hurt yourself.
- As your comfort level rises, increase your exercise intensity level.
- Work out regularly, so that it becomes a habit. After a while, you'll find that you actually miss exercising on the days that you skip it.
- After exercising, stretch again and then cool off by walking slowly for as much as one-quarter mile, whether indoors or out.

A stronger body builds a stronger mind and improves eye health. Exercise decreases stress and regulates hormones, including those that influence the brain. But it's vital to exercise safely. Know the signs that warn against continued exercise:

- Continuous pain
- Any chest pain or pain radiating from neck or jaw
- Shortness of breath
- Irregular heartbeat
- Nausea
- Discomfort in joints or muscles

If your symptoms make you suspect you may be having a heart attack—if you have chest pain, shortness of breath, or an irregular heartbeat—call your physician, call 911, or go to an emergency room immediately.

If you need to learn how to stretch your muscles safely, I suggest reading a good book on the subject like Bob Anderson's *Stretching*. Most books about stretching explain which to use before different types of exercises.

Remember to breathe in slow, rhythmic breaths. This will provide oxygen, create a rhythm in your thinking as well as your breathing, and relax your mind. I can't emphasize too strongly the value of deep, slow, breathing and its contribution to relaxation.

Weight resistance exercise strengthens the whole body. Because it generally employs some form of weight lifting—employing a Nautilus machine, hand-held weights, or even dumbbells—you need to learn how to perform this type of exercise properly. That doesn't mean you need to spend a fortune hiring a personal trainer or even joining a gym. There are centers that teach people to perform weight resistance exercises safely for little or no money (free centers generally serve only older people). Aerobic exercise—like walking, jogging, playing tennis—can usually be performed without supervision, unless you are elderly, disabled, or in poor health.

Miriam E. Nelson, Ph.D., Tufts University professor and author of *Strong Women Stay Young*, points out that inactivity causes both men and women to lose muscle and bone mass by the age of 55. If this situation is not corrected, it can lead to depression, balance loss (which can cause falls), frailty, and increased risk for chronic illnesses like diabetes and heart disease.

Dr. Nelson recommends twenty minutes of aerobic exercise daily, accompanied by strength-training techniques using weight or strength-training equipment, or even just hand-held weights. Her research examined women between the ages of 50 and 79, comparing those who were sedentary with those who followed her exercise regimen. One year later, the women who hadn't exercised had lost muscle and bone density, gained body fat, and were less active overall. Those who exercised not only replaced fat with muscle, but gained small amounts of bone density, strength, and balance. Balance is harmony, and harmony promotes health.

Tai Chi Chu'an and Yoga

Chi is the energy that flows through our bodies and moves, if unimpeded, as we move.

Tai Chi Chuan (pronounced "tie chee choowan") was created by Chang San-feng during the Sung Dynasty (960–1279 A.D.) as a form of movement that creates health and serves as a method of self-defense. It is a disguised martial art that exercises joints and tendons without acutely exerting muscles.

In Tai Chi, movements are slow and smooth and synchronized with breathing. Directed by conscious intention, the movements are usually circular and relax tension. Over time, as you repeat the Tai Chi movements thousands of times, they becomes unconscious, supporting all your movements. Because of Tai Chi's complexity, novice practitioners need a teacher to show them how to pay attention, relax the tension in their joints and do the movements without strain.

In one of my favorite books about Tai Chi, *Ride the Tiger to the Mountain: Tai Chi for Health*, Jo Ann Johnstone Chace writes that each of its movements, like everything in nature, has a firm side and a soft side, an empty aspect and a solid one, corresponding to the Chinese concepts of yin and yang.

I began practicing Tai Chi when I was 46 years old. Every time I perform a Tai Chi form, it is a different experience. Often by the time the form is completed, I find that I have drifted away to a more comfortable and relaxed space, away from thinking about everything I did not do today and my obligations for tomorrow. When I finish, I return to my daily life.

Yoga is part of a 6000-year-old Hindu religious philosophy that combines physicality with the spiritual belief that mind, body, and spirit cannot be separated. Like other Eastern forms of exercise/meditation, yoga emphasizes breathing and posture while moving through various poses. Yoga's poses (asanas) build strength and flexibility in muscles, while stretching ligaments and joints gently. Yoga's concentration on deep breathing slows the heart rate, resulting in a state of deep relaxation that helps you find a quiet space that can always be visited. "If you look after the root of the tree, the fragrance and flowering will come by itself. If you look after the body, the fragrance of the mind and spirit will come of itself," Yoga Master B. K. S. Iyengar writes in Yoga the Iyengar Way.

There are many books, magazines, and videotapes that can teach you the basic yoga positions and can help you stretch and strengthen your body. As with any of the Eastern disciplines discussed here, it is in your best interest to find an experienced yoga teacher.

Summary

Don't stand still! Walk, do aerobic exercises if you're able and your doctor approves, perform weight-resistance exercises. Be sure to replace the water-soluble vitamins you lose when you sweat, including B, C, magnesium, and other minerals. Drink lots of water, especially when you're exercising, and avoid saunas, which can overheat the eyes.

While all of this may seem a little far afield in a book about eyes, remember our mantra—the eyes are connected to the body. Postexercise relaxation, meditation, and a calmer approach to life will improve your vision as well as your general health. Each one of us is capable of fully utilizing his or her powers to enhance physical, mental, and spiritual health.

California psychiatrist William Glasser, M.D., developed the concept of a "positive addiction" from his experience of working with addictive personalities and transforming their destructive habits into health-promoting ones. If we exercise often enough, we'll feel good about it, and even begin to need it. Scientists now understand that endorphins, which create a scense of euphoria, are produced by exercise. The chemistry of exercise is far more complicated than we previously thought; more hormonal and psychological states benefit from regular exercise. This tangible aspect of the mind-body relationship requires no one else's intervention—it just requires you. If you're elderly, sedentary, or ill, exercise slowly or find a center to assist you. If you're able to, walk briskly, and go on a march every day for your own health. If you establish an exercise routine, you'll be less likely to hurt yourself performing daily tasks. I'd love to be able to do it for you, to provide you with a magic bullet, a food or supplement that would give you the same benefits as exercise, but it does not exist. You just have to get up and do it yourself.

CHAPTER 17

The Healing Touch

• *Jo is a 40-year-old hospital employee who had long suffered with chronic back, neck, and headaches. She lived on ibuprofen. The chronic pain interfered with her every movement, even walking, and she couldn't wait for 5:00* P.M. to arrive every day so she could go home to relative comfort. Knowing my interest in alternative medicine, she asked my advice about how to lessen her pain and her need for so many painkillers. I pressed on a couple of spots on her neck and back muscles and identified several that elicited pain. I referred her to a chiropractor who also performs massage and suggested that she try just three chiropractic treatments for alignment and softening the contracted muscles to see if they helped her. Two weeks later, Jo rushed up to me in the operating room to tell me she hadn't felt so good in years and has stopped taking her ibuprofen.

• *An acquaintance of mine from high school whom I'd not seen in thirty-five years called me from Philadelphia. He had developed weakness in both hands after a neck injury and, one year later, continued to have numbness and tingling and hadn't recovered much strength. His caregivers in Philadelphia had told him that nothing more could be done. I recommended a combination of nerve-supportive supplements and a series of acupuncture treatments, which he underwent. Three months later, he called to invite my wife and me to dinner in Philadelphia to celebrate his incredible improvement.*

Ancient Ways to Release Healing Energy

In 1972, *New York Times* correspondent James Reston required an emergency appendectomy while accompanying President Richard Nixon to China. While Reston was in the hospital, he watched many procedures performed with acupuncture, and also observed postoperative pain relieved by application of these slender needles.

According to Chinese traditional medicine, energy, or *chi* moves through the body along channels, or *meridiens*. In *acupuncture*, fine needles are inserted at appropriate points along these meridiens. In *acupressure*, massage is used in the place of needles to stimulate these points and influence the flow of chi. Practitioners of acupuncture and acupressure are knowledgeable about the location of every acupuncture or acupressure point, the function of each, and how to treat disease by stimulating the points to remove blockages to the flow of energy.

Acupuncture

Subhuti Dharmananda, Ph.D., director of the Institute for Traditional Medicine in Portland, Oregon, suggests that acupuncture stimulates cellular signaling systems to increase the rate of healing. Studies show that endorphins (natural painkillers) and other neurotransmitters are produced not only at the site of stimulation, but also in other parts of the nervous system and corresponding internal organs. This is a classic example of an ancient therapy whose biological and neurophysiological effectiveness has been measured, tested, and proved in our own modern laboratories and clinics.

The results of acupuncture in animals also show that it produces a physiological effect. Since animals don't understand what to expect, they are immune to the placebo effect, yet they appear to experience significant arthritis pain relief from acupuncture treatment.

Acupuncture is also used to treat a variety of eye conditions. In the May-June 1996 issue of *Natural Health* magazine, health care provider and writer Carole Jones described her battle with retinitis complicated by a tear in her retina (a potentially blinding condition), and its reversal following acupuncture and Chinese herbal treatments. Four years after undergoing acupuncture in place of the laser treatment recommended by her ophthalmologist, Jones reported that the condition of her retinas is "excellent" and her vision restored.

Laser therapy, of course, would probably have worked as well and, although retinal specialists don't treat every hole in the retina, a retinal tear is often a medical emergency. Do not seek alternative care for such a serious condition without first consulting an ophthalmic specialist.

In March 1998, Z. H. Cho, M.D., and colleagues reported a correlation between acupuncture stimulation of an area related to the eye and a response in the occipital cortex of the brain where vision processing occurs. The vision-related acupuncture point (VA1) is located on the outside edge of the foot. When stimulation is applied, functional MRI brain scans reveal activation in the occipital lobe, as Dr. Cho reported in the *Proceedings of the National Academy of Sciences USA.*

This remarkable finding demonstrates why it's important to listen to our Asian colleagues, who employ treatments that have been used for thousands of years. I have many patients whose pain around the eyes has been relieved by acupuncture and who even state that their vision has improved, so I recommend it in appropriate cases.

A modern variation on these ancient Chinese therapies is called color-puncture, a noninvasive technique that uses colored lights to stimulate acupoints in a way similar to acupuncture's use of needles and acupressure's use of massage. Colorpuncture was developed by German naturopath and acupuncturist Peter Mandel in the early 1980s. Mandel based his work on Chinese and Russian studies suggesting that the meridiens guide light through the body. He believes that different colored lights can influence the body's energy vibrations. A flashlight-type tool that has interchange-able, colored glass tips is used to stimulate acupoints with six basic colors of light. The yang (energy-producing) colors are red, orange, and yellow. The yin (energy-reducing or calming) colors are blue, green, and violet. Green is used to treat eye diseases, according to California acupuncturist Helga Prosak.

Colorpuncture may turn out to be another example of modern science catching up with ancient theory. In January 1998, it was discovered that a blue light, focused on the back of the knee, influences melatonin produc-tion just as effectively as daylight striking the retina. In both these areas, blood vessels are very close to the surface, and the blue light apparently interacts with a chemical in the blood. Blue-light therapy was suggested by the scientists who made the discovery as a possible treatment for jet lag, seasonal affective disorder (SAD syndrome), and other melatonin-regulated body functions. According to colorpuncture, blue light not only eases pain, congestion, and symptoms of menopause, it also treats sleep-lessness. If blue light focused on the retina or the back of the knee stimulates melatonin production, it would also induce sleep. Although it may sound incredible, this groundbreaking research was published in the century-old and well-respected journal *Science*. As the twenty-first century progresses, more and more legitimate science may sound like science fiction.

Acupressure

Acupressure, like acupuncture, regulates the flow of energy, or *chi*, through the body. Pressure is used just like acupuncture's needles to remove blockages and open the channels correlating with specific disharmonies in the body to facilitate chi's flow. Acupressure does not have the same electrical energy as acupuncture.

I've begun recommending an acupuncture exercise to reduce bags under the eyes that's been reported by Julia Busch, publisher of the Anti-Aging Press Inc. (800-SO-YOUNG). Two acupressure points can also be gently massaged. The first is at the outside of the eye's orbit, just outside the bony rim and level with the eye. The second point is under the center of the eye, in the notch of the lower orbital rim. Before pressing on these trigger points, rub your hands together several times to warm and energize them. Then apply gentle pressure in the spots I've described with the index (first) or middle finger to the first point for seven seconds. Release the pressure without moving your finger, and repeat two more times for seven-second counts.

Then find the notch under the eye socket (the second point I described), and repeat the same process. When finished, tap gently 360 degrees around the eye on the bony rim with one or two fingers, several times, never pressing on the eyeball itself. This is an easy way to unload unnecessary "baggage." If it doesn't work for you, you may not have found the right points. If you want to investigate acupressure or other meridien-stimulating techniques further, you may wish to find an instructor.

Body Work

Body work is another name for various types of massage and touch therapy, such as reflexology, acupressure, shiatsu, therapeutic touch, craniosacral manipulation, myofascial release, and chiropractic. Massage has been used to relieve stress, pain, and fatigue for centuries. Julius Caesar reportedly received a daily massage for his headaches. Socrates said, "Rubbing is just slightly less important than food itself." And Hippocrates instructed, "The physician must be experienced in many things, but most assuredly in rubbing." As modern day physicians and patients have begun to investigate natural ways of addressing health problems, these techniques have regained their popularity and respect.

Massage

Massage releases toxins from muscles, loosens ligaments and muscles, improves lymphatic flow, lowers blood pressure, and is relaxing.

When properly performed by a trained, licensed massage therapist, massage can have positive effects on a wide variety of physical and emotional problems. I can personally attest that it's good for all that ails you, since I get a massage twice a month. There are times, however, when you should ask your physician whether it's okay for you to have a massage. Check first with your doctor if you have:

- Skin or lymphatic cancer
- A skin injury, infection, or condition like psoriasis
- A recently broken bone or bad sprain
- A heart condition
- Areas of unexplained heavy bruising or hemorrhage
- An infectious illness (like the flu) or a fever
- High blood pressure, or any other serious illness

Make sure that your massage therapist is properly trained. Don't ever be too shy to ask about a health practitioner's education and experience. Many states require massage therapists to be licensed. In addition to local resources, the American Massage Therapy Association has state chapters all around the country that can refer you to a licensed therapist (see Resource Guide).

Reiki

Reiki is another method of realigning the channels of energy flow. When toxins and aches dissipate, pain may be felt elsewhere before the patient feels better. Two informative books are Walter Lubec's *The Complete Reiki Handbook* and Diane Stein's *Essential Reiki: A Complete Guide to an Ancient Healing Art.*

Chiropractic and Osteopathy

Chiropractic and osteopathy both began in the late 1800s in the midwestern United States. The term *osteopathy* derives from the Greek word *osteon,* which means healing (not from the word *osteo,* for bone). Osteopathy was started by Andrew Taylor Still, M.D., in Oklahoma, who realized that the process of healing required manipulation of the body. He opened schools that taught anatomy and specific mechanical techniques that moved not only the bones but the internal organs as well. The number of osteopathic schools increased and still thrive today. Osteopaths are physicians and part of mainstream medicine. Although differences still exist between osteopathic and allopathic medicine, these two branches of Western medicine have sufficiently merged to enable osteopathic physicians to practice in all hospitals and be eligible to take specialty training in most states.

Daniel David Palmer, M.D., started chiropractic in Davenport, Iowa, around 1895. He practiced Asian healing methods and felt that this body-manipulation technique was a derivative of them. Palmer believed that all disease originates from an imbalance in the musculoskeletal system. Although we realize today that that is not the case, we've learned that proper body alignment is important to maintaining good health. Chiropractors' services are generally covered by insurance providers when needed for rehabilitation. Some people find improvement in certain types of back pain as effectively through chiropractic manipulation as through surgery.

My personal experience is that alignment can be accomplished through either chiropractic manipulation or deep-tissue massage, but the therapist or chiropractor must be well trained, so that he or she can recognize an underlying neurological condition if one is present.

Other Techniques

There are almost as many different body-work techniques as there are berries and fruits. Some, like myofascial release and craniosacral massage, may be part of complete body massage. Others are separate techniques, such as shiatsu, rolfing, and therapeutic touch. Some, like reflexology, may work on only a part of the body (i.e., the feet) to achieve relaxation at remote and deeper areas. Likewise, massaging, stimulating, or relaxing one part of the body may have a corresponding effect elsewhere. Reflexology stimulates the occipital lobe of the brain and doubles lymphatic flow.

I feel certain that some of these techniques will prove to have scientific bases and will become part of mainstream medicine. Others may be changed or discarded as we learn more about them. Therapeutic touch—which isn't actually body work since it does not involve direct touching—has recently come under scrutiny. Therapeutic touch practitioners swear by its beneficial effects especially in treating pain, while others are more cautious. Time and testing will clarify exactly how it works and how best to use it.

Of course, any therapeutic modality may have an effect if the recipient believes that it will. A crucial part of any healing technique is the active participation of the patient as well as the healer.

The success of various body-work techniques has clearly demonstrated to me that no profession has a monopoly on the healing arts.

CHAPTER 18

Improving Your Eyes' Environment

If you are unable to live in this moment, what will you do with another thirty years?

The way you live your life can have a very positive impact on your health, because the well-being of both your body and your eyes greatly depends on your lifestyle. Should you ever be diagnosed with a medical condition, however serious, find out its risk factors and causes. Environment, which *you* can influence, may play a central role here. Risk factors for macular degeneration, for instance, include having a family history of this condition, blue eyes, high blood pressure, and a tendency to go out in the sun without sunglasses. You can't do anything about your blue eyes or your family history, but you can certainly do something about reducing your blood pressure and protecting your eyes from strong sunlight. You can also improve the health of your body—and your eyes—by ceasing to smoke (if you still do), by taking the appropriate supplements, by exercising regularly, and by ensuring that you get enough rest and genuine relaxation.

Seventy-eight-year-old Sarah came in to my office with her daughter because she had experienced a sudden hemorrhage (bleeding) in her right retina, associated with her macular degeneration. The hemorrhage caused Sarah to lose the central vision in that eye quite suddenly. She told me she'd never had any problems with her vision before, and asked, "Why did this happen to me?" After examining her and recognizing early, dry-form macular degeneration changes even in her good eye, I asked Sarah about her fine, close vision—the vision that is slowly lost in macular degeneration. She told me that she'd given up sewing and could no longer read the telephone book;

in other words, her vision changes were not so sudden. After the examination, I asked her (as I do all my patients in similar situations), "Why do you think this happened?" When she didn't have an immediate answer, I suggested, "Let me help you look at some of the factors that contributed to your vision loss and determine how to protect the other eye."

Unfortunately, not much can be done to restore vision following a hemorrhage and destruction of the retina; the goal of therapy at this point is to identify personal and environmental risk factors and change as many as possible while improving nutrition and digestion, and adding the appropriate supplements (see Chapter 8). I pointed out to Sarah and her daughter that we all have choices, and even after vision-robbing damage has occurred, we can take steps to limit it. As an interactive physician, I try to use an acute illness like Sarah's to awaken patients to the necessity of taking control of their own health.

Mood-control is a very important component in a disease-prevention lifestyle. Illness, isolation, stress, and repeated criticism can lower self-esteem. We have a natural cycle of ups and downs, but sometimes we can get into a rut of negativity. If you've been feeling isolated, join a local group, like one working on beautifying your community, for example, or do something else you enjoy with others who enjoy it as well.

Humor transforms. Laughter is a vital emotional tool for adapting to life's dilemmas. Laughing clears the lungs, enhances breathing, and is almost a form of exercise. Laughter has helped some notable people, including author Norman Cousins, conquer disease. Harvey Becker wrote a book-length comic book during his battle with cancer. Try to laugh minor problems away—it might just work.

Music is a spirit-lifter that is readily available to almost everyone, as is dancing. If no one else is around, dance alone. Pets allow us to share love and trust with another living being, and walking them opens our eyes to the world around us.

Although you can address short-term depression by any of these methods, unrelieved depression is another matter entirely. If you are depressed, don't hesitate to seek professional help.

I've always believed that our bodies can and often do heal themselves if we help and encourage them to do so. I'm not alone in holding this view of health and healing. In his book *Spontaneous Healing*, Andrew Weil, M.D., describes our bodies' inherent ability to heal. Dr. Weil feels that patient and doctor must both believe that a cure is possible. I feel that it can be beneficial to share this belief with other people who are important to you, not just your doctor.

There is no one prescription for good health. You are the doctor of your own body—you will take care of yourself better than anyone else would.

Obesity

Although being overweight is extremely difficult for some people to control, it is a major lifestyle factor contributing to many illnesses. The Institute of Medicine estimates that the cost of obesity is now $70 billion a year. Obesity is increasing in all ethnic groups in the United States (male and female), and underlies many cases of high blood pressure, elevated cholesterol, diabetes, gallbladder disease, cancer, heart disease, and eye problems. Twenty-five percent of today's children are overweight. To combat this trend, some schools are combining exercise with health education, and encouraging thirty minutes of vigorous physical activity a day.

Don't take any weight-loss–inducing supplement without asking your physician or herbalist's advice. As we learned from the Fen-Phen disaster, "natural" does not always mean "safe." A new weight-loss pill, MAX 10, is a combination of the Chinese herb ma huang (or *ephedra*), the herb kola (which contains a great deal of caffeine), and other herbs. Ephedra itself is a stimulant and, coupled with the high concentration of caffeine in kola, can produce health problems for people with heart disease, diabetes, high blood pressure, or thyroid disease. Of course, children should never take any sort of weight-loss preparation except under the close supervision of a physician. Sadly, there is no magic bullet for effortless weight loss—we just have to burn more calories than we consume.

Dr. Abel's Tip

Exercise aerobically. Instead of processed foods, eat raw salads and cooked vegetables every day.

Going up in Smoke

England's King James I knew that smoking was bad for your health. The king, in fact, wrote a treatise warning against tobacco use in 1604. Tobacco was not used habitually by the American Indians, but only for ceremonial and ritual purposes. When European colonists picked up smoking, it became an addiction (especially later, once additives were added to commercially produced cigarettes).

Smoking definitely increases the incidence of cataracts, glaucoma, macular degeneration, and diabetic retinopathy, among other ills. Secondhand smoke, according to a study published in the *Journal of the American Medical Association*, raises blood pressure and contributes to the development of clogged and narrowed arteries (atherosclerosis), especially in diabetics who smoke. Vascular damage from both diabetes and smoking definitely increases the risk of eye disease among diabetics. Nicotine is not the only toxin in cigarettes; they also contain toxic gasses and addictive chemicals that are passed on to anyone within breathing distance—one reason smoking has been banned in most public places in the United States.

Infection and Immunity

As overall health declines, epidemics occur more frequently. Yes, there are new strains of organisms that we cannot foresee or deflect in time. We can try to make vaccines to combat them (an arduous and expensive process), but infections for which there are no effective vaccines—staph, tuberculosis, influenza, SARS and even HIV—require that we respond individually by building up our immune systems.

With decreasing immunity generally, however, innocuous organisms can cause serious illness. Candida can overrun the bowel; an ordinary plant fungus can infect a wound; an operation can seed bacteria. Bacteria can grow wherever there is mucus or obstruction. Even cleaning your teeth can spread bacteria, which build up in the plaque between the tooth and the gum. Brushing can send bacteria into the bloodstream, resulting in infections in remote places, such as the heart.

We learned from the Hungarian physician Ignaz Semmelweis a century-and-a-half ago that washing one's hands radically reduces the incidence of infection. This simple trick was first taught by the Arabs in the Middle Ages; it remains the most effective way to reduce the spread of bacteria and viruses and even decrease colds.

The eye is an important, but often overlooked, port of entry for infectious agents. Pinkeye can cause colds if you spread the infection to your nasal passages by touching the infected eye. Viruses may be breathed in, but infected tears also run into the nose, helping the virus spread. The monkey herpes B virus and the Hong Kong "bird flu" both caused fatal infections after entering the body through people's eyes. Even hemophilus and pneumococcus, two bacterial organisms more commonly diagnosed in children, can enter the body through the eyes.

Longevity

In Japan, there are more than 6000 centenarians—people over the age of 100. In the United States, there are ten times that many, and there will undoubtedly be many more, because the fastest-growing age group in this country is people over 65. This group already accounts for 14 percent of the population, and will increase to 20 percent by the middle of this century, with women comprising 79 percent of those over 100.

Older Americans develop more degenerative eye problems than younger ones do. Senior Americans want to keep driving, but not only does visual acuity often decrease as we get older, visual processing in the brain may also be impaired. Some of my suggestions involve ways to help older Americans see better and drive more safely.

Hearing also declines with age, and it is not as easily corrected as vision. The elderly also take a lot of drugs, often prescribed by more than one physician, and up to 41 percent of patients experience an adverse drug reaction. We need to examine the total nutrient requirements of senior citizens. The recommended daily allowances (RDAs) are finally being increased for seniors, including those for thiamine (B_1), riboflavin (B_6), folic acid (B_{12}), and vitamin D.

For memory, I recommend taking a good multivitamin, *ginkgo biloba*, *gotu kola* from India (now being tested as a possible Alzheimer's treatment), phosphatidyl serine, L-carotene, CoQ10, and magnesium. If you are having memory problems, consult your physician.

Other supplements have also been shown to contribute to good health in the elderly. A five-year study in China examined the rate of stroke among 29,000 elderly individuals in the province of Linxian. Those who consumed supplements including vitamins A and E, beta-carotene, selenium, and zinc experienced a 29 percent decrease in the number of strokes suffered (as of 1998). People who supplemented with selenium alone had a 13 percent decrease in cancer-related deaths and a 9 percent decrease in death from all causes.

Sleep

At least one-third of Americans battle insomnia periodically. The disruption of a good night's sleep or the inability to fall asleep in the first place adds frustration to the listlessness we feel after sleeping poorly. Many people take sleep-inducing medications, not knowing that they may become counterproductive after a week. Their long-term effects are unknown, and they may be addictive. People subsequently consume more caffeine, then experience rebound fatigue, which is not the same as feeling ready to sleep. Adding sugar produces highs and lows in blood sugar, fatiguing the pancreas and adrenal glands.

We've long thought that sleep rests the body. Studies of brain wave patterns, however, tell us something else: the mind is just as active when we're sleeping as when we're awake. We need deep levels of sleep to enter the rapid-eye-movement (REM) sleep during which we dream. Some experts are beginning to believe that, during REM sleep, the unconscious mind clears away emotional stress.

Exercising regularly will help you sleep better. Tension is not relieved by just lying down. We need to be limber to be relaxed.

Melatonin, now recommended for jet lag, may be useful in the short term (three days) to restore a normal sleep cycle. A number of herbal teas—chamomile, valerian, and others—can help people fall asleep. A glass of red wine or grape juice, taken about an hour before bedtime (assuming you don't get headaches from sulfites in red wine) helps induce sleep and also provides some important antioxidants.

Discover a pre-bed routine that's good for you, and stick to it. Whether you have physical discomforts or too much on your mind, it's time to clean house and approach your symptoms or problems using natural means.

Water

Few of us really drink our eight full glasses (64–80 ounces) of water a day. We're too busy and we forget. If we remembered, we'd hate to be excusing ourselves for bathroom breaks all the time. Nevertheless, water is the most necessary element (after air) for our survival. The body and the mind need to be hydrated. All the salt in our diet needs to be diluted and excreted. Otherwise, our kidneys can't do all their work, and leave it to the liver which, like the kidneys, processes toxins. If the liver is overwhelmed by toxins, it doesn't transport fat, and there's no chance we can lose weight or have sufficient energy. Drinking an adequate amount of water helps the liver and kidneys rid the body of toxins.

If you have a medical condition like high blood pressure, kidney disease, or are already on a diuretic, this advice may not apply to you. You may actually have to restrict your water, and you should ask your physician's advice. If you have bladder or prostate problems, you should try to drink the majority of your fluids before dinner, so you're not up all night. If you have a loose bladder from childbearing, ask your doctor for help—it's available.

Washing a little bit of anxiety out of our lives will make for better health. Let's drink to that.

Stress

Stress seems to be the watchword of our lives. We can't avoid it in our conversations with others or with ourselves. Our rush to arrive at work, deal with the bottom-line requirements of our jobs, and be wonderful to everybody is occasionally overwhelming. We all have cycles of exhilaration and depression which are normal, but chronic stress reduces self-esteem. Depression can become sustained, resulting in withdrawal, overeating, and looking for help in a bottle.

Help is available from other people, whether it's psychotherapy, maintaining relationships with friends or family, doing good deeds, or walking your dog. These activities not only get you out of the house, they get you out of yourself. Once you realize you can't be superman or superwoman, you have to establish priorities especially in regard to your health.

Excessive amounts of cortisol produced in response to extreme stress may also contribute to a serious eye disease called *retinitis pigmentosa*, which has long been thought to be a genetic disease. At a medical conference in March 1998, immunologist Alfred Sapse, M.D., announced that not only do elevated levels of cortisol contribute to the development of retinitis pigmentosa; treating people with anti-cortisol drugs improves their condition. Dr. Sapse, who left the University of California Los Angeles to start his own company (Steroidogenesis Inhibitors, Inc.), is developing such drugs. Reducing stress, Dr. Sapse points out, also lowers dangerously high cortisol levels.

Stress reduction comes in many forms, including laughing, crying, playing, getting distracted, sleeping, exercising, day-dreaming, and even deep breathing. Breathing patterns reflect both our mood, and our level of stress/relaxation. Don't we stop and count to ten, take a deep breath, or even sigh, when we want to change emotional frequencies?

The field of psychoimmunology studies how using our minds to relax changes our chemical balance. The mind can both cure and potentiate disease. If the body is tense, antioxidants and other "good guys" are fighting tension instead of maintaining good metabolism. If we smoke, drink to excess, or are obese, we are diluting our resources. We are therefore more susceptible to toxins and contagions, including viral infections like flu or herpes, ulcers, and long-term diseases that rob us of years of vigorous, happy life.

Environmental Contaminants

One out of every eight plant species on our planet is now threatened with extinction. All animals, including ourselves, will also be endangered if we don't protect the environment. Short-term economic gain for some may cause long-term health loss for all of us. Chemical pollution is undermining many species' health and ability to reproduce. In Delaware, more than 50 percent of frogs are born with three legs instead of four. The porous skin of this water-bound amphibian allows rapid absorption of pollution, and so we see its effects earlier. Frogs give warning that more complex species are at risk as well.

The evidence linking pesticides, certain plastics, and solvents to the increased incidence of cancer is mounting. Of the 100,000 synthetic chemicals commercially available today, nearly one-quarter have been listed as hazardous. Pesticides have been implicated as having a role in breast cancer (some act as pseudoestrogens). The Harvard nurses' study, which looked for PCB and DDE (a metabolite of DDT), found these potentially carcinogenic chemicals stored in all its subjects' fat samples. Poor nutrition and bad sanitation, along with exposure to pesticides, greatly increase the vulnerability of farm workers in developing countries. In addition, chemical and other plants are disposing of toxic waste by selling it to fertilizer companies—so it becomes part of the food chain.

Power plants may also be linked to disease-causing pollution. After years of denying any possible connection between the electric and magnetic fields surrounding power lines and increased cancer rates, a panel at the National Institutes of Health concluded that these fields should be considered possible cancer-causers.

The level of ozone (a clear odorless gas that forms from chemicals emitted in car exhaust, fluorocarbon refrigerants, and petroleum products) increases in the summer when pollutants react with sunlight, heat, and stagnant air. Refineries emit benzene, chlorine, chlorobenzine, and other pollutants into the air. In the areas within a hundred miles of Chernobyl there has already been at least a doubling in the usual number of breast cancer cases reported. People exposed to passive smoke for twenty or more hours a week at home or at work will have distinctly lower levels of vitamin C in their blood. I won't enumerate all the potential toxicities of each of these pollutants, but the more I know about them, the more I wish to remove myself from them.

Contaminants in our food are also a great concern. (I hope you're not reading this just after eating a meal.) Pesticides may stay on washed fruit even after it's peeled. The California Safe Drinking Water Initiative is trying to prohibit fluoridation, which may be linked to bone pathology, neurologic impairment, lowered IQ in children, and even cancers. Tap water may also contain lead and mercury. Fungicides, which may contain mercury, are used on seeds and grains and may get into our bread. Canned tuna can contain small amounts of lead, but there's more in the can, especially if it's been soldered. Grapefruit skin can contain lead. Even some popular hair coloring products contain lead.

Consider what we add to food: artificial sweeteners, cold tars with arsenic, benzoic acid, preservatives, chemical coloring agents, and dye. These ingredients are not innocuous. Think about what we cook it in: aluminum cookware can contaminate food (a concern in the search for the cause of Alzheimer's) and can destroy vitamin C. Heated plastics cause respiratory dysfunction when the fumes are breathed. Packaged meat like hot dogs and bacon contain nitrates and nitrites. Charcoal grilling produces nitrosamine and other carcinogenic compounds that accumulate over time.

Be aware that household products and appliances can make you sick. Forget the microscopic spores that lurk everywhere—that innocuous container in the basement could contain antifreeze, which is poisonous to breathe as well as to drink. Formaldehyde (found in thousands of building and consumer products) and benzene are toxic to the nervous system when breathed or absorbed through the skin. It can also cause asthma, respiratory allergies, and skin disease. Benzene, a cause of leukemia, is found in tires, gasoline, paint strippers, and varnishes.

Many household products—including paint, building materials like particleboard, carpets, and the chemicals applied to them—contain *volatile organic compounds* (like formaldehyde, benzene, and toluene, abbreviated as VOCs). Poorly ventilated buildings do not allow VOCs or other toxins to be expelled. It's no coincidence that sick-building syndrome—a condition characterized by fatigue, confusion, and respiratory problems—arose at the same time as the architectural fad of hermetically sealed buildings that allow no outdoor ventilation. VOCs can be generated in the workplace by heaters, laser printers, photocopying machines, tile, linoleum, carpeting, and video display terminals on computers.

Both at work and at home, additional VOCs can include air fresheners, deodorizers, disinfectants, moth repellents, pesticides, and biological contaminants like dust mites, mildew, and mold. Instead of using a chemical air freshener, try placing an open box or jar of baking soda in an enclosed space (like under the sink), or place flowers around the room. Instead of harsh chemical cleaners, buy natural products, which are now widely available. To rid your home or workplace of mold and mildew, use a dehumidifier and dispose of pieces of furniture, carpeting, or bedding that you suspect of harboring mites or mold.

If you have airborne allergies, you should also consider that dogs and/ or cats may be the source of them. The dander and allergens from these animals' sebaceous glands can be significantly reduced by weekly baths.

Protect your children against exposure to chemicals. Children, with their developing brains and nervous systems, are very susceptible to pesticides. Organophosphates are found even in baby foods (especially fruits and vegetables), and Gerber, Heinz, and other baby food manufacturers are now producing organic baby food lines. Bug sprays have toxins in them that can be inhaled by infants. Instead, use Buzz Away, manufactured by Quantum, which is a natural, plant-oil bug repellent.

Instead of chemicals, use nature's own air purifiers, plants. According to retired NASA scientist William Wolverton, Ph.D. (author of *How to Grow Clean Air: 50 Houseplants That Purify Your Home or Office*), many ordinary houseplants remove air pollutants, including:

Aloe vera *(Aloe vera)*
Arrowhead plant *(Syngonium)*
Bamboo palm *(Chamaedorea)*
Banana *(Musa)*
Boston fern *(Nephrolepis exalta Bostoniensis)*
Chinese evergreen *(Aglaonema)*
Corn plant *(Dracaena fragrans massangeana)*
Devil's ivy *(Epipremum aureum)*
English ivy *(Hedera helix)*

Philodendron *(Philodendron cordatum)*
Janet Craig *(Dracaena deremensis)*
Madagascar dragon tree *(Dracaena marginata)*
Mum *(Chrysanthemum)*
Peace lily *(Spathiphyllum)*
Snake plant *(Sanseveria)*
Spider plant *(Chlorophytum)*
Umbrella plant *(Schefflera)*
Split-leaf philodendron *(Pepperomia Philodendron pertusum)*

These plants are able to remove chemicals like benzene and formaldehyde because they resemble chemicals naturally found in plant leaves and the microbes around plants.

Cosmetics

Why do you think more women than men have cataracts? It might be because many women have coated their faces and hair every day for years with cosmetics containing damaging ingredients, thinking that the skin is a vinyl covering instead of the largest organ in the body.

Skin, of course, is more than an envelope for our bodies. It also absorbs and excretes. It is not only the body's largest organ, it's the liver's backup in terms of excreting waste (that's what whiteheads and acne are). Skin is also the mantle that's exposed to sunlight and absorbs toxic ultraviolet (UV) rays day in and day out. UV damage can result in loss of collagen, which causes wrinkles, and pigment changes, which cause age spots. And, of course, UV light damage is implicated as a cause of skin cancers.

The skin is really an acid mantle, because its pH is less than that of water (a high pH is alkaline; a low pH is acidic; water is neutral). The oil glands secrete sebum, which is composed of fatty acids, to keep the skin supple and partially immune from the environment. The jojoba plant exudes a natural fatty ingredient, actually a wax, that protects it from becoming desiccated in the harsh environment of the desert. Cold-water fish are loaded with essential fatty acids (EFAs) to keep their skin from absorbing water. People, however, who live in more temperate climates have less of a protective layer. Therefore, we need to protect and rehydrate our outer body.

The skin has two major components: the epidermis and the underlying dermis. Both are composed of layers of cells with protein fibers, carbohydrate matrix, and fat membranes and surface sealers. Skin contains essential fatty acids, carbohydrate, protein (i.e., collagen), hyaluronic acid, and elastic fibers named *elastin*. The skin's underlying dermis also has connective tissue, copious blood vessels, nerves, and hyaluronic acid. Elastin and collagen are two very prominent protein fibers in the epidermis. They make our skin flexible in youth. With age, as the body runs out of cysteine and methionine, elastin and collagen fibers become inflexible, and wrinkles result. Collagen (like the cornea) is made in part of hydroxyproline, which is derived from ascorbic acid (vitamin C). Essential fatty acids and hydroxyproline work together to help collagen keep its shape.

Skin disorders can be reflected in the eye. People with dry skin can develop conjunctivitis, people with acne can get red eyes and even corneal ulcers; too much oil, too little oil, and dehydration can all be reflected in the external ocular surface and cornea.

Many people think that skin, hair, and nails are dead. Nothing could be further from the truth. Fingernails, hair, and skin all have their own life cycles.

Anything that's good for the body is also good for the skin and nails. For healthy nails, hair, and skin, you need to consume adequate amounts of essential fatty acids, zinc, silica, the B vitamins (especially pantothine), calcium, magnesium, and protein (to build collagen and keratin). Vitamin E rubbed into nails, strengthens them, as does white camellia oil (available from Aubrey Organics; see Resource Guide for this and other natural nail-savers).

You also need to protect your skin from the sun by using sunscreens. We can be irradiated by reflected light off water, sand, and flat surfaces. Believe it or not, car windows may not filter out all of the UVA. It's no surprise that there are roughly one million cases of skin cancer a year in the U.S. Even if you don't get cancer, your skin will age faster without protection.

While sunscreens are important to the life of the skin, those that contain PABA and its derivatives shouldn't be used by people allergic to sulfonamides, thiazide diuretics, or local anesthetics. Equally effective sunscreens can be purchased that contain benzophenones and cinnamates, as well as pastes made of zinc oxide, titanium dioxide, and red petrolatum (petrochemical). Obviously, wearing a sunscreen with an SPF (sun protection factor) of 30 or more is best and, of course, remember to wear your broad-brimmed hat and sunglasses. If you don't protect your skin from the sun, at least protect your retina, which is less forgiving of damage than skin.

Cosmetics have been used at least since the ancient Egyptians. Having left the agricultural age and entered the chemical/industrial age, we've developed inexpensive synthetic products.

Preservatives, which can be toxic to the skin, are put in cosmetics so they won't break down and become contaminated by microbes. Most cosmetics made of natural components don't become contaminated; however, the synthetic ones need EDTA, parabens, and ammonium salts, which are actually toxic to skin.

Don't let your cosmetics—particularly eye makeup—age or become contaminated. I've treated corneal ulcers resulting from *Pseudomonus*-contaminated eye makeup. *Pseudomonus* can contaminate water; if you dip a mascara brush in water (to thin the mascara and make it last longer), it can become contaminated, causing an eye infection. So don't dilute mascara with water and be sure to discard it every three months.

Cosmetics are more easily contaminated in the summer than in the winter, and putting your finger into lotions also contaminates them, so wash your hands first. Makeup brushes should be washed weekly in an antibacterial solutions; discard makeup sponges after use. These products are a breeding ground for microbes.

Wrinkles are caused by the loss of elastic tissue and cross-linking of collagen. When we lose collagen, the flexible becomes inflexible. The eyelids wrinkle easily because they're so thin, have a good blood supply, and reflect environmental changes, especially cold, fatigue, and lack of sleep. Smoking causes wrinkles because nicotine constricts blood vessels, restricting circulation to collagen fibers. Sun also causes collagen breakdown.

New vitamin C–rich creams reduce wrinkling and age spots. One is Cellex, which was invented at Duke University and contains a tremendous amount of absorbable vitamin C.

Botox—a toxin made from the *Cholestridia bostulida* bacteria—is now being used to eradicate eyelid and facial wrinkles, after being used for years to treat twitching eyelids (blepharospasm). It should be remembered that botox is, as its name indicates, a toxin that weakens muscle function and muscle sphincter actions (i.e., winking and puckering). I suggest trying less toxic methods of reducing wrinkles first.

Lying on your stomach when you sleep allows fluid to accumulate around your eyes. Dark circles can result from melanin deposits (in response to sunlight), but may also result from engorged blood vessels when the eyes are rubbed, sleep deficient, or allergic.

One trick to ease swollen eyes is to place herbal tea bags, especially chamomile tea bags on your eyes (after the tea bags cool, of course), for a couple of minutes. Arnica, a homeopathic and naturopathic remedy, can be massaged around the lids (not *in* the eye) to help reduce swelling. Some of my patients have told me they successfully use Preparation H to decrease puffiness around their eyes. I do not normally recommend this but if you choose to do so, be careful not to get it in your eyes.

Hair is made from keratin, which contains eighteen amino acids, the most abundant of which is cysteine (the sulfonated amino acid). Hair is made up of spirals of these protein strands, and its coloring is determined by the amount and size of melanin-type pigments.

The essential fatty acids, as well as the B vitamins (especially folic acid, biotin, and pantothine), help to eliminate dandruff as well as improving cuticles. Allantoin (isolated from comfrey root in 1910) is a natural sun protector often found in shampoos, lip balms, and deodorants. It works well with selenium and methionine to reconstitute the protein content of damaged hair. All these herbs and nutrients refresh the hair and prevent loss of vital antioxidants.

Hair has a natural growth cycle; larger hairs, surprisingly, grow faster than short hairs, but they all fall out and are replenished. Stress can cause hair loss even months later. Relaxation, exercise, nutrition, and hydration, therefore, are all as important to healthy hair as they are to healthy eyes. You may also want to treat yourself to a scalp massage, using essential oils like jojoba, chamomile, or rosemary.

Shampoo ingredients like jojoba oil, selenium, avocado, aloe, vitamin

A, and carotene stimulate hair growth. Rogaine (minoxidil) actually supports the hairs that remain rather than encouraging new growth in most individuals. However, once the treatment is stopped, the hair returns to its original condition, and some individuals actually have experienced no effect from minoxidil, continuing to lose hair.

Why do we turn gray? Experts believe that it is primarily a copper deficiency that catches up with us, but it could be due to low levels of cysteine, glutathione, or zinc. A diet or even hair ingredients that have copper, zinc, PABA, and pantothine—which facilitate the enzyme tyrosinase, which binds copper—help to maintain pigment. Many hair dyes contain toxic and cancer-causing chemicals, including antifreeze (PEG, polyethylene glycol, or PPG, polypropylene glycol); sodium laurel sulfate; DEA (diethaneolamanine); and TEA (triethaneolamine). They may even be contaminated by nitrosamines or dioxane, which are carcinogens. (See the Resource Guide for natural hair dyes.) And, of course, getting hair dye in your eyes can cause serious, even permanent, damage.

Summary

Try to achieve and maintain an optimal weight by balancing diet, exercise, and mood. What you consume contributes to your biochemistry, so be sure to drink eight glasses of filtered water a day. This helps hydrate your kidneys, flush out the toxins, and improve circulation to remote areas, including your eyes. Develop a good sleep pattern, because we heal at night. A glass of red wine, or doing some yoga exercise or light reading before bedtime, will help induce sleep. Don't make your To Do list at the end of the day. Reduce stress by using music, nature, pets, friends, and relationships. The mind can cure as well as harm the body and the soul. The most important thing you can do is forgive yourself and start each day anew—a healthy body and an improved environment will not be achieved overnight. What's good for your eyes is good for all of you, including your spiritual self. Appreciate yourself, and make better health your self-fulfilling prophecy.

PART VII

INTERACTIVE MEDICINE

CHAPTER 19

No Magic Bullet: Drug Interactions and Toxicity to the Eyes

• *I saw a patient who'd been treated with beta-blocker eyedrops for the previous five years in order to control her intraocular pressure. Although she denied having any problems while on it, I asked her about her very hoarse voice, which she said she'd developed only after using the eyedrops. I suggested that she discontinue them for two months, substitute natural alternatives, and begin an exercise program. By the end of the two-month period, her hoarseness and phlegm had disappeared.*

• For my father's eightieth birthday, I gave him a copy of the Physician's Desk Reference, *which lists, describes, and pictures all approved prescription drugs and their side effects. Upon receiving his very own copy of the* PDR, *my father thanked me, and then said, "It's about time you gave me this."*

When I was an intern and resident from 1969 to 1973, at least one out of every four night calls I was awakened to deal with resulted from a medication problem. My son completed his internship in 1998 and, judging by his experience, the situation has not improved over the intervening decades. In fact, it seems to be worse. I want to impress you with the importance of paying attention to your body and recognizing drug-related symptoms early to avoid serious consequences from drug reactions, which are just waiting to happen. Don't let them happen to you.

All drugs have side effects. Even herbs, food, and vitamins can have side effects, although we're usually unaware of them. We have become a culture that expects and demands pharmaceutical preparations to treat every symptom, no matter how slight. Some of these pharmaceutical agents are thought to be so safe they can be purchased over the counter to treat headache, fatigue, insomnia, allergies, colds, diarrhea, and even obesity.

Even prescription drugs are not completely safe in all circumstances. In 1993, there were over 100,000 deaths due to adverse effects from drugs. In June 1998, the FDA recalled two prescription drugs because of potentially fatal side effects, including interactions with other drugs. The heart drug Posicor, used to treat high blood pressure and chest pain (angina), had many negative, potentially lethal reactions with other medications, and was withdrawn on June 8, 1998. Only two weeks later, the FDA recalled the painkiller Duract, which was implicated in about a dozen cases of liver failure during the year since it had been approved, four of which were fatal, and eight of which required liver transplants.

Drug reactions are not always recognized immediately. Some medications produce gradual symptoms that necessitate a visit to a physician (perhaps in a specialty different from that of the doctor who prescribed the drug in the first place), who may unknowingly prescribe two or three other drugs to counteract the side effects of the first drug.

We are courting disaster, as Thomas J. Moore (author of *Prescription for Disaster: The Hidden Dangers in Your Medicine Cabinet*) has stated. He points out that drugs kill more people than gun violence, cigarettes, or even automobile or plane crashes in a single year. The lifetime risk of developing lung cancer is one-third that of being severely harmed by a prescription drug.

Our sophisticated modern pharmaceuticals have been designed to act in subtle ways. They are rapidly disseminated throughout our bodies and flip multiple switches that can throw our systems out of balance. Did you know that there are 287 drugs that can cause hair loss, including some of those that are prescribed to grow it? Did you know that sleeping medications can alter behavior so significantly that the person taking them becomes even more dependent on them?

One of the roots of our society's legal drug problem is the overprescription of antibiotics, antidepressants, cholesterol-lowering drugs, and other common pharmaceuticals. Overuse of prescription drugs:

1. Contributes to the development of microbial (viral and bacterial) drug resistance
2. Overtreats conditions that may be sensitive to lower doses or natural remedies
3. Counteracts the effect of other drugs that patients are already taking

4. Treats conditions that are merely temporary or episodic (like "white-coat hypertension," a temporary rise in blood pressure caused by the stress of visiting the doctor)

5. Keeps the patients on medications for too long by assuming that their conditions don't vary and their tolerance doesn't change.

Medicines have effects on multiple systems besides the targeted one. Remember, there are hidden connections between many parts of our bodies that we don't usually think about—and some we haven't yet identified. A drug applied topically may have a remote effect, because it can enter the bloodstream through the skin and travel to a different area of the body. For example, Clindamycin, used in the treatment of skin infections, has been reported to cause abdominal pain and diarrhea.

Even over-the-counter drugs have side effects about which you need to be aware. Analgesics (painkillers) like ibuprofen (Motrin, Aleve, and Advil), acetaminophen (Tylenol), and even aspirin can have eye, as well as total-body, side effects. It's rare for these drugs to cause serious side effects, but they can occur at therapeutic levels. One study found that people who take more than two ibuprofen tablets a day for seven years have a nine times higher risk of developing kidney failure than people who take only two tablets a week. This study also estimated that up to 10 percent of new cases of kidney failure (about 5000 a year) could be prevented by limiting ibuprofen use.

Most people know that taking excessive amounts of aspirin can harm the stomach and intestinal lining, sometimes resulting in internal bleeding. To avoid this aspirin effect, many people have switched to taking Tylenol (acetaminophen). High doses of Tylenol, however, not only cause the same type of gastric problems, but have been linked to liver failure. *This is another case in which you must read the label.* Many over-the-counter cold and cough medications contain Tylenol (acetaminophen). Rare cases have been reported in which people unknowingly took more than one type of cold medication containing acetaminophen combined with a cough medication containing acetaminophen, along with extra acetaminophen to treat the cold's headache or general aches and pains, and their livers were so severely damaged that they required liver transplants to save their lives.

Antacids can cause subconjunctival hemorrhage (bleeding in the white of the eye), corneal deposits, skin changes, and, at toxic levels, visual hallucinations. They also may contain aluminum.

Prescription drugs are even more powerful than over-the-counter drugs, and they can cause more severe side effects. During the first weeks after its approval by the FDA, a record number of prescriptions were written for the anti-impotence drug Viagra. Its eye side effects were the most frequently observed. Many individuals with disturbed vision had exceeded the recommended dosage of 50 mg in four hours—which the literature accompanying the drug says a patient can exceed if necessary. Michael F. Marmor, M.D., and colleagues at Stanford University reported the eye side effects of Viagra to be bluish-color vision (that is, a blue haze over the vision), light sensitivity, and a drop in retinal electrical measurements of 30–50 percent, lasting for a number of hours. As a result of Dr. Marmor's findings, the American Academy of Ophthalmology issued a news release on May 11, 1998, warning ophthalmologists to follow patients with macular degeneration, retinitis pigmentosa, or diabetic retinopathy carefully if they are taking Viagra, or advise them to avoid the drug altogether if they experience any eye side effects. Viagra is unlikely to cause permanent alteration in vision. The chemical pathway, however, that is changed by Viagra to allow normal erections to occur is the same pathway used by cells in the eye to change light into a signal sent to the brain, and the effects on vision of repeatedly interrupting this chemical pathway are unknown.

This is another example of the eye acting as a sentinel for the rest of the body. The eyes often herald a problem with a drug before it becomes apparent in other places in the body.

Cholesterol-lowering drugs can also have significant side effects, such as accelerating cataracts, producing fatigue, and decreasing memory. For this reason, if you have high cholesterol, you should explore natural methods of controlling it, such as the following:

1. Consume monounsaturated fats, such as olive oil.

2. Eat oatmeal in the morning (but don't take your minerals with your oatmeal or it will bind them so you can't use them).

3. Include soy, garlic, onions, and even peppers and shiitake mushrooms in your diet.

4. Take supplements of vitamins C, E, niacin, and the essential fatty acids.

A patient with both high cholesterol and cataracts came to see me and mentioned that he hadn't needed to have his cataracts checked for three years. I discovered he was right when I checked his vision, which had improved from 20/25 to 20/20. During those three years, this gentleman had been taking a supplement eye formula containing lutein and extra vitamin C and E. Also, he began eating oatmeal for breakfast. In addition to his improved vision, he had lost twenty points on his total cholesterol count in each of the three years, and his good cholesterol (HDL) had risen.

The optic nerve can suffer a kind of stroke if it doesn't receive enough blood at night, which can happen when people take blood-pressure–lowering drugs. Sohan Singh Heyreh, M.D., has done research at the University of Iowa College of Medicine, indicating that taking blood pressure medications before going to bed precipitously lowers blood flow to the optic nerve. This can cause an optic nerve stroke, called *arteritic ischemic optic neuropathy* (AION), which can cause permanent vision loss. Its primary symptom is blurred vision upon waking, including blackness or grayness in a portion of the vision, or blurring in one portion of the vision (the lower half, for instance). Dr. Heyreh urges anyone on blood pressure–lowering medication who wakens with any type of blurred vision to seek medical care immediately, because the earlier AION is identified, the less vision will be lost.

Many different kinds of drug reactions surface at night because people are not distracted by work or other activities and so are able to feel what is happening in their bodies. In hospitals, more drug reactions are identified at night because the nursing staff has more time to investigate patients' problems.

The same dose of a medication does not affect people equally. Some people—especially the elderly—are very sensitive to drugs. Heavy drinkers and smokers metabolize drugs rapidly and require higher doses than people who don't smoke and drink. Therefore, a one-dose-fits-all method of prescribing drugs is worrisome. Specific medications may need to be titrated by patients. For instance, I've advised you to build up to taking 3000 mg of vitamin C a day. Likewise, your doctor might tell you to build up to taking 20 mg of blood pressure medication a day.

The cumulative effects of a drug may be very different from the daily effect. Over a long period of time (several weeks, for instance), the drug may build up to a level in your bloodstream that causes side effects such as blurred vision, memory loss, or lethargy. You don't eat one food every day, but vary your diet. You should consider medication as being a temporary fix and, at three or six months down the road, realize that your body may be different and require a different approach.

It's very important to know the differences between an idiosyncratic reaction to a drug (an example might be Valium causing agitation rather than acting as a tranquilizer), an intolerance (which can give you an upset stomach, dizziness, and inability to urinate), and a true drug allergy, which can be severe.

A drug allergy or hypersensitivy causes itching, sometimes even in the top of your mouth (palate), rash or hives, and sinus congestion. Allergies tend to become worse with each administration of the drug, and can lead to low blood pressure, flushing, severe asthma attack, swelling in the throat (which impedes breathing), and even anaphylaxis (which is potentially fatal).

If you are taking a new medication (or even a new dosage of an old medication), and develop symptoms that could signal a drug-drug interaction, a drug-food interaction, a drug-herb interaction, or a possible allergic reaction, call your doctor immediately. (See Tables 28 and 29.) If you are having trouble breathing because of severe asthma or throat swelling, go immediately to the emergency room.

Symptoms of Possible Drug Toxicity or Allergy

If you or any family member experiences any of the following symptoms and suspect they are related to a new drug or taking a different dose of an old drug, call your physician immediately: rash, fever, unexplained nausea, unexplained diarrhea, difficulty breathing, dizziness, mental confusion, somnolence (inability to stay awake), and coma.

Eye symptoms of drug toxicity or allergy include: tearing, light sensitivity, itching, eyelid swelling, blurred or distorted vision, abnormal color vision, double vision, development of cataracts, and development of glaucoma.

Among the commonly used drugs with well-known side effects that often cause emergency situations are: analgesics (gastric ulceration), anti-diabetes drugs (low blood sugar), and blood pressure medications (dizziness, especially upon arising). You must be alert to all new sensations and report them immediately to your doctor. It may be necessary to discontinue a medication to determine the cause of your symptoms. It amazes me that people can experience the same side effect every day right after taking their medication and not realize that their symptoms are related to that medication.

When the FDA evaluates drug safety, it tries to determine whether a new drug is habit-forming, causes cancer, is unusually toxic, or is harmful to the heart, before investigating whether it works. Of the fifty best-selling prescription drugs, many cause at least one of these problems.

Who's to blame? We all are. Doctors don't like to discuss the risk of medicines. In some cases, they have neither the time nor the interest. In others, they're afraid that mentioning the risks will keep their patients from taking their medicines or diminish the healing impact of their patients' belief in their benefits.

As patients, we are responsible because we often visit the doctor and demand a prescription. After an expensive examination and the briefest discussion of your diagnosis, you are handed a prescription and shown the door. Something is wrong here; and you need to ask questions. It's both your ethical and legal right to be a participant in an interactive partnership with your doctor. Ask the doctor, ask the pharmacist, do research on the Internet or at your library, and read the *Physician's Desk Reference*.

F. T. Fraunfelder, M.D., wrote *Drug-Induced Ocular Side Effects* (an immensely popular book among ophthalmologists and the seminal work in this field), and has started a registry of drug-induced eye side effects. Among the drugs that Dr. Fraunfelder has identified as having frequent and/or serious eye side effects are:

• Ergotamine and methysergide, often used to treat migraine headaches. These drugs can change vision and visual field.

• Captapril and Enalapril are angiotensin-converting enzyme inhibitors of high blood pressure. They can cause eyelid swelling, decreased vision, light sensitivity, subconjunctival changes, and visual hallucinations. Fortunately, these side effects occur rarely and are reversible.

• Furosemide (Lasix) reduces blood pressure and removes fluid. Besides washing out minerals and water-soluble vitamins, however, it can decrease vision, change color vision, and decrease tolerance to contact lenses. It is also a photosensitizer and causes hallucinations.

• Digitalis preparations (used to treat heart disease). These drugs, in excess, can change color vision. Amiodarone, an important anti-arrhythmia drug, causes changes in the cornea, lens, retina, ciliary body, and choroid of the eye, none of which is visually significant.

• Minoxidil, a vasodilator used to treat high blood pressure. This drug can cause optic neuritis. Even applying it to the scalp to grow hair can cause the side effects of dry skin, keratitis (corneal disease), and decreased vision.

• The anti-acne drug Acutane (isoretinoin) can cause depression and is contraindicated in pregnancy because of its potential for causing birth defects. These side effects were not identified until it had been on the market for some time.

• Systemic adrenal corticosteroids (pills) and corticosteroid eyedrops have nearly one hundred side effects, including cataracts, glaucoma, ptosis, dilated pupils, conjunctival reaction, corneal deposits, vision changes, color vision changes, and optic nerve changes. Even corticosteroid cream applied to the skin can cause cataracts, light sensitivity, and swelling of the optic nerve head.

Following is the number of prescription medications (as of mid-1998) that can cause specific eye side effects:

Eyelid and conjunctival allergies	340
Double vision	267
Focus problems	255
Light sensitivity (which lead to cataracts eventually)	250
Severe allergies	250
Change in color vision	140
Optic nerve atrophy	135
Myopia	100+
Optic nerve swelling	100
Optic nerve toxicity	100
Cataracts	95
Tearing	78
Loss of lashes or brows	75
Optic nerve swelling due to swelling in the brain	60
Uveitis (all intraocular inflammation)	51
Pigment in the retina	43
Macular edema	41
Dry eye	28
Eye muscle abnormality	25
Iritis	23
Macular degeneration	8

Many topical eye medications cause localized side effects. Eyedrops are concentrated medications; when you visit other doctors, let them know what eyedrops you are taking. The most notorious for causing side effects are the cortisone eyedrops, which are more likely to cause cataracts and glaucoma in susceptible people than are oral steroids. Over time, some glaucoma eyedrops may increase the probability of developing cataracts. All eyedrops can cause allergy or chemical irritation, which is often due to their preservatives. Many artificial tears also have irritating preservatives in them.

Following is a list of side effects from topical timolol, a beta-blocker glaucoma medication. Beta-blockers cause bronchial spasm, which accelerates asthma, an effect that often occurs after exertion. A very careful history is required to determine whether these breathing problems are being caused by an eyedrop, so if you have glaucoma and asthma, be aware of this possible effect. Beta-blocker drugs should not be prescribed for the very old or for individuals with known lung and heart disease.

Some ophthalmologists recommend that mean-flow breathing tests be performed for all patients using beta-blocker eyedrops to catch this side effect. Patients should be aware of this potential problem and of any abnormal effect during their regular exercise routines.

Possible Side Effects of Timolol Eyedrops
asthma and shortness of breath
bradycardia (heart arrhythmia)
congestive heart failure
depression
dilated pupils
fatigue and reduced exercise tolerance
hair loss
impotence
increase in cholesterol and other blood lipids
memory loss
red eyes

Even herbs, which are usually harmless, can cause side effects, especially when mixed and taken with drugs. Additionally, it's not advisable to take herbs for an extended length of time without consulting your herbalist or physician.

Summary

You can help prevent prescription mistakes and avoid suffering their serious side effects. Learn about the prescribed medication, how you take it (with food or on an empty stomach), at what time of day, for how long, its possible side effects, and which are most likely for you. Is this drug compatible with your other medications? Are there any foods or herbs that should be avoided? Is there any written information available to you about this drug?

Never take medicine prescribed for someone else. If you or a loved one has trouble remembering whether the proper dose of a drug has been taken, inexpensive plastic containers are available that are designed to contain pills counted out in advance for each day of the week. If you or a relative can't swallow a pill, ask if there's a liquid form. If you're taking pain relievers for a time period that seems excessive—more than one day for a headache, three days for a toothache, a week for a muscle sprain—consult your doctor. Remember my modified Murphy's Law: Anything can happen to anybody. Don't be a drug statistic.

Many common medications may deplete our cells of necessary vitamins. Ross Pelton, R.Ph., wrote the *Drug Induced, Nutrient Depletion Handbook*, which provides amazing information about drugs that we thought were safe. For instance, artificial estrogens (birth control pills) deplete riboflavin, pyridoxine, folic acid, vitamin B_{12}, vitamin C, and zinc. Furthermore, oral contraceptive use results in increased vitamin K, iron, and copper. Vitamin K can increase bleeding, and iron and copper are both prooxidants.

Drugs such as the statin family of drugs, which reduce cholesterol, also decrease the production of CoQ10, and possibly glutathione in the liver. Consumption of sugar-laden soft drinks during the formative teenage years increases urinary calcium excretion and decreases the amount of calcium laid down in bone. People who drink a lot of soft drinks in their teens and twenties are more prone to osteoporosis and fractures in their later years.

One of Hippocrates' most important rules for physicians was, "First do no harm" *("Nil nocere,"* in Latin). You can take an active part in helping your physician to do no harm by educating yourself about the drugs you need to take.

Although they occur less frequently than drug-drug interactions, dangerous interactions between drugs and foods can also occur. Many foods and herbs have active chemicals in them, but they are usually balanced by the fact that the whole food contains a combination of phytochemicals. You, the patient, must be watchful and wise at all times. It is your body, your life, and your vision.

Table 28. Natural Alternatives to Commonly Used Drugs

Symptom Treated (Type of Drug)	Brand Names	Natural Alternative
Allergy (antihistamine)	Benadryl, Contac, Sudafed	Bee pollen, feverfew, pycnogenol, vitamin C
Constipation (laxatives)	Ex-Lax, Metamucil	Aloe vera, vegetables high in fiber, vitamin C, water
Depression (antidepressants)	Prozac, Zoloft	St. John's wort, vitamin B_1
Gas (antacids or antigas)	Pepcid AC, Tagamet, Zantac	Ginger root, probiotics, vitamin C
High blood pressure (antihypertensives)	Vasotec	Calcium, garlic, magnesium, potassium
Menopausal symptoms (estrogen replacement)	Premarin	Black cohosh, soy
Insomnia	Halcion	5-hydroxytryptophane and Kava Kava
Elevated cholesterol	Lopid, Mevacor	Garlic, soy, vitamins C, E, niacin, gugulipid, and essential fats

Table 29. Drug-Food Supplement Interactions to Be Wary of

Brand Name Drug	Food or Supplement	Interaction
Heart Medications Digoxin, Lanoxin	• Magnesium supplements; bran fiber; licorice • Vitamin D	• Can decrease the medication's effectiveness • Can cause overdose
Quinidine	• Citrus fruits (in large amounts)	• Can cause overdose
Antidepressants Marplan, Isocarbaxazid	• Aged cheese; smoked and aged meat; red wines; Brewers yeast	• Can cause elevation of blood pressure
Anticonvulsants Phenyltoin, Dilantin	• Folic Acid • Vitamin D	• Can decrease drug absorption and/or deplete vitamins
High Blood Pressure Lasix	• High-salt foods; natural licorice; bacon; olives; processed meats	• Can lead to too much sodium in the blood. Increase potassium (to counteract sodium) by eating these foods: oranges, bananas, apricots, potatoes
Osteoporosis Etidronate Sodium, Didronel	• Dairy products high in calcium	• Dairy products and/or calcium supplements should not be consumed at the same time as the medication
ACE Inhibitors (for high blood pressure) Capoten, Vaso-tec	• Foods high in potassium: bananas, oranges, apricots, potatoes	• Will produce too much potassium in blood
Thyroid Medications Cholaxin	• Dark greens (cabbage, cauliflower, kale, mustard greens); rutabaga, turnips.	• Can decrease drug's effectiveness
Propylthiouracil, Methimazone, Levothyroxine	• Foods containing iodine (seafood, table salt) • Ensure Liquid Supplement	• May cause low thyroid • May cause low thyroid

CHAPTER 20

Does Your Doctor Care? Your Health Includes You!

Each patient carries his own doctor inside him. They come to us not knowing that truth. We are at our best when we give the doctor who resides in each patient a chance to go to work.

—*Dr. Albert Schweitzer*

As Albert Schweitzer understood, each of us is in charge of our own body, often has our own answers, and should have a say in our own care. With a little bit of reflection, we can present our own history better than any doctor's chart. Sir William Osler, an internationally known physician at the turn of the century, commented that 80 percent of diagnoses can be made by the patients themselves. Osler also urged his fellow physicians to listen to their patients. Whole textbooks have been based upon patients' histories and examinations.

There is an art and a science to being a patient, as there is to being a doctor. You feel, and the doctor listens; you listen, and the doctor feels. You both draw observations and share them with each other. When both partners understand this, they are practicing what I call *interactive medicine*, which is the best kind of medicine we have.

In *Spontaneous Healing*, Andrew Weil, M.D., emphasizes the tendency for each of us to heal ourselves. That's why so many people get better without going to the doctor. Patient and doctor must share the belief that a cure is possible.

Something is Wrong

- *A dear friend of mine, Judy, went to the doctor for an abdominal imaging procedure and was told, on a Friday afternoon, that she had a malignant tumor of the kidney. Only on Monday after the CAT scan had been reevalu-*

ated was her tumor pronounced to be benign. If the CAT scan had been double-checked initially, Judy could have avoided a weekend from hell.

- Another acquaintance who was treated for many years with cortisone complained of abdominal pain for about three months. When abdominal surgery was finally performed, the amount of destruction in her bowel from a chronic circulation disorder—due to long-term cortisone use—was too great to repair. She died several days later.

- A friend, whose ophthalmologist I've been for years, is now over 90. He's developing decreased memory, slower speech, and double vision. I was not willing to accept that his physical decline was due simply to age. So I asked his cardiologist to discontinue one of his heart medications (a beta-blocker) to see if his symptoms improved. They did.

- Another friend had the same tumor removed three different times, from the same area.

Each of these stories illustrates a syndrome I call *myopic medicine*, whereby we treat a symptom and fail to look for the real cause of the disease, only to be surprised when the symptoms bloom again. That's why you need to be a medical detective. It's time to stop, look, listen, and change.

Interactive Medicine

What is interactive medicine? It is comprehensive care with the goal that you, your physicians, and other caregivers can work together in deciding what's best for you, and whether your symptoms and conditions can be allayed. In interactive medicine, Western scientific techniques can be combined with holistic or Eastern medical practices, like herbal medicine and acupuncture. Under the guidance of a physician-coordinator, you get the best blend of the Eastern and Western medical worlds.

Some call this *complementary* or *integrative* medicine. I prefer the term *interactive*, because that's what it really is: a dialogue.

First you must believe that you are valuable, even if you are scared of cancer, coronary disease, or cataracts. You need a sense of responsibility to get past helplessness. You can make a difference in your own care.

Second, formulate a plan. Find a doctor, make your appointment, write a list of questions. Even interview the doctor on your first visit.

Third, once you have seen the doctor and received a diagnosis, continue to ask questions. Ask what the second-most-likely diagnosis is. Ask for a second option for treating the diagnosis you were given. Are there side effects to the treatment that's recommended? If you're given a prescription, ask about its risks, benefits, and natural alternatives. Medication is often prescribed as a placebo because both patient and doctor believe in it as part of the program. If you're given information about a test result, such as a CAT scan, find out how accurate the reading of this test generally is. Should it be repeated? How will you learn the results of a test? You want to avoid having a breast biopsy and learning from a message on your answering machine New Year's Eve that you have cancer. All these questions mean that both you and your doctor must be constantly vigilant and equally involved in your health.

When the doctor shares your loved one's condition with you, is it described in Latin and Greek? These languages create a professional mystique but are usually too disguised for us to make any sense out of them. Even very young doctors use the same kind of verbiage: They say "peds" or "pediatrics" instead of "children," and "orthopod" instead of "bone doctor." Then there's "ophthalmology"—nobody can even spell it!

We need to restructure the eye and medical exams. I call the current system HEAP: The first part of the exam is the *History*; then you are given your actual *Examination*. Afterwards, the doctor pulls together what he's learned into an *Assessment* (or diagnosis), and lastly he forms a *Plan*. Doctors are compensated for the *H* and *E*, but not very much for *A* and *P*. But the *A* and the *P* are the most important parts for you. They must be based on solid information, but you need to know your options, both short and long term, and what you can expect from different choices. Surgery or drugs may be necessary, but do not accept them without an explanation.

The Roadblocks to Achieving Interactive Medicine

The symbol of the medical profession is the caduseus, a sword with two entwined snakes. One snake represents science and rationality; the other, art and intuition. Healing requires both science and intuition.

If you think about people you've met whom you would term a healer— people who are inspiring, whose touch can transform, whose listening is profound, and whose words make you feel better in minutes—few are physicians. We don't have many Albert Schweitzers in our communities. The healer is more likely to be a native shaman, a natural medicine practitioner, or a nurse.

I don't mean to be harsh in judging my fellow physicians, on whom there are many pressures, some of which begin in medical school.

Medicine is now packaged as a business. Relative value units are applied to everything we doctors do (whether it makes money or not). Insurance companies and HMOs claim that they look at quality of care, but they definitely evaluate levels of care. Doctors are being pressed into being efficient and adding to the bottom line. There is a tendency for the doctor to be more concerned about cost than cure.

Reflex treating is also encouraged by drug companies. Who do you think gives the doctor his or her black bag, stethoscope, and free dinners?

Doctors also begin identifying patients with their diagnoses, and don't spend much time looking for other possible causes or related problems. A study of one million residents of Ontario published in the New England Journal of Medicine in 1998 found that physicians treating older patients with serious chronic illnesses—diabetes, emphysema, and emotional diseases—often overlooked other chronic diseases that were also present in those patients.

Doctors usually don't have the time to spend with patients discussing the diagnosis, other possible diagnoses, treatment options, side effects of the medicines they're prescribing, or options to treat naturally.

Western biomedicine fragments the body into compartments, and before the resurgence of family practice, specialists had developed different turfs, viewing only that part of the body of concern to their specialty. As a result, many pains and diseases are referred from one place to another. If you have a sinus headache from either poor digestion or tight muscles, the ear, nose, and throat doctor may not be able to make that connection. Physicians must develop a sense of cooperation among themselves to allow new treatment possibilities, because a patient often has many doctors.

It is interesting that doctors call me about alternative medicine options when they or a member of their family is sick, but are not willing to expose their ignorance regarding a patient. Fortunately, this is changing, and colleagues of mine are speaking out. More and more physicians are visiting the developing world, learning about indigenous therapies, and sharing the knowledge they gain not only with their patients but also with other doctors.

Innovation is difficult. Physicians often don't respond when great ideas are first broached and are slow to accept new ways of practicing medicine because they represent risks. Proof in practice, over time, changes many minds. In 1949, Harold Ridley, M.D., first put plastic intraocular lenses into the eyes of cataract patients to rehabilitate their sight. At first, he was a maverick; now, lenses are placed in the eyes of cataract patients all over the world. In Canada, the Shute brothers espoused the virtues of vitamin E, while Nobel Laureate Linus Pauling tried to educate us about the importance of vitamin C. It was decades before physicians accepted these innovations in treatment—even though they involved mere vitamins.

You, the Patient

Wellness requires change—it is not just the absence of disease. The patient needs to take responsibility, and use disease as an opportunity for transformation.

A 1995 article in *Consumer Reports* polled 70,000 readers about their relationship with their physicians. One-third said their doctors did not seek their opinion. Over one-fifth said their doctors did not require a thorough history. Nearly the same number said their doctors didn't encourage them to ask questions. Most physicians want to help their patients, but it is often up to patients to keep their doctors involved.

Patients need to have choices in order to participate. People explore options when orthodox medicine doesn't have a ready answer and they're not ready to give up—but we might be able to improve our own health even more by exploring alternative options sooner.

It's important to plan ahead. You must be the one to create effective communication with your doctor. Here are some tips:

- Write down any new symptoms or recent illnesses. Take your questions to your appointment or mail them to your doctor ahead of time.
- Keep a list of all your past medications and therapies, including surgery. Include not only your prescription medications, but also the over-the-counter drugs, supplements, and the vitamins you take regularly.
- Make a list of lifestyle changes, including those involving smoking, drinking, exercise, and diet.
- Take a friend or family member with you to your doctor's appointment if you need an extra set of eyes and ears to help you remember.
- Ask for a copy of any letters your doctor sends to a consulting physician regarding you.
- If necessary, ask for a copy of your records (to the best of my knowledge, in all fifty states, you have a right to your medical records).
- If you are selecting a new doctor, talk to other people and then

call the doctor for an interview (for which you will pay). Can you get an appointment within two weeks? If there is an emergency at night or over the weekend, is your doctor or an associate available? Can you call the doctor's nurse or technician to ask routine questions? Does your doctor speak in plain English and listen to your questions? Is your doctor board certified in his or her specialty? Does he or she prescribe medication without examining you thoroughly? Or is medication withheld so as not to overtreat? Are you allowed to refuse certain treatments? Is there confidentiality in all matters concerning your health care? Are you considered as a person, or just an illness that's walked through the door?

HMO Survival Guide

Do your homework before joining an HMO or selecting a doctor. Know your rights. Read the membership information. Hedge your bets by choosing the option of fee-for-service, if you can, so you can select your own doctors (this will come at a higher price). If your doctor is not enrolled in such a program, that may be important in making the decision whether to participate.

Check out the doctor panel in the HMO and make sure that it has the specialists important to you. Inexpensive may not be best. Free services may mean half-hour waits on the phone before you speak to a human. What is the paperwork like? How can you reverse a denial? What are prescription benefits? Are there options for long-term care? Are there limitations for costs over a certain amount? Will any alternative therapies be covered?

Medicine will continue to change in response to society. When people demand dietary management before bypass surgery, supplementation with saw palmetto before prostatectomy, oatmeal before cholesterol-lowering drugs, doctors and the medical system will listen.

Partnership with your physician can bring greater satisfaction with your health care system and can reduce costs. I say that it can be done. If you catch diseases earlier, while they are deficiencies or degenerations instead of acute problems, everyone will benefit. This is one reason that Eastern medical concepts must be incorporated into the Western medical system. Illness can then be viewed as an opportunity for transformation.

PART VIII

LOOKING FORWARD
TO
BETTER HEALTH

CHAPTER 21

Let's Get Started!

To understand life, you must look at it backwards, but unfortunately, you have to live it going forwards.

—*Søren Kierkegaard*

Don't wait for a medical scare to break you out of your old pattern. You must form an intention to make changes in your life to improve your sight and your total body health.

Begin by forgiving yourself for the past and empowering yourself for the future. The journey starts with the right attitude.

Take Inventory

What particular physical problems do you have? Make a list, and start a personal calendar, because you'll want to look back and see how you did in dealing with these problems. What is your wish list for your body, your health, and your attitude? Now is as good a time as any to write it down.

The goal is to make things simple. I like to think of a life-changing strategy as NEWBARS: Nutrition, Exercise, Water, Breathing, Alternative options, Relaxation, and Spirituality.

- *Nutrition:* Begin by cleaning the fridge. I enjoy snacking as much as anyone, but if the cookies aren't there, it makes forgoing them much easier. Use my food pyramid (see Chapter 14) to plan a balanced diet composed of appropriate amounts of natural meat, fresh fruit and vegetables, dairy and eggs, fish, soy products and water. Avoid refined, packaged foods containing white sugar and white flour. Remember, you're making deposits in your antioxidant bank account. If you're not putting in enough nutrients, you are debiting your account all the time.

• *Exercise:* Exercise not only burns calories, it fuels the mind. It can even be fun and make you feel good. Exercise can be as simple as walking at a regular time, perhaps even on your lunch hour, several days a week. Exercising for 100 days in a row will cause you to miss it if you forget. Exercise improves posture, cardiovascular health, and eye pressure. It also reduces stress.

• *Water:* Drink your eight glasses every day. Make sure it's healthful water, either spring, bottled or filtered.

• *Breathing:* For ten minutes each day, perhaps after a shower, on getting home from work, or before going to bed, take the time to breathe as a prelude to relaxing. Lie on the floor, stretch, take a few good, deep breaths, then get into a sitting or standing position, close your eyes, let your arms hang at your side, breathe deeply with your belly expanding out for inhalation and contracting in for exhalation. Do this for five or ten minutes. Your breathing will become deep and slow, and your mind will get more oxygen because your body is beginning to relax.

• *Alternative options:* These are not restricted to finding a guru. Look at your home, for instance. Are the lights in your house adequate? Where is the evidence of nature inside or outside? Do you have plants that not only give some color to your surroundings but actually help to detoxify the chemicals in the air? These changes are easy to make and manage, and provide a sense of cheer without great expense.

• *Relaxation:* Do you listen to music? If you frequently dine alone, develop a social group. We come into the world alone, we go out alone, but it's sure nice to have company in between. Make some time to enjoy the outdoors. Do you have a pet? Studies have found that pets improve the mental and physical health of people who live alone.

• *Spirituality:* As you change your life in the next 100 days, perhaps you'll consider meditation and visual imagery, or other such techniques particularly to target a problem like macular degeneration, a weak heart, or arthritis.

Beginning a Supplementation Program

It's my conviction that most of the antioxidants that enrich our bodies, fill our antioxidant bank accounts, and reduce toxins should come from the food we eat. That said, there are plenty of times and reasons that call for the addition of nutritional supplements:

- At the beginning of your new program, before you have found an adviser in East/West or interactive medicine.
- As short-term therapy for general health; this may become long term, depending on your particular needs and how your body reacts.
- If you live in an area where fresh fruits and vegetables are not available year-round, where the soil is minerally depleted, and/or where you do not have access to natural meat, poultry, and organic produce.
- If you already have an eye problem, a risk factor for one, or a relative with macular degeneration, cataracts, or glaucoma.
- If you have a medical disease known to respond well to specific vitamin or phytonutrient supplementation (heart disease, diabetes, Alzheimer's, MS, cancer, and many others).
- If, after receiving your physician's advice, you are trying a therapeutic dose of a vitamin as an alternative to a prescription drug or surgery (e.g., B_6 for carpal tunnel syndrome, multinutrient package instead of bypass surgery, magnesium instead of calcium channel-blockers for blood pressure).

Dr. Abel's A List

- Eat a balanced diet and make sure you include fish, dark greens, carrots, and wine, if appropriate.
- Exercise regularly.
- Evaluate the drugs you are taking. Are there natural alternatives to any of them?
- Do you have an interactive doctor and health care system?
- Take supplements to build up your antioxidant bank account:
  Vitamin A
  Vitamin B complex
  Vitamin C
  Vitamin D
  Vitamin E
  Selenium, Chromium
  Multivitamin with taurine and cysteine
  Bilberry and other bioflavonoids
  Alpha Lipoic Acid
  Omega-3 essential fatty acids

Remember, you're establishing a set of habits for 100 days at least. They are not fixed in stone; you must feel your body, know your limits, know your attitude. Reevaluate your supplements every three to six months. Learn from the past but plan for future.

CHAPTER 22

A View of the Future Through Your Eyes

In every generation, there has to be some fool who will speak the truth as he sees it.

—Boris Pasternak

My goal is to empower you to take control of your health. Life is a circle. I'm always amazed that the best therapy is also the best prevention. In particular, we now know that good nutrition can prevent and reverse eye (and other) diseases. Since we know that certain phytochemicals in food help prevent eye diseases, why not use them as preventatives before we need to treat disease?

We are also beginning to understand the true extent of the innerconnectedness of each part of the body to every other part; that's why it's impossible for me to write only about eyes. We must stop treating isolated symptoms without knowing how they connect with the whole.

A 1998 MacArthur Foundation twin study concluded that, while 30 percent of our overall health may be genetically determined, as much as 70 percent may be determined by what we eat and how we live.

Although good health must be built on the foundation of proper nutrition, supplements can be used as extra insurance. In times of ill health, supplements may be needed in higher doses for short periods of time.

Begin the journey with a complete physical examination and appropriate laboratory tests. You should have a blood clotting test, because a number of foods and supplements recommended here may thin the blood—a good thing for most people, but not for those taking certain medications.

Of course, good nutrition consists of making deposits in your antioxidant bank account by consuming foods rich in antioxidants to nourish your eyes and provide support for your whole body, but especially for your liver. It's also important to improve digestion by adding tonifying herbs, lactobacillus, and other digestive aids, as well as having a test for stomach acid, if it appears you should. Remember that poor digestion contributes to the development of macular degeneration, cataracts, and glaucoma. The eyes don't like a constipated colon, so keep your colon active by drinking plenty of good water, eating foods rich in fiber, and supplementing with digestive aids, if it's necessary from time to time.

Eat foods that specifically nourish the eyes and vision. Dark fruits, like blueberries and grapes, nourish night vision; light fruits high in vitamin C, like kiwis, oranges, and papaya, nourish day vision. Bioflavonoids in the skin of plants protect the growing fruits and berries from the sun's ultraviolet light. We need these compounds to protect our skin, lens, and retina. While using bioflavonoids to protect from within, don't forget to protect yourself from without, too, by wearing good, UV-blocking sunglasses.

Design a diet based on sound nutritional principles. Avoid the harmful fats, processed foods, nitrates, and refined flour and sugar. Increase your intake of fresh fruits and vegetables, fish, spinach, grapes, whole grains, Omega-3 essential fatty acids, fiber, and good water. Sit down and eat slowly. Make each meal a time for rebuilding, not just another period of stress in an already congested day.

The "French paradox"—consuming red meat and wine without a concomitant rise in the rate of heart disease—applies to eyesight as well as to the heart. Studies show that the natural substances in red wine prevent, and may even repair, dry macular degeneration. I have never been a drinker, but I now have one glass of wine at night, which my children find highly amusing. If you can't or don't want to drink alcohol, however, grape juice will provide you with the same nutrients as red wine.

Supplement wisely and remember that supplements, drugs, and herbs work in more than one area in your body. Reevaluate any supplement you add to your regular regime after 100 days to see if it is helping you. Seek out a knowledgeable practitioner to advise you (an alternative physician or an herbal practitioner) and do your own research.

At the same time, take a drug inventory. Ask yourself how many drugs are you taking and why? Do any of them have side effects that could cause a vision problem? How do they interact with each other? And most important, do all your doctors, including your eye doctor, know about every drug that you're taking?

Don't forget to exercise for good health. Stretch, perform some aerobic exercise, and lift weights for your upper body if possible, breathe deeply, and relax as you work your body. Weight-resistance exercise—push-ups and mild weight lifting—will increase muscle tone, improve circulation, and even help prevent osteoporosis. Stretch and massage your neck, your

TMJ (jaw joint), and bend or twist at the waist to stimulate your liver. Remember that you need a flexible and erect spine, not only to stay healthy and youthful, but to allow for creative energy to reach the brain and eyes. A healthy spine will encourage good circulation to the brain as well. Consider adding "eye aerobics" to your workplace breaks, to rest and refresh your eyes and avoid developing the computer charley horse.

Regular exercise can help you to remain vigorous and flexible as you age. My father started doing Royal Canadian Mounted Police exercises (which include sit-ups, push-ups, and isometric or weight-resistance exercises) 35 years ago and, at the age of 86, he still does them regularly. He remains youthful, still plays both golf and tennis, and has 20/20 vision.

Eye exercises may have great value in both your personal and professional lives as well. Moving your eyes around helps you feel good and relaxes the convergence that causes computer stress. Eye movements also unlock the unconscious and enhance both vision and perception. Most important, they relieve stress in general (see Appendix F to learn more about eye exercises).

Remember that our earliest eyedrops came from fruits and berries— not only the antiglaucoma drug pilocarpine, but also berberine for conjunctivitis and trifola for glaucoma. Nevertheless, if you have an eye infection, you'll probably need to use strong medicine—an antibiotic or antiviral drug—and not rely on natural approaches alone. In the future, iodine eyedrops (which kill several kinds of organisms) may become available, since at least two companies are now developing them. Eye infections must be treated early to preserve both your tear film and your cornea. If you nurture your parasympathetic nervous system, it will keep your tears flushing and normal tear ingredients like the antibacterial compound lysozyme circulating, further protecting your eye against infection.

If you wear glasses, make sure they work properly, because you're the one who has to live with them. If you're having headaches, consider your glasses as a possible first cause. If the headaches persist, you may need a new eye exam. And if you do get the exam, make sure it's a complete exam and that you're satisfied with the results. The same goes for an exam for any other kind of eye condition. Know what questions you want to ask of the doctor; make a list of questions if you wish to; get a definitive diagnosis if possible; ask what the other possible causes of your problem are; and learn about your treatment options, including natural treatment options.

Above all, if you are diagnosed as having a serious eye disease, don't despair and never accept "nothing can be done" as a response by any doctor. We are learning that vision may improve in some conditions, including multiple sclerosis (an acute inflammation), macular degeneration, cataract, glaucoma (a chronic disease), and other retinal nerve disorders. Who knows what we may soon be able to accomplish in treating optic atrophy or retinitis pigmentosa? It's not just high-tech medicine that will achieve these advances in therapy; some will probably arise from using herbal therapies.

We don't go from being well to being ill in an instant—all diseases are essentially imbalances. The Chinese label these imbalances as deficiencies or excesses of yin or yang, alterations in the balance of the five elements, or insufficient *chi*. We should use both Eastern and Western medicine to evaluate these imbalances. Different people require different therapies, which is why I look askance at treating all people with cataracts, heart disease, or arthritis with the same dosage of the same medication. Chinese medical therapy is based on administering a mixture of herbs, determined by an individual's dynamics, for ten days to two weeks, and then adjusting it. Perhaps we should take all of our medication this way, adjusting them as the patient feels changes taking place in the body and relating those changes to his or her medical advisers.

In the 21st century, medicine is going to be radically different. The patient will contribute to his or her own cure. The power of placebo is educating medical experts to realize that the body can heal itself. Patients will have to use their own belief systems—and physicians will have to allow them to—so that medical conditions will improve. Additionally, patients taking control of their own diet and nutrition will be viewed as a necessary step.

For the sake of your vision and your body, be sure to select interactive care givers. After all, if you don't take care of your body, where will you live?

If your doctor doesn't listen to you, start looking for another doctor. When you start taking supplements or seeing alternative healers, tell your doctor.

In addition to finding an interactive physician who will be a partner to you in your medical care, you need to take responsibility for your own health. If you have an eye disease for which you need to take a medication (such as glaucoma), compliance is important—and you can't take a "drug holiday" if you expect your condition to improve in a timely fashion.

There is no magic bullet that can pull you out of every health crisis. High-tech medicine is helpful—Western medicine can save your sight and even your life in an emergency—but you must design a day-to-day health maintenance program for yourself. The difference between making a good start and achieving success is *you*. You are both the barrier and the key to your own improved vision and health. We must heal ourselves from within and without; true healing requires you, your doctor, and whatever deity in whom you put faith.

The eye is close to the center of the self and the soul. It reveals your energy level and reflects changes in your mood. Just look in the mirror, and see how you look to yourself. Are your eyes sparkling and full of energy, or dull and defeated?

I have tried to use all the therapies that are both effective and available to me, whether from China, India, Africa, Europe, or Native Americans. I seek answers from both East and West, and so should you. I want the best in vision and health for my family, my friends, my patients, you, my reader, and myself. From my patients, I've learned how emotions can affect both eyes and vision. Your emotional outlook contributes to determining your vision and your total-body health. People with a positive outlook achieve the best results in transforming their lives and health. People who are negative find fault with almost everything—especially themselves. Believe in self-fulfilling prophecies. Imagine yourself achieving better health, step by step, over the next 100 days. If you haven't achieved every goal you set for yourself within that time frame, pause, appreciate the good you have accomplished for your body, and set new, achievable goals for the next 100 days.

I cannot accept it when people are told that nothing can be done to save or improve their vision. Whatever a patient's previous complaints are, I start with the assumption that I can improve his or her health. Nothing can be done if people *think* nothing can be done. I refuse to hear that "nothing can be done," when I see miracles happening every day.

Some 1500 years ago, Hippocrates instructed his students, "Let food be your medicine, and medicine be your food." Many of the "new" therapies to which we are now turning have been known since the beginning of Western civilization. As patients and doctors, let's honor our medical-botanical heritage by using these ancient wisdoms to attain the best health we can. Take charge, know that you can do it, and perhaps this book will lead you to your own miracle.

Discovery never stops. I plan on providing new information as it is uncovered on my Web site (www.eyeadvisory.com).

CHAPTER 23

What's New and What's True

Every month more information comes out of research institutions and off the press. Some of these exciting new studies have confirmed the role of oxidative stress in the development of common eye diseases and affirm the role of antioxidants. In this chapter, I will mention the Nutritional Research Center on Aging, the Beaver Dam Study Group, the Australian Blue Mountains Study, and Dr. Stuart Richer's research over the past couple of years. I will mention nutrition, genetics, and even a combination of the two. However, the emphasis of *The Eye Care Revolution* remains exploring natural options first and leaving the more invasive techniques for more difficult situations.

Nutrition and Eye Health

The big news is the incontrovertible evidence that vitamins can help some people with age-related macular degeneration (AMD), which we learned from the 2001 ARED Study. This randomized perspective study, sponsored by the National Institutes of Health, was completed early because the more than 3600 patients demonstrated that vitamin supplementation can reduce the risk of progression in moderate and advanced cases of AMD. Beta-carotene (15 mg), vitamin C (500 mg), and vitamin E (400 IU) reduced the risk by 20 percent; zinc (80 mg) reduced the risk by 25 percent; and taken together, these nutrients reduced the risk by 28 percent. Not only can something now be done about this dreaded disease, but the paradigm has shifted in the blink of an eye. Most ophthalmologists are now prescribing vitamins for their patients with AMD.

Dr. Abel's Tip

The 2001 ARED Study provides hope that several time-heralded vitamins can prevent future patients with AMD from losing vision. The use of the Amsler Grid and periodic eye examinations remain important.

The Best Supplements for Your Health, which I coauthored with Donald P. Goldberg, R.Ph., and Arnold Gitomer, R.Ph. (Kensington, 2002), gives some basic information about vitamins as well as mentioning drugs that can deplete vitamins. More has been learned about the role of DHA, the long-chain Omega-3 fatty acid that is the backbone of every cell membrane and comprises 30 percent of the retina and brain. DHA is being used to help people with learning disabilities, AMD, depression, high cholesterol, and schizophrenia.

Lights, Lasers, and Glasses

It has been known that melatonin in the skin of frogs responds to blue wavelengths of light and can change the frog's twenty-four-hour circadian rhythm. But now researchers have identified a new type of retina receptor (other than a rod or a cone) that responds similarly. This receptor connects to the pineal gland, which makes melatonin and stimulates wakefulness. By wearing special glasses for an hour each day, people will stay awake for twelve to thirteen hours and then will want to fall asleep. (For example, by wearing the glasses at 10 A.M. every day, a person will stay awake until about 10 or 11 P.M., at which time he or she will become sleepy.) This blue light technology (not strong blue light, which can damage the receptors) can normalize the biological clock for those with jet lag, SAD syndrome, chronic pain, or insomnia. Once available, these glasses will be sold or rented in optical shops and may be covered under Medicare.

SAD syndrome, which stands for Seasonal Affective Disorder, is not confined only to people exposed to long dark winters; a few people have it during the bright summer, too. The winter depression is linked to insufficient production of melatonin because of lack of sunlight; natural lighting solves the condition for many. For those who get depressed in the summer and stay indoors, the trigger mechanism is less well understood.

Dr. Abel's Tip

Blue light technology will redefine how we treat insomnia, jet lag, and the SAD syndrome.

Laser treatments for refractive errors such as nearsightedness, farsightedness, and astigmatism are becoming routine. LASIK has proven safe and effective for people with a wide range of refractive errors (as long as they haven't worn hard contact lenses or had corneal problems in the preceding year). There are tracking lasers (known as LADAR), wavefront technologies (like those that control cruise missiles), and even a few new gimmicks around LASIK. But the procedure with the current lasers is excellent for those with a stable spectacle correction when performed by a well-trained surgeon. I've become more enthusiastic because I have witnessed the excellent results achieved by my colleague, Andrew Barrett, M.D.

Surgical incisions and laser procedures for presbyopia have been far from predictable in leaving a lasting and satisfying correction. Therefore, I recommend presbyopic people stay with the weakest bifocal or reading glasses possible. Good nutrition in conjunction with simple eye exercises may hold off the deterioration of the focusing process of the eye; however, our accommodation naturally declines through the years which becomes most noticeable in the forties and fifties.

Contact lenses and glasses (plastic ones too!) continue to provide more options to more people. Contact lenses can be daily wear, weekly wear, or extended wear. Spectacle options include transition from light to dark (although not 100 percent UV blocking), progressive from far to near, and specialty lenses. Essilor, the company that created Varilux, has improved glare resistance, created the interview lens for computer users (middle and near distances), and improved drugstore reading glasses (those lenses haven't been measured for your eyes).

Scanning lasers have gone from NASA to eye care. There are laser devices that scan the optic nerve and retina for use in glaucoma and AMD patients (mentioned later on). They can tell the thickness of the retina or the nerve fiber layer alone, or the density of the macula pigment (RPE is often the first to deteriorate in AMD).

Tom Cruise's character in *Minority Report* had to avoid laser scanning of his iris. This new technique using iris identification is accomplished by making a rapid photo of the iris and placing it on a grid to generate a distinctive bar code that can be matched in less than half a second. So iris and even retina patterns can be used for security purposes.

Dr. Abel's Tip

There are so many lasers in ophthalmology that you need to ask which particular laser your doctor may be considering.

It has been learned that the movement of the pupil, or the pupil pulse, is a measurement of cognitive activity, and thermal imaging of the eyes can therefore see through the face of deception. Apparently the blood flow around the eyes increases instantly with fear or lying. This technique is more practical and is as accurate as a polygraph (lie detector) test. It seems that the eyes are the key to the body, the soul, and all falsehoods.

Computers, Migraines, and Surviving in the Dark

Computer vision syndrome is not new but is becoming more prevalent with the proliferation of and reliance on computers. My advice remains the same: Practice good ergonomics, reduce peripheral glare, use proper lighting to avoid fatigue, raise the flicker rate to 70 or above, wear corrective glasses if necessary, and take breaks. Blink frequently, use eye drops, stretch out, rub your neck and shoulders, and drink lots of water, which will foster more breaks.

The incidence of migraine phenomena with and without headaches is on the upswing. Some investigators say 18 percent of women and 6 percent of men are afflicted. Even though migraines are considered a neurological disease, you can still try to avoid your particular trigger event. Taking magnesium (500 mg) at bedtime or parthenolides twice a day (see Chapter 5) and avoiding constant sunlight or fluorescent light in the eye may very well prevent migraines. There are several medications that are now available but prevention remains the best option. If migraines persist, then an MRI may be necessary to rule out a brain tumor or an aneurysm.

Night vision or adaptation to the dark dwindles with every decade in life. Christian and colleagues have demonstrated that zinc (25 mg) alone will not help until vitamin A is administered as well; then night vision will be restored to normal. I have created an eye supplement (Able Eyes™) that includes all five of the nutrients that improve night vision: DHA, lutein, zinc, vitamin A, and bilberry. So even people with eye conditions like cataracts, glaucoma, or AMD may experience rapid improvement in their night vision.

> **Dr. Abel's Tip**
>
> Dark adaptation, or getting used to vision under low illumination, diminishes with each decade of life. Improved nutrition or taking specific vitamins may improve your driving after dark.

Cataracts

Cataracts continue to be a major concern for all people around the world. A decreasing ozone layer, reduced water intake, diets heavy in refined products and saturated fats, and ignorance about UV protection contribute to the fact that most seniors around the world can develop vision-impairing cataracts.

Prevention is based on lifestyle modification and nutrition. In the past four years, multiple studies have documented the value of vitamins in reducing the risk of cataracts. The Beaver Dam Eye Study showed a 60 percent reduction in cataracts in those people taking vitamin C or E or a multivitamin for ten years or more. Taylor and colleagues (2002) at the Tufts Nutrition Research Center on Aging demonstrated a similar decreased risk of cortical cataracts in females taking at least 362 mg vitamin C daily. They had reported up to 77 percent protection in a previous study. Jacques and colleagues (2001) showed similar protection with vitamin C and multivitamins while demonstrating a slight protective effect from vitamin E.

Lutein is one of the carotenoids that has received increasing attention since it was reported in 1994 to confer a 20 percent protection against lens opacities. Gale (2001) showed that lutein decreased the risk of posterior subcapsular cataracts by 50 percent while lycopene decreased the risk of cortical cataracts and high levels of alpha- and beta-carotene decreased levels of nuclear cataracts. Similarly Taylor's group confirmed that carotenoids (which maintain cell membrane integrity and facilitate nutrient transport) protect against posterior subcapsular cataracts. Individuals who consume high carotenoids also have high folic acid levels.

Saturated fat intake has been associated with increased risk of cataract and AMD, whereas fish intake has been proven beneficial to ocular health. Obesity increases the risk of both cataracts and AMD; fat tends to absorb fat-soluble antioxidants so higher levels are required. Also, evidence suggests that estrogen therapy decreases the risk of cataracts in postmenopausal women.

Wang and colleagues reported the correlation of cataract development with decreased lifespan. Therefore, it is fair to say that factors that reduce the risk of cataracts would tend to promote health in general. Furthermore, as you may expect, cataracts increase the chance of automotive accidents. Owsley reported, in the four-to-six-year follow-up on 277 patients in twelve Alabama clinics, that those with cataracts had twice the rate of motor vehicle accidents.

So I continue to recommend taking vitamin C (2000 mg per day) and sulfur-containing glutathione boosters (ALA, MSM, or NAC, 200 mg per day) and eating onions, garlic, asparagus, eggs, and avocados. Also patients with early cataracts should drink lots of water and wear UV-blocking sunglasses.

Although there is a cascade of evidence that antioxidants can stop cataracts, many patients do not get this information until it is too late. Therefore, surgery remains the only treatment option for many. But it is important to know that the decision for cataract surgery is determined by the patient after his vision can no longer be corrected with glasses.

Dr. Abel's Tip

The development of cataracts may be related to the quality of nutrition, general health, and longevity. Let's stop cataracts early if we can.

The surgical technique of phaco emulsification remains the standard procedure for removing cataracts. Until smaller intraocular implanted lenses (IOLs) are available, there is no reason to make a smaller incision than the current 2.5 to 3.0 mm, which doesn't require a suture. In terms of IOLs, silicone is favored over acrylic (folded plastic), while PMMA (nonfoldable plastic) is infrequently used. The Collamer synthetic collagen lens from Staar is rising in popularity because of its flexibility. Multifocal IOLs, which provide some distance and near vision, are reserved for people who don't drive much at night.

Laser cataract surgery (with laser probe in the eye) has been approved by the FDA but is rarely used. The laser technique is highly expensive and prolongs surgery time. So we will continue to look for cheaper, safer, and more effective techniques. Stopping cataracts before they form remains the best choice.

Research continues to be done on an accommodative IOL such as injection of a hydrogel material into the cataract bag, which can allow people to focus. Also phakic IOLs are being approved for people with very high refractive errors; in these cases the normal lens is not removed. Lastly some surgeons are removing the clear crystalline lens as a refractive procedure to alter the power of the eye without ever having to worry about developing a cataract later; since this is a refractive procedure, it is not covered by conventional health insurance companies.

Glaucoma

Several new avenues of diagnosis and treatment for glaucoma have opened up as the factors that cause the disease are better understood. The role of systemic disease has received more attention since Gottfredsdottir and colleagues indicated the coexistence of diseases such as diabetes, hypertension, and hypothyroidism with glaucoma.

We have known that the measurement of IOP may vary throughout the twenty-four-hour cycle; the IOP is often highest at night, when the melatonin level is low. The optic nerve is even more vulnerable at nighttime because blood pressure is often at its lowest (and even lower if antihypertensive medication is being used).

Kountouras reported a high prevalence of heliobacter pylori infection (gastric ulcers) in patients with glaucoma. These were detected in 88 percent of 41 patients with glaucoma and 47 percent of 30 age-matched normal people. Two years after treatment the glaucoma patients had not only improved IOP control but also demonstrated improved visual fields. Other researchers felt that this study is flawed, but nonetheless, it points to a previously undiscovered and very treatable factor in glaucoma.

Laser scanning of the optic nerve and retina have become standard tests for following the course of glaucoma and can tell which therapies are the best for individual patients. Viewing of the optic nerve (now with scanning devices over conventional observation or photography), IOP measurements, and visual fields are still the three yardsticks of diagnosis and therapy. Also it has been documented that IOP measurements can be artificially higher in patients with thicker corneas, such as farsighted people or those who have had cataract or corneal surgery.

There are new techniques to evaluate the optic nerve, and the HRT (Heidelberg Retina Tomography) is witnessing increased popularity. Other scanning devices are the GDx, which views the nerve fiber layer; OCT (optical coherence tomography); and Retinal Thickness Analyzer. Most up-to-date glaucoma specialists will use one of these for an annual evaluation.

Dr. Abel's Tip

The treatment of glaucoma is directed at
·Lowering IOP
·Improving blood flow to the optic nerve (and the retina)
·Protecting the nerve fibers against chemicals, proteins, hormones, etc.

Ophthalmologic therapy is generally aimed at lowering eye pressure, which is the easiest to measure and control with the more effective eyedrops at our disposal. There is an increased reliance on long-term medical therapy and fewer surgeries. The first lines of eyedrop therapy are the prostamides, which are actually derivatives of essential fatty acids, and bromonidine, an epinephrine-type drug. The beta-blockers, which can lower pulse and blood pressure (after many years in the elderly), are used as supporting therapy.

The current prostamides or prostaglandin-type drugs are latanoprost .005 (xalatan), travoprost .004 (travatan), and bimatoprost .003 percent (lumigan). These drugs increase outflow and, being applied at bedtime, counteract the period in which IOP may be at its highest. Rescula, a derivative of the essential fatty acid DHA, is a weaker agent that seems to lubricate the outflow channels.

I recommend improving circulation to the optic nerve by practicing total body relaxation and stimulation of the parasympathetic nervous system (see Chapter 7). Deep breathing relaxes the body and allows increased blood flow, which is necessary for the retina, which has the highest level of metabolism in the body. Chung and colleagues found ginkgo biloba increased the ocular blood flow in volunteers and in some glaucoma patients. Dr. Robert Ritch of New York Eye and Ear Infirmary uses it in all of his glaucoma patients. Ginkgo is a bioflavonoid that may increase anxiety or alter blood pressure, so inform your doctor of what you are taking. An alternative is salvia miltirhizia, a calming Chinese herb that also dilates blood vessels.

I have used trifola or triphala (a combination of three fruits) in 100 patients, 80 percent of whom remain on it because it has been successful in helping stabilize their glaucoma condition. Although trifola's IOP reduction may be short lasting, the supplement also improves circulation and relaxes the body. Always make sure you are seeing a competent herbalist and that the herbs are standardized. Also tell your doctor to rule out the remote chance of any interactions.

Lastly, genetic research may cast some light on the third aspect of glaucoma therapy, neuroprotection. Some investigators now feel that glaucoma is a disease of preprogrammed cell death, i.e., cells die before their time. The gene OPTN (which makes a protein called optineurin) has been isolated. The normal gene makes optineurin and protects the cells around the optic nerve from free radical damage. The abnormal gene makes a defective smaller protein that doesn't do the job. Who knows where this existing avenue of research can lead.

Macular Degeneration

There are many new things happening in the fields of AMD and retina diseases in general. The eight-year multicenter ARED Study produced some definitive results. Not only did this landmark study document that the combination of beta-carotene, vitamins C and E, and zinc spares vision loss, but it also confirmed certain predisposing factors. The study broke the development of AMD into five stages, with the fifth being the most severe. Obesity, farsightedness, being Caucasion, use of thyroid hormones, and use of antacids were associated with the development of end-stage macular degeneration. Smoking was associated with stages 3 and 5. Meanwhile the Beaver Dam Eye Study showed that the greater the unprotected exposure to sunlight, the greater the risk of AMD.

Since the ARED formula proved so successful, Bausch and Lomb has created Ocuvite PreserVision™ to provide patients with the same formula. It has recently been noted that beta-carotene conversion to vitamin A is very unreliable. Therefore, taking vitamin A, which is the active nutrient, may be the wiser choice. Some studies indicate that high levels of zinc (e.g., 80 mg) may interfere with the absorption of calcium, magnesium, selenium, copper, and other two-valance minerals. My recommendation is to take less than 50 mg a day.

But other nutrients are proving effective in counteracting the free radicals produced by light and oxidative stress. At the top of the list is lutein (the FloraGLO® purified lutein). Hammond demonstrated 2.4 mg of lutein doubles the blood level. Other groups showed that 10 to 30 mg per day increase the pigment levels in the macula area significantly.

Bone and colleages demonstrated in autopsy eyes that those eyes with the highest lutein and zeoxanthin levels in the retina were 82 percent less likely to have AMD. This parallels Seddon et al.'s 1994 results showing those with the highest blood levels of carotenoids were 86 percent less likely to develop AMD. In fact, Bernstein has found that there is more lutein in the eye than beta-carotene or vitamin A. It's astonishing to think that spinach is better for your eyes than Bugs Bunny's carrots.

Since I have been recommending a multivitamin (including vitamins

A, C, and E), lutein, DHA, and a B-complex, I have seen very few AMD patients worsen over the years and 10 percent of those with dry type improve. Starvation of the retina can be rectified by supporting the liver, eliminating antacids, minimizing prescription drugs, and eating well whenever possible. Wear sunglasses, since the amount of solar radiation hitting the eyes plays a role in the development of AMD.

Dr. Abel's Tip

Keep your antioxidant bank account full: choose a healthy lifestyle and maintain a positive attitude.

Well, there is also hope for people who develop the wet form of macular degeneration. Photodynamic therapy using an intravenous dye that clings to leaky blood vessels beneath the retina (verteporfin) is activated by a "cold" laser, which is far less destructive to the overlaying fragile retinal receptors. The procedure is effective and safe and may have to be repeated. Novartis has been approved for early retreatment of the neovascular membrane beneath the macula. Photodynamic therapy is currently the most available therapy for wet macular degeneration when promptly detected.

Several companies have produced drugs that can be injected onto the surface of the retina to stop the bleeding of AMD. Genetech's RhuFab™ and Eyetech Pharmaceutical's Macujen™ counter new blood-vessel growth into the retina. As these trials proceed, more retina specialists will have the drugs available for their patients.

Other Retina Conditions

The treatment of macular holes and epiretinal membranes consists of removing the vitreous fluid and scar tissue in the retina; this procedure is called a virectomy and has become standard for all retina surgeons. This surgical technique has been expanded to include new options for patients with AMD and retinal disease. These new experimental options consist of replacing the RPE, translocating the retina in severe cases, and injecting pigment epithelium derived factor in wet AMD patients. Other investigators are inserting silicone chips either above or in the retina. Such chips are placed in poor-seeing eyes with possibly a second one (to stimulate it) located in the glasses. These devices have a role in treating retinitis pigmentosa (RP) patients, since many of the layers in the retina are not involved in this degenerative disease.

Research is continuing into the placement of electrodes near or into the visual cortex at the back of the brain. The risks of infection and the generation of heat remain the two barriers to be surmounted before this technique becomes clinically available.

Imagine that placing genes in the eye has become a reality. The RPE 65 gene makes a protein that transports vitamin A into the retina receptors. This is missing in Leber's congenital optic neuropathy. By injecting a virus containing RPE 65 into the eyes of dogs with a variant of Leber's disease, some vision has been restored. This therapy is also being studied for patients with RP, AMD, and retinablastoma tumor.

Diabetes

The incidence of diabetes is skyrocketing, with 16 million adults and at least 300,000 children now diagnosed with type II diabetes. Diabetes mellitus is another area in which researchers are studying how to prevent abnormal new blood vessel growth. Many factors that inhibit blood vessel growth have been identified in animal models. Frank reported an enzyme that facilitates the development of diabetic retinopathy; here is another area that is being actively studied.

People must pay attention to the glycemic index, or rather the glycemic load, of their food. Nutritionists are in agreement that you should choose vegetables, fish, and whole grains over red meat, refined products, coffee, and soft drinks. But the vending machines in schools are not placed there by organic farmers. A 7 percent weight loss combined with 2.5 hours of brisk walking per week are enough to lower blood sugar and HbA1c.

Consider that even a short duration of diabetes may be associated with increased occlusion of retinal capillaries. Therefore, the American Diabetes Association recommends an aspirin tablet a day. Alpha-lipoic acid (250 mg twice daily) will lower blood sugar by making cell membranes more sensitive to insulin. In fact, Coleman states that alpha-lipoic acid protects people from full-blown diabetes, and I have found that vitamin C (1000 to 2000 mg) and quercetin (1000 mg) can strengthen blood vessels. DHA and other selective supplements and lifestyle changes are imperative for managing diabetes. Prevention starts at the dining room table.

Dry Eyes

More of my colleagues are talking about the good results they are seeing in their dry eye patients since they have begun recommending Omega-3 essential fatty acids. The end product of the Omega-3 fatty acids is DHA, which stabilizes membranes, reduces inflammation, and makes for more stable meiborman (oil) gland secretions. For more information on the subject of essential fatty acids and DHA in particular, see my book *The DHA Story* (Basic Health Publications, 2002).

Lee and colleages reported that as much as 23 percent of patients had reduced Scheirmer tests, i.e. more ocular dryness, up to six months after LASIK surgery. This is why I recommend vitamin C (2000 mg) and DHA (400 to 600 mg) with vitamin E (400 IU) to support the tear film and the cornea after laser surgery. Wavefront technology should lessen dry eyes.

Hormone replacement therapy, once thought to protect the heart and prevent dry eye in postmenopausal females, has proved a failure on both counts. Women who used estrogen alone were found to be 69 percent more likely to have dry eyes than women who did not use hormones. Those women who used estrogen and progesterone together had a 29 percent greater risk of dry eyes. I recommend that you consider taking human estrogen and progesterone, obtainable from compounding pharmacies, but discuss this with your doctor first.

In the cornea field there have been few advances. Implanting healthy cells in the internal lining of the cornea is making slow progress. There is a new artificial cornea from Australia, but corneal prostheses remain for those people who have failed human donor corneal transplants.

Children's Eye Problems

Essential fatty acids are mandatory for the development of a child's retina and brain in utero. The placenta selectively pumps DHA and the Omega-6 arachidonic acid, which together comprise almost 60 percent of the brain. Martek Biosciences Corporation has developed an infant formula blending these two essential fatty acids, DHA and arachidonic acid, which are normally found in breast milk. This formula has received FDA approval for use with pregnant women, lactating mother, and infants.

Dr. Abel's Tip

Studies show breastfed infants whose mothers took DHA from a vegetarian source scored higher on psychomotor development tests than infants whose mothers did not supplement with DHA. Infants who have these two compounds added to their formula experience faster mental and visual development, much like breastfed infants, than those with ordinary formulas.

Why do I bring this up? Well, infants who have the highest DHA levels will grow up with less chance of having a learning disability. Pregnant women and mothers of infants and small children should consider DHA supplementation. Omega-6 fatty acids are abundantly available in terrestrial plants so are frequently consumed in our diets. But the long-chain Omega-3 fatty acids found primarily in algae and cold-water fatty fish are not often included in our diet.

Patching the good (seeing) eye has been the standard for treating infants with amblyopia, or lazy eye. Repka and colleagues have demonstrated that both parents and children prefer to blur the good eye with atropine drops and that this method is just as effective as patching.

Autism in children may now be detected as early as 3 months with new eye-tracking technology. It appears that children with autism focus on people's mouths rather than their eyes. Earlier diagnosis and treatment for this little-understood neurological condition can make a great difference, since it is often undetected until the age of 3 or 4.

Other Eye Diseases

Optic neuritis is a cause of sudden visual loss that may appear as an isolated condition or as part of a recurrent dermyelinating disorder, multiple sclerosis. The CHAMPS (Controlled High Risk Subjects Avonex MS Prevention Study) has indicated that interferon beta-1A decreases the chance of patients with optic neuritis developing MS in the future. For those individuals with more advanced disease, DHA and Myelin Sheath Support Formula™ may be supportive and help stabilize the disease.

Uveitis and iritis are acute, chronic, or episodic disorders often without a recognized underlying cause. Topical dilating drops and steroids remain the conventional treatment, although long-term steroid therapy can have side effects. Tumeric root extract (also known as curcumin) has long been used in Chinese medicine for its anti-inflammatory effect, which has recently been scientifically studied. Gail reported that curcumin (378 mg three times daily) in thirty-two patients with chronic iritis provided improvement comparable to that seen with similar cortisone doses.

Foods for Eye Health

Hippocrates continues to be correct when he said we should let food be our medicine. The starting point for eye and total body health remains the diet: balancing food groups, reducing saturated fat, and eliminating transfats. Below is my list for the top ten foods for sight:

1. *Cold-water fish (sardines, cod, mackerel, tuna)* are excellent sources of DHA, which provides structural support to the cell membrane and is recommended for dry eyes, macular degeneration, and sight preservation. Farm-raised fish is not as good.

2. *Spinach, kale, and green leafy vegetables* are rich in the carotenoids, especially lutein and zeaxanthin. Lutein, a yellow pigment, protects the macula from sun damage and from blue light.

3. *Eggs* are rich in cysteine, sulfur, lecithin, amino acids, and lutein. Sulfur-containing compounds protect the lens of the eye from cataract formation.

4. *Garlic, onions, shallots, and capers* are also rich in sulfur, which is necessary for the production of glutathoine, an important antioxidant for the lens of the eye and for the whole body as well.

5. *Soy,* low in fat and rich in protein, has become a staple in vegetarian diets. Soy contains essential fatty acids, phytoestrogens, vitamin E, and natural anti-inflammatory agents.

6. *Fruits and vegetables high in vitamins A, C, and E, and beta-carotene* are important for vision. The yellow vegetables, such as carrots and squash, are important for daytime vision. The green leafy vegetables are rich in lutein. Tomatoes and tomato paste are high in lycopene.

7. *Blueberries and grapes* contain anthocyanins, which improve night vision. A cup of blueberries, huckleberry jam, or a 100 mg bilberry supplement should improve dark adaptation within thirty minutes.

8. *Wine,* known to have cardioprotective effects, has many important nutrients that protect the vision, the heart, and blood flow. Needless to say, moderation is always important. Also *green tea* is high in catechins, bioflavonoids that are cardioprotective.

9. *Nuts and berries* are nature's most concentrated food sources. *Seeds,* such as flaxseed, are high in the beneficial Omega-3 fatty acids, which help lower cholesterol and stabilize cell membranes. But DHA from algae and fish is a much better source.

10. *Virgin olive oil,* a monounsaturated oil, is a healthy alternative to butter, margarine, and other cooking oils.

In addition to increasing your consumption of these beneficial foods, be sure to minimize your use of refined flour, sugar, artificial sweeteners, processed hydrogenated foods, and hormone-fed meat products.

Supplements

Over the past few years there have been several negative articles about certain supplements. I feel that a balanced approach to the subject of supplementation is necessary. The Finnish Smokers Study reported that beta-carotene users had a higher incidence of lung cancer than the control group. Well, it turns out that synthetic beta-carotene, a very ineffective version of the true provitamin A compound, was used for the study, which featured a high-risk group of subjects. Vitamin A at doses of 17,000 IU daily has been established as safe.

Reading the label is important. Natural vitamin E is delta-alpha-tocopherol, the active form. Synthetic vitamin E is made with the delta and levo forms, which almost neutralize each other. Vitamin C is either praised or disregarded. Well, a 2001 *Lancet* article correlated high blood levels of ascorbic acid with greater longevity. Similarly vitamin C use was shown to decreases the risk of cataracts and the development of cataracts in the Australian Blue Mountain Study.

Vitamin C should also be used in the prevention of diabetic retinopathy, says the University of Aachen team that showed vitamin C, a basic component of the vitreous humor, maintains the health of the retinal pigment epithelial cells.

Ginkgo biloba (120 mg per day) showed no cognitive benefits in a 2002 study conducted by Solomon and colleagues at Williams College. However, there are more than 125 clinical trials spanning two decades that have indicated ginkgo's effectiveness at improving memory or cognitive activity. Ginkgo certainly must have some effect when it increases the blood flow to the eye. At any rate, this ancient nostrum remains the top-selling herbal supplement in the United States, edging out panax ginseng, whose claims are more disputed.

Remember, our bodies produce glutathione, which prevents oxidative stress and delays aging. Gluthathione is a combination of three amino acids that trap free radicals, serve as enzymes, bind with Tylenol to remove it from the body, and keep the lens of the eye clear. Knight has shown that the levels of serum glutathione correlate with the speed of aging. So eat the sulfur-containing foods or supplement with NAC (600 mg twice daily), MSM (1000 mg daily), or alpha-lipoic acid (250 mg twice daily).

For the best supplements for your vision, refer to Chapter 15.

Aging Gracefully

A 1999 PBS program on aging moderated by Bill Moyers highlighted five factors that enable the elderly to maintain good memory. These factors are:

1. A changing social environment (socializing with others)
2. Cardiopulmonary health (the ability to avoid serious heart or lung disease)
3. Plenty of exercise (walking a minium of four to seven times a week)
4. Fine motor control (for example, using a computer or playing chess or darts)
5. A flexible personality (the ability to cope with change)

You could also add two more factors to this list: the dietary choices your mother made before, during, and after her pregnancy; and your current dietary habits.

Environment Awareness

Cosmetics with caffeine? Check the label. If it has caffeine, look for another product.

By-products of animal production, fertilizers, and manure are full of nitrogen and phosphorous, which do not biodegrade. They run into streams, causing algae plumes that change the ecosystem. We are using up water faster than it is being replenished due to overirrigating, excessive lawn watering, removal of trees, and erosion from our natural habitat.

Pollution doesn't affect just one part of the body. We need to practice conservation so we can get our six to eight glasses in!

Nature Versus Nurture: Uncovering Genetics

A great deal of attention and research is being focused on unraveling the role of genetic susceptibility in certain common diseases. For instance, a gene called Apo E has three different forms: E2, E3, and E4. A patient with Apo E4 has a greater risk of heart disease. Conversely, people with Apo E2 and Apo E3 will not be able to alter their cholesterol levels by diet, but are at less risk of heart disease.

There is a growing field called nutrigenomics that looks at the way food interacts with heredity. Researchers have found that only 15 percent of the population has high blood pressure caused by salt (sodium) retention. Therefore, only 15 percent of hypertensives will derive any benefit from salt restriction. So why treat all hypertensives with low-sodium diets?

Soon people will be able to obtain a genetic profile (currently on 300 or so genes) to predict how they personally might benefit from different diets. Ultimately the answer to nature versus nurture is that you cannot pick your parents, but you can choose your food. In addition, researchers are examining how various medications affect people differently.

Summary

A recent neurobiological study reported the response of baby owls to wearing prism glasses that diverted their vision. Since owls combine their seeing and hearing to localize their prey, the prism goggles, which threw off their sight 17 degrees, interrupted their ability to hunt. However, within days the baby owls were able to readjust their sensory orientation and hunt again. On the other hand, adult owls upon wearing the prism glasses were unable to adapt and thus became depressed; the goggles had to be removed to avoid their starving. The study reported that shifting the vision by 6-degree increments allowed adult owls to adjust as well as the juveniles.

This lesson from nature may not be as remote as it first seems. Flexibility and adaptability enable these nocturnal carnivores to adapt and survive. We also need to recognize that occasionally we wear blinders and must remain flexible in our approaches to adversity. One of the important messages of The Eye Care Revolution is to always look for options while you protect the health of your eyes and your body. In fact, if you remain proactive in taking care of yourself, you will manage early symptoms and may avoid medications and surgery when symptoms become full blown.

Lastly, discovery never stops. There are many helpful resources on the path of wellness. My wish is that you always remain the shepherd of your own body and partner in its care.

Resource Guide

Throughout this book, I have made the connection between the necessity of total body health in achieving eye health. To that end, this resource guide includes companies and organizations with superior products and useful information for achieving eye and body health.

Allergy Research Group
30806 Santana Street
Hayward, CA 94544
1-800-545-9960
510-487-8526

Carlson® Laboratories
15 College Drive
Arlington Heights, IL 60004-1985
1-800-323-4141
1-847-255-1600

Cooper Concepts
12200 Preston Road
Dallas, TX 75230
1-888-393-2221

Gaia Herbs, Inc.
1-800-831-7780

Jarrow Formulas, Inc.™
1824 South Robertson Blvd.
Los Angeles, CA 90035-4317
1-800-726-0886
1-310-204-6936

Natrol®
21411 Prairie St.

Chatsworth, CA 91311
1-800-326-1520
818-739-6000
http://www.natrol.com

Nature's Plus
548 Broadhollow Road
Melville, NY 11747
1-800-937-0500

Nature's Way
1-800-962-8873

NEEDS
1-800-634-1380
This is a total resource for every type of environmental product (air cleaners, water filters, etc.).

NutriCology (subsidiary of Scottsdale Scientific, Inc.)
418 Mission Street
San Rafael, CA 94901
888-563-1506

OncoLogics, Inc.
1-800-724-5566

Plantetary Formula
23 Janis Way
Scotts Valley, CA 95066
408-438-1144

ScienceBased Health Co.
3579 Highway 50 East
Carson City, NV 89701
888-433-4726
http://www.sciencebasedhealth.com

Solaray (Nutraceutical Corp.)
1-800-669-8877

Solgar Vitamin & Herb
500 Willow Tree Road
Leonia, NJ 07605
1-800-645-2246

Source Naturals®
23 Janis Way
Scotts Valley, CA 96066
1-800-777-5677
http://www.sourcenaturals.com
Products available at fine healthfood stores everywhere.

Twin Laboratories, Inc.
150 Motor Parkway
Hauppauge, NY 11788
1-800-645-5626

Wakunaga of America
Mission Viejo, CA 92691
1-800-421-2998

Eye Formulations
(The following companies have excellent composite formulations designed specifically for eye health:)

Carlson®
PRODUCT NAME: Abel Eyes
CONTAINS: Vitamin C, Vitamin A, Vitamin E, Lutein, Magnesium, Chromium, Quercetin, Bilberry, Rutin, Silymarin, and Zinc. In soft gel form. Created as a basic eye supplement, these essential ingredients were formulated by Dr. Robert Abel.

PRODUCT NAME: Eye-Rite™
CONTAINS: Lutein, Bilberry Extract, Cranberry Extract, Grape Seed Extract, Citrus Bioflavonoid Complex, Quercetin, Soy Isoflavone Concentrate, Alpha Lipoic, Vitamin E, Vitamin C, Vitamin A, Zinc, Chromium, and Spirulina-Algae. In capsule form.

PRODUCT NAME: Moistur-Eyes™
CONTAINS: Salmon Oil (supplying EPA and DHA), Borage Oil (supplying GLA), Vitamin E, Vitamin A, Vitamin D, Vitamin B-6, Biotin, Vitamin C, and Zinc. In softgel form.

Biometrics
PRODUCT NAME: Macula
CONTAINS: Vitamins A, C and E, Vitamin B2, Beta-Carotene Lycopene, Lutein, Zeaxanthin, Zinc, Selenium, NAC, and Bilberry. In tablet form.

Healthy Impact
PRODUCT NAME: Nutrition for Your Eyes
CONTAINS: Vitamin C, MSM, Vitamin E, Beta-Carotene, N-Acetyl Cysteine, Alpha Lipoic Acid, Taurine, Cysteine, Lutein, Grape Seed Extract, Dilphindrin, and Selenium. In capsule form.

Natrol™
PRODUCT NAME: Eye Support w/Bilberry
CONTAINS: Bilberry Fruit Extract, Blueberry Leaf, Eyebright Leaf, Rasberry Leaf, Barberry Leaf, and Pulsatilla Leaf. In capsule form.

NutriCology®
PRODUCT NAME: OcuDyne II with Lutein
CONTAINS: NAC, Bilberry Extract, Ginko Biloba, Quercetin, Taurine, L-Methionine, Silicon, Lutein, and important minerals and B Vitamins. In capsule form.

Planetary Formula (Michael Tierra, C.A., N.D.)
PRODUCT NAME: Bilberry Eye Complex
Available in 643mg tablets

PRODUCT NAME: Bilberry Vision
CONTAINS: Bilberry Extract, yielding 37% Anthocyanosides
Available in 100mg tablets

ScienceBased Health
PRODUCT NAME: HydroEye™
Formulation for dry eye syndrome, containing a blend of Omega-6 fatty acids,
    mucim/sialic acid complex, and nutrient cofactors. In softgel form.

PRODUCT NAME: MaculaRx™
CONTAINS: Bilberry Extract, Carotenoids, Beta Carotene, Xanthophylls,
    Zeazanthin & Cryotoxanthin, Ginkgo Biloba Extract, Inositol, Lipoic Acid, NAC, and
    Taurine. Includes other compatible vitamins such as Vitamins A, C and E. In
    capsule form.

PRODUCT NAME: OculaRx™
CONTAINS: Bilberry Extract, Carotenoids, Beta Carotene, Xanthophylls, Lutein,
    Zeaxanthin & Cryptoxanthin, Choline, Ginkgo Biloba Extract, Grape Seed Extract,
    Hesperidin Bioflavonoid Complex, Lipoic Acid, NAC, Rutin, and Taurine. Also
    includes a total multivitamin and multimineral formulation. In capsule form.

PRODUCT NAME: Optic Nerve Formula™
A synergistic combination of neuroprotective agents, ocular antioxidants, and vaso
    neuronal activators
Available in capsule form.

PRODUCT NAME: SBH Ocular Essentials™
A complete multivitamin/mineral with special eye formulations: Carotenoids,
    Carotenes, Alpha-Carotene, Beta-Carotene, Gamma-Carotene, Lycopene,
    Xanthophylls, Lutein, Zeaxanthin and Cryptoxanthin, Taurine, and Bilberry
    Extract. Available in capsules.

Solgar
PRODUCT NAME: Bilberry Ginkgo Eyebright Complex Plus Lutein
CONTAINS: Vitamin A, Natural Beta Carotene/Carotenoid Mix, Lutein, Vitamin
    C, and Vitamin E
Available in Vegicaps®

Source Naturals
PRODUCT NAME: Visual-Eyes
Multi-Nutrient Complex
CONTAINS: Bilberry Extract, Lipoic Acid, Lutein, Ginkgo Biloba, Quercetin, NAC,
    Taurine, and Inositol. Includes other synergistic vitamins and minerals.
Available in tablet form

Twin Laboratories, Inc.
PRODUCT NAME: OcuGuard® Plus
CONTAINS: (in 2 capsules) Vitamins A, C; E, Riboflavin, Zinc, Selenium,
    Chromium, Lutein, Citrus Bioflavonoid Complex, NAC, Taurine, Quercetin, Rutin,
    Bilberry Extract, and L-glutathione

Vitamin A
Available from the following companies:

Carlson®
PRODUCT NAME: ACES

PRODUCT NAME: Vitamin A
Available in various forms

Source Naturals™
PRODUCT NAME: Vitamin A
CONTAINS: 10,000 i.u. in tablet form

Allergy Control
Available from the following company:
Biometrics
PRODUCT NAME: Aller Clear
CONTAINS: Vitamin C, Pantothenic Acid, Quercetin, and Stinging Nettles
Available in capsule form

Aplha Lipoic Acid
Available from the following companies:
Allergy Research Group
PRODUCT NAME: ThioDox™
CONTAINS: N-Acetyl-Cysteine, Glutathione, Lipoic Acid, TTFD, Riboflavin 5
    Phosphate, Ascorbic Acid, and L-Selenomethionine. Available in tablets.

Carlson®
PRODUCT NAME: Alpha Lipoic Acid
Available in 100mg tablets

Jarrow Formulas™
PRODUCT NAME: Alpha Lipoic Acid
Available in 100mg capsules

PRODUCT NAME: Alpha Lipoic Sustain 300
Sustained released tablets, 300mg each

Source Naturals™
PRODUCT NAME: Lipoic Acid
Available in 200mg tablets

Amino Acids
Available from the following company:
Allergy Research Group
PRODUCT NAME: Free Aminos™
CONTAINS: 17 naturally occurring amino acids in their free forms, including 9
    essential amino acids. Does not contain tryptophan. Available in capsules or powder.

Antioxidants
Available from the following companies:

Carlson®
PRODUCT NAME: Aces Gold™
CONTAINS: Vitamin E, Zinc, Selenium, Co-Q10, Glutathione, N-Acetyl Cysteine,
    Alpha Lipoic, Citrus Bioflavonoids, Quercetin, Garlic, Grape Seed Extract,
    Green Tea, and others.
RECOMMENDED: 2 tablets daily at mealtime

Natrol®
PRODUCT NAME: The Ultimate Anti-Oxidant Formula
CONTAINS: Vitamins A, C and E, Niacinamide, Copper, and Zinc
Available in capsules

Source Naturals
PRODUCT NAME: Super Beta Carotene
CONTAINS: 20,000 i.u. in softgel form

B-Complex (contains all of the individual B Vitamins)
Available from the following companies:

Carlson®
PRODUCT NAME: B-50 Gel
Balanced B-Complex in softgel form

PRODUCT NAME: Time-B®
Timed-Release: 50mg tablets

Jarrow Formulas™
PRODUCT NAME: B-Right™
Balanced B-Complex in capsule form

Source Naturals
PRODUCT NAME: CoEnzymate™ B Complex
Sublingual (dissolves under the tongue and goes directly into bloodstream) tablets
    in peppermint and orange flavors with Co-Q10

PRODUCT NAME: B-12
Dibencozide Sublingual CoEnzymated™ B-12

Beta Carotene
Available from the following companies:

Carlson®
PRODUCT NAME: Super Beta Carotene 25,000 i.u.

Jarrow Formulas™
PRODUCT NAME: Marine Beta Carotene™
Available in 15mg softgels

Available in softgels

PRODUCT NAME: Marine Carotene
100% Natural D. Salina, 25,000 I.U.
Available in softgels

PRODUCT NAME:Multi Carotene
CONTAINS: Beta Carotene, Alpha Carotene, Lycopene, Lutein and Zeaxanthin
Available in capsules

Source Naturals®
PRODUCT NAME: Beta Carotene
Pro-Vitamin A
CONTAINS: 20,000 i.u. Vitamin A in softgel form

PRODUCT NAME: SuperBeta Carotene™
All-natural, derived from single-cell algae, available in softgel form

Bilberry (contains active ingredients which affect proper eye function)
Available from the following companies:

Carlson®
PRODUCT NAME: Bilberry
CONTAINS: Potent Standardized Bilberry plus Vitamins A and E
In 25mg softgels

Jarrow Formulas™
PRODUCT NAME: Bilberry 100:1 and Grapeskin Polyphenols
Available in 280 mg capsules

Natrol®
PRODUCT NAME: Bilberry 25%
CONTAINS: 100:1 Bilberry Extract in capsule form

Solgar
PRODUCT NAME: Bilberry
Available in 260mg Vegicaps®

Source Naturals™
PRODUCT NAME: Bilberry Extract
Standardized to 25% Anthocyanosides
Available in 100mg tablets

Borage (oil)
Available from the following company:

Jarrow Formulas™
PRODUCT NAME: Borage GLA-240 and Ganna Tocopherol
240mg Gammalinolenic Acid (GLA) in softgel form

Vitamin C and Ester C©
Available from the following companies:

Carlson®
PRODUCT NAME: Buffered Vitamin C
Also other vitamin C formulations. Available in caps

Natrol®
PRODUCT NAME: Ester-C® 500 Mg with Bioflavonoids
Available in 500mg capsules and tablets

Source Naturals
PRODUCT NAME: Vitamin C
Available in crystals in varying doses

Cod Liver Oil
Available from the following companies:

Carlson®:
PRODUCT NAME: Norwegian Cod Liver Oil
CONTAINS: 500-550mg DHA, 460-500mg EPA, and 46-50mg ALA
In liquid form and also available in lemon flavored.

Co-Q10
Available from the following companies:

Carlson®
PRODUCT NAME: Coenzyme Q10
Different strengths available up to 300 mg

Solgar
PRODUCT NAME: Coenzyme Q-10
Available in 30mg and 100mg softgels

Source Naturals®
PRODUCT NAME: Coenzyme Q10 with Bioperinerm
Available in 30mg capsules

PRODUCT NAME: Coenzyme Q10 Lipoic Acid
Available in 30mg capsules

PRODUCT NAME: Ultra Potency Coenzyme Q10
Available in 125mg capsules

DHA (necessary for tissue building in the brain and retina)
Available from the following companies:

Carlson®
PRODUCT NAME: Super DHA™
Available in 500mg softgels. An excellent product

PRODUCT NAME: Liquid Omega 3 oil
500 mg DHA and 500 mg EPA
Available in softgels; an excellent product.

Jarrow Formulas™
PRODUCT NAME: Max DHA™
Available in 505mg softgels

Neuromins® DHA (from non-fish micro-algae sources, in softgel form)

Source Naturals®: available in 100 and 200mg softgels, by an excellent company.

Digestive Enzymes
Available from the following companies:

Natrol®
PRODUCT NAME: Digest Support™
CONTAINS: Proteolytic Enzymes, Amylolytic Enzymes, Lipolytic Enzymes, and
    Anti-Gas Factor
Available in capsules

Source Naturals®
PRODUCT NAME: Essential Enzymes™
Available in 500mg capsules

Twin Laboratories, Inc.
PRODUCT NAME: Digestease
Available in capsules

Vitamin E
Available from the following company:

Carlson®
PRODUCT NAME: E-Gems®
Available in 30-1200 i.u. softgels

PRODUCT NAME: E-Sel
CONTAINS: Vitamin E 400 I.U.
Available in softgels

Echinacea
Available from the following companies:

Carlson®
PRODUCT NAME: Echinacea plus Vitamin C
CONTAINS: 100mg Echinacea Extract and 250mg Vitamin C
In softgel form

Jarrow Formulas™
PRODUCT NAME: Echinacea Super 3
Made with super concentrates, available in 226mg capsules

Flaxseed Oil
Available from the following companies:

Allergy Research Group
PRODUCT NAME: Flax Seed Oil
Cold pressed, organic, in liquid form

Jarrow Formulas™
PRODUCT NAME: Flaxseed Oil™
Certified organic vegetarian Omega-3, available in 1000mg capsules

Source Naturals®
PRODUCT NAME: Flax Seed-Primrose Oil
ALA and GLA complex
Available in 1300mg softgels

Folic Acid
Available from the following company:

Jarrow Formulas™
PRODUCT NAME: Folic Acid
Available in 800mg capsules

Garlic
Available from the following companies:

Carlson®
PRODUCT NAME: Garlic-600
Odorless garlic supplement, available in 600mg tablets

Wakunaga of America
PRODUCT NAME: KyolicR Aged Garlic Extract™
Organically grown, 100% odorless

Ginger
Available from the following company:

Jarrow Formulas™
PRODUCT NAME: Freeze Dried Ginger
6:1 Concentrate, available in 500mg capsules

Ginkgo Biloba
Available from the following companies:

Carlson®
PRODUCT NAME: Ginkgo Biloba plus L-Glutamine
In softgel form

Jarrow Formulas™
PRODUCT NAME: Ginkgo Biloba 50:1
Available in 40mg and 60mg capsules and tablets

Glucosamine
Available from the following company:
Jarrow Formulas™
PRODUCT NAME: Glucosamine Sulfate 500
Sodium free, available in 670mg capsules

Glutathione
Available from the following companies:
Allergy Research Group
PRODUCT NAME: ThioDox™
CONTAINS: Lipoic Acid, NAC, and Glutathione, in tablet form

Carlson®
PRODUCT NAME: Glutathione Booster™
Available in capsule form

Grape Seed
Available from the following companies:
Carlson®
PRODUCT NAME: Grape Seed extract: 130 MG
Available in softgel form

Jarrow Formulas™
PRODUCT NAME: OPC + 95
Grape Seed Extract: 100:1, available in 50mg and 100mg capsules

L-Carnitine
Available from the following company:
Jarrow Formulas™
PRODUCT NAME: L-Carnitine 250
Sodium free, available in 250mg capsules

PRODUCT NAME: L-Canitine 500
Sodium Free, available in 500mg capsules

L-Carnosine
Available from the following company:
Source Naturals®
PRODUCT NAME: L-Carnosine 500mg
Available in tablets

Lutein
Available from the following company:

Solgar
PRODUCT NAME: Lutein Carotenoid Complex
Available in 15mg Vegicaps®

Lycopene
Available from the following companies:

Carlson®
PRODUCT NAME: Lycopene
Available in 5mg softgels

Source Naturals®
PRODUCT NAME: Lycopene
Antioxidant Carotenoid
Available in 5mg softgels

Magnesium
Available from the following company:

Jarrow Formulas™
PRODUCT NAME: Magnesium Optimizer
CONTAINS: Magnesium Citrate, Potassium Chloride, and Taurine.
Available in Quik-Solv™ tablets

Multivitamin and Mineral Formulas—for Adults
Available from the following companies:

Carlson®
PRODUCT NAME: Super-1-Daily
In tablet form
Nutrients and excipients derived from sources other than animal, fish or fowl.
    Formulated to contain extra Vitamin B-12.

Cooper Concepts
PRODUCT NAME: Cooper Complete
A scientifically proven formula with multiple health benefits that has been
    reformulated for eye health as well
Designed by Kenneth H. Cooper, M.D., MPH

Mariposa
PRODUCT NAME: In Vite™ Formula
Designed by Andrew Weil, M.D., and Samuel Benjamin, M.D.
Multivitamin formula with Co-Q10, in a 1-softgel, 1-coated tablet combination

ScienceBased Health
PRODUCT NAME: OptimumRx™
Multivitamin, multimineral, antioxidant formula in capsule form

Solgar
PRODUCT NAME: Omnium Multiple
A complete multiple including Alpha Lipoic Acid and Co-Q10.
Available in tablet form. Also available in iron and iodine free tablets.

Source Naturals®
PRODUCT NAME: Life Force™ Multiple
Metabolic Activator, iron-free, in tablet form

Twin Laboratories, Inc.
PRODUCT NAME: OcuGuard Plus
A multivitamin with clinically proven ingredients for eye health

Twin Laboratories, Inc.
PRODUCT NAME: Dia-Balance
5 formulations for diabetics. The eye health formula consists of ocuguard plus
pyenogenol.

Multivitamin and Mineral Formulas—for Children
Available from the following companies:

Allergy Research Group
PRODUCT NAME: Children's Multi—Vi—Min
Developed by Stephen A. Levine, Ph.D. Also available without copper or iron.
In capsule form

PRODUCT NAME: ProBalance™ for Kids
For children who hate swallowing pills. A great tasting combination powdered
nutritional supplement. Blends with any liquid easily for maximum
absorption. An excellent source of Soy.

Carlson®
PRODUCT NAME: Scooter Rabbit
Chewable and tasty tablets containing 13 natural vitamins and 12 organic minerals.
Sucrose-free.

Natrol®
PRODUCT NAME: My Favorite Multiple®
Available in capsules and tablets, also iron-free

Source Naturals®
PRODUCT NAME: Mega-Kid™
A delicious chewable multivitamin for children ages 1-10. Contains a full complement
of vitamins and minerals, and also includes Bioflavanoids, Bee Pollen, Papaya
and Rutin.
See bottle for correct dosage according to age.

N-Acetyl Cysteine
Available from the following companies:

Allergy Research Group
PRODUCT NAME: ThioDox™
CONTAINS: N-Acetyl-Cysteine, Glutathione, Lipoic Acid, TTFD, Riboflavin 5
Phosphate, Ascorbic Acid, and L-Selenomethionine. Available in tablets.

Carlson®
PRODUCT NAME: N•A•C•
Available in 500mg capsules and powder

Solgar
PRODUCT NAME: NAC
Available in 600mg Vegicaps®

Olive Leaf Extract
Available from the following companies:

Nature's Plus
PRODUCT NAME: Herbal Actives
Standardized Olive Leaf Extract with 6% Oleuropein
Available in 250mg capsules

Source Naturals®
PRODUCT NAME: Wellness Olive Leaf Extract
Superior product

Probiotics (including Acidophilus)
Available from the following companies:

Allergy Research Group
PRODUCT NAME: Symbiotics
CONTAINS: acidophilus group, bifidophilus group, sporogenes, in powdered form.
RECOMMENDED: ½-1 teaspoon daily

PRODUCT NAME: ProGreens with Advanced Probiotic Formula
CONTAINS: organic gluten-free barley, wheat, alfalfa grasses, Spirulina, Chlorella
Dairy-free probiotic cultures
RECOMMENDED: 1 capsule per day

Jarrow Formulas™
PRODUCT NAME: Jarro-Dophilus™ + FOS
CONTAINS: 7 species, high potency, non-dairy probiotics. Hypoallergenic.
Available in capsule or powder form

Wakunaga
PRODUCT NAME: Kyo-Dophilus®
CONTAINS: L. acidophilus, B. bifidum, and B. longum, 1.5 billion live cells per
  capsule
RECOMMENDED: 1 capsule twice daily with meals

Quercetin
Available from the following companies:

Jarrow Formulas™
PRODUCT NAME: Quercetin 500™
Available in 500mg capsules

Source Naturals
PRODUCT NAME: Activated Quercetin
non-allergenic Bioflavonoid Complex with Bromelain
Available in 1000mg tablets

Resveratrol
Available from the following companies:

Natrol®
PRODUCT NAME: Protykin™/Reservatrol
Available in capsules

Source Naturals®
PRODUCT NAME: Reservatrol
Available in 10mg tablets

Selenium
Available from the following companies:

Carlson®
PRODUCT NAME: Selenium
Available in 200mcg tablets

Jarrow Formulas™
PRODUCT NAME: Selenium Synergy™
Selenium with Vitamin B2, Vitamin E, and garlic in capsule form

Natrol®
PRODUCT NAME: Selenium 200 Mcg
Available in 200mcg tablets

Source Naturals®
PRODUCT NAME: Selenomax®
High Selenium Yeast
Available in 200mcg tablets

Silymarin
Available from the following company:

Source Naturals®
PRODUCT NAME: Milk Thistle Seed Extract
Available in 474 mg tablets

Turmeric
Available from the following company:

Solgar
PRODUCT NAME: Turmeric Root Extract
CONTAINS: turmeric extract and raw turmeric powder
Available in 450mg Vegicaps®

Zinc
Available from the following companies:

Source Naturals®
PRODUCT NAME: Zinc
Amino Acid Chelate, 50mg

Twin Laboratories, Inc.
PRODUCT NAME: Zinc
Available in 30mg and 50mg in capsules

PRODUCT NAME:Zinc Picolinate
Available in 25mg capsules

Special Resource Section

OncoLogics, Inc. (800-724-5566): Thera-Greens IPP contains over 50 ingredients, including antioxidants, phytonutrients, and nutritional food extracts. Available in jars and capsules. Recommended: 2 scoops daily.

NutriCology (888-563-1506): ProGreens® with Advanced Probiotic Formula is an all-natural, synergistically blended Super Green Food with adaptogenic herbs, active probiotics, and enzyme-rich ingredients. Recommended daily serving: 1 scoop.

Fish
Dr. Abel recommends certain seafood as a wonderful source of DHA and essential fatty acids.

Crown Prince, Inc.: 800-323-4141 (all canned fish):
Brisling Sardines in Pure Olive Oil
Brisling Sardines in Water
Skinless & Boneless Sardines in Pure Olive Oil
Skinless & Boneless Sardines in Water
Salmon without coloring agents
Albacore Tuna in Spring Water
Albacore Tuna in Spring Water—Low Sodium

Herbs
Chrysalis Natural Medicine Clinic & Herbal Pharmacy: Over 1,000 herbal medicines and nutrients from around the world, including hard-to-find Ayurvedic and Chinese herbs. (302-994-0565)

Juicing Machine
Omega Products, Inc.: Omega's "New" Model 8000 Juicer with Twin Gears is designed to efficiently juice wheatgrass, carrots and most other fruits and vegetables. Runs at a low 90 rpms to retain the healthful enzymes needed for a healthy diet. Comes with a 5-year warranty.
(1-800-633-3401/717-561-1105)

Natural Cosmetics

Desert Essence: Vitamin E Therapy and other skin care products with Eco-Harvest
   Tea Tree Oil
(888-476-8647)

Carlson® (800-323-4141);
E Gem Shampoo with Natural Vitamin E
E Gem Glycerine Soap with Vitamins E and A and no animal ingredients
ADE® Intensive Moisturizing Cream with Natural Vitamin E
Key•E® Moisturizing Cream with Natural Vitamin E
Key•E® Soothing Ointment with Natural Vitamin E

Organic Foods
Goldmine Natural Food Company: Wide selection of hard-to-find organic grains,
   beans, and seeds; wheat-free pastas, soy products, sea products, sea vegetables,
   and Japanese green teas.
(1-800-475-3663/1-800-863-2347)*http://www.goldminenaturalfood.com*

Wine
Frey Vineyards: Organic wines with no sulfites added. (1-800-760-3739)
Organic Wineworks: Producers of 100% organic wines. (1-800-699-9463) *http://
   www.organic.com*

Health Care Organizations

American Academy of Environmental Medicine
P.O. Box 5001-8001
New Hope, PA 18938
1-215-862-4544

American Academy of Ophthalmology
P.O. Box 429098
San Francisco, CA 94142-9098
National Care Eye Project: 1-800-222-EYES (3937)
Glaucoma 2001: 1-800-391-EYES (3937)

American Academy of Optometry
6110 Executive Boulevard, Suite 506
Rockville, MD 20852
1-301-984-1441
www.aaopt.org

American Cancer Society
1599 Clifton Road, NE
Atlanta, GA 30329
1-800-ACS-2345

American Diabetes Association
1660 Duke Street
Alexandria, VA 22314
1-800-232-3472
www.diabetes.org
   (*Provides information about diabetes.*)

American Foundation for the Blind
15 West 16th Street
New York, NY 10011
1-800-232-5463
> *(Helps people with restricted vision
> identify helpful visual aids and
> large-print books.)*

American Medical Association
www.ama-assn.org

American Printing House for the Blind
1839 Frankfort Avenue
P.O. Box 6085
Louisville, KY 40206
1-800-223-1839
> *(Publishes large-print books.)*

Arthritis Foundation of America
1330 West Peachtree Street
Atlanta, GA 30309
1-404-872-7100

Centers for Disease Control and Prevention
www.cdc.gov

Crohn's and Colitis Foundation of America
386 Park Avenue South
New York, NY 10016
1-212-685-3440

Foundation Fighting Blindness
Executive Plaza 1, Suite 800
11350 McCormick Road
Hunt Valley, MD 21031
1-888-394-3937
> *(Publishes* Update, *an informational newsletter on eye health.)*

Glaucoma Foundation
1-800-GLAUCOMA (452-8266)
www.glaucomafoundation.org/info

Glaucoma Research Foundation
490 Post Street
San Francisco, CA 94102
1-800-826-6693

Howe Press of Perkins School for the Blind
175 North Beacon Street
Watertown, MA 02172
1-617-924-3434
> *(Helps people with restricted vision
> identify helpful visual aids and
> large-print books.)*

The Juvenile Diabetes Foundation
www.jdfcure.com

Library of Congress
National Library Service for the Blind and Physically Handicapped
1291 Taylor Street NW
Washington, DC 20542
1-800-424-8567
   (Publishes recorded and braille books and magazines as well as music.)

Lighthouse International Center for Vision and Aging
111 East 59th Street, 12th floor
New York, NY 10022
1-800-334-5497

Macular Degeneration Foundation, Inc.
P.O. Box 9752
San Jose, CA 95157
1-408-260-1335
   (Publishes informational newsletter.)

National Association for the Visually Handicapped
22 West 21st Street
New York, NY 10010
1-212-889-3141

National College for Certification of Accupuncture
Arlington, Virginia
1-202-232-1404

National Diabetes Information Clearinghouse
1 Information Way
Bethesda, MD 20892
1-301-654-3397
   (Provides information about diabetes.)

National Eye Institute
National Institutes of Health
Building 31, Room 6A32
Bethesda, MD 20892-2510
1-301-496-5248

National Headache Foundation
www.headaches.org

National Institute of Arthritis and Musculoskeletal and Skin Diseases
Building 31, Room 4CO5
31 Center Drive MSC 2350
Bethesda, MD 20892
1-301-496-8188

National Institute of Diabetes and Digestive and Kidney Diseases
31 Center Drive, Room 9A04
Bethesda, MD 20892
1-301-496-3583

National Institutes of Health
Bethesda, MD 20892
www.nih.gov

New York Times Large-Print Weekly
1-800-631-2580
> *(Publishes large-print editions of the New York Times.)*

Prevent Blindness America
1-800-331-2020
www.preventblindness.org
> *(Promotes glaucoma awareness.)*

Reader's Digest Large-Print Editions
P.O. Box 241
Mount Morris, IL 61054
1-800-877-5293

Suggested Reading

Abel, R., Jr. *The DHA Story*. Basic Health Publ. (North Bergen, NJ), 2002.

Arvigo, Rosita, ND and Michael Balick, Ph.D. *Rainforest Remedies*. Lotus Press (Twin Lakes, MI), 1992.

Berne, Samuel A. *Creating Your Personal Vision: A Mind-Body Guide for Better Eyesight*. Color Stone (Santa Fe, NM), 1998.

Carper, Jean. *Food, Your Miracle Medicine*. Harper Perennial (New York City), 1993.

Cassel, Gary H., M.D., Michael D. Billig, O.D., and Harry G. Randall, M.D. *The Eye Book: A Complete Guide to Eye Disorders and Health*. Johns Hopkins University (Baltimore, MD), 1998.

Cohen, Kenneth. *The Way of Qigong*. Ballantine (New York), 1997.

Dossey, Larry, M.D. *Healing Words: The Power of Prayer and the Practice of Medicine*. HarperCollins, 1997.

Duke, James. *The Green Collins Pharmacy*. Rodale Press (Emmaus, PA), 1997.

Ehling, Dagmar, with Stuart Schwartz. *The Chinese Herbalist's Handbook*. In Word (Santa Fe, NM), 1996.

Erasmus, Udo. *Fats That Heal Fats That Kill*. Alive (Vancouver, Canada), 1993. Available by mail order from Flora (1-800-498-3610).

Galland, Leo. *The Four Pillars of Healing*. Random House (New York), 1997.

Haas, Elson M., M.D. *The Detox Diet*. Celestial Arts, 1996.

Hadady, Letha. *Asian Health Secrets*. Three Rivers (New York), 1996.

Hampton, Aubrey. *Natural Organic Hair and Skin Care*. Organic (Tampa, FL), 1987.

Ketham, Katherine, and Jason Elias. *The Five Elements of Self-Healing*. Harmony (New York), 1998.

Keuneke, Robin. *Total Breast Health: The Power Food Solution for Protection and Wellness*. Kensington (New York), 1998.

King, Shirley. *Fish the Basics*. Chapters (Shelburne, VT), 1996.

Lee, J. R. *Progesterone: The Multiple Roles of a Remarkable Hormone*. BLL (Sebastapol, CA), 1993.

Lee, Martin, Emily Lee, and Jo Ann Johnstone. *Ride the Tiger to the Mountain: Tai Chi for Health*. Stanford University (Stanford, CA).

Liang, Master T. T. *T'ai Chi Chu'an For Health and Self-Defense*. Vintage (New York), 1977.

Lu, Henry C. *Chinese System of Food Cures*. Sterling (New York), 1986.

Matthews, Dale, M.D.; *The Faith Factor: Proof of the Healing Power of Prayer*. Viking (New York), 1998.

McCully, Kilmer, M.D. *The Homocysteine Revolution*. Keats (New Canaan, CT), 1997.

Mehta, Silva, Mira Mehta, and Shayam Mehta. *Yoga the Iyengar Way*. Alfred Knopf (New York), 1996.

Moore, Thomas J. *Prescription for Disaster: The Hidden Dangers in Your Medicine Cabinet*. Simon & Schuster (New York), 1998.

Morgan, Brian L.G. *Nutrition Prescription*. Crown (New York), 1987.

Ornish, Dean, M.D. *Love and Survival: The Scientific Basis for the Healing Power of Intimacy*. HarperCollins (New York), 1998.

Oz, Mehmet, M.D. *Healing from the Heart.* Dutton (New York), 1998.

Pierpaoli, Walter, M.D. and William Regenson, M.D., with Carol Colman. *The Melatonin Miracle.* Simon & Schuster (New York), 1995.

Roy, Marilyn. *EyeRobics: How to Improve Your Vision.* Peanut Butter (Seattle, WA).

Schulick, Paul. *Ginger: Common Spice and Wonder Drug.* Herbal Free Press (Brattleboro, VT), 1993 (1-800-903-9104).

Simopoulos, Artemis P., M.D., and Jo Robinson. *The Omega Plan.* HarperCollins (New York), 1998.

Steinman, David. *The Safe Shopper's Bible: A Consumer's Guide to Nontoxic Household Products, Cosmetics and Food.* Macmillan (New York), 1995.

Tillotson, Alan K., Naishin, Hu, and Abel, Robert, Jr. *The One Earth Herbal Sourcebook.* Kensington (New York), 2001.

Unschuld, Paul U. *Medicine in China.* University of California (Berkeley), 1985.

Waters, Alice. *Chez Panisse Vegetables.* HarperCollins (New York), 1996.

Weil, Andrew, M.D. *Spontaneous Healing.* Ballantine (New York), 1995.

Wolverton, William. *How to Grow Clean Air: 50 Houseplants That Purify Your Home or Office,* Penguin (New York), 1998.

Appendices

Appendices A–E contain supplemental information for Chapters 4, 6, 7, 8, and 9 (which discuss light, cataracts, glaucoma, macular degeneration, and diabetes). Appendix F, "Eye Aerobics," describes how eye movements relate to health. This information, perhaps too technical for the general reader, may be of interest to readers with scientific curiosity or those who want to gain a more detailed understanding of a therapy or procedure they may be undergoing. Appendices G and H present comparisons of the RDIs, RDAs, and DRIs of vitamins and minerals over the years.

Appendix A: Light and the Eye (Chapter 4)

Ultraviolet (UV) light is composed of wavelengths that are shorter than the light our eyes perceive, which is called the visual spectrum. The visual spectrum falls between 400 and 700 nanometers (nm); UV light, which makes up 5 percent of solar radiation (i.e., sunlight), falls below the visual spectrum. *UVA light*—the type used in tanning booths—is the closest to the visual spectrum (320 to 400 nm), falling near the purple and blue wavelengths. Prolonged exposure to near-UV-containing sunlight at high altitudes or reflected off sand, snow, or water at low altitudes may result in *snow blindness,* in which the profound amount of UV rays in the reflected light washes the purple colors out of the retina, leaving a telltale pink afterimage.

When UV radiation penetrates the lens, it can burn the retina, a condition called *solar retinopathy*. Solar retinopathy can develop from actually staring at the sun—possibly the reason that Galileo became blind in his later years. Like UV light, lasers can also damage eyes. While they produce no heat, they possess damaging ionizing radiation. Blue light (in the 400–500 nm range) is also toxic to the retina, especially in individuals exposed to high altitude reflection. The surgical microscope used to perform eye operations emanates a lot of blue light, and procedures requiring it should therefore be done as quickly as possible.

Certain medications—called *photosensitizing drugs*—make the eye more sensitive to light by adhering to the lens protein and causing cataracts. These drugs also bind with the skin, which is why the pharmacist will tell you not to be in the sunlight for at least ten days after you've discontinued such a drug. Eight hundred international units (IU) of vitamin E has been found to decrease the toxicity of UV light in animal models; vitamin C (1000 mg) will do the same.

Although excessive exposure to UV light can be toxic, we require a certain amount for both vision and good health. In addition to producing vitamin D in response to light, our bodies manufacture numerous chemicals that regulate our *circadian* (daily) rhythm. One is melatonin, a supplement that induces sleep and governs time zone–related rhythms (i.e., jet lag), which results from the short-circuiting of the circadian rhythm and disruption of melatonin production. Taking a supplemental dose of as little as 0.3 mg of melatonin (which is far lower than the doses in which it is marketed) before bed can induce sleep. However, I caution my patients that melatonin and other hormones and hormone-like substances may have wide-reaching and unexpected effects on body systems, and should be used wisely and only for short periods of time. For example, we may have hormone-regulated periods at which our eyes are more sensitive to damage by UV light, and disturbing those periods by taking excessive amounts of melatonin could produce unknown long-term consequences.

While melatonin is primarily tied to inducing sleep, it has other interesting characteristics, including some suspected anticancer properties. A 1997 study showed that, in test tube experiments, melatonin stops breast cancer cells from growing. Melatonin appears to protect the retina from glaucoma. It also reduces the production of cortisol, a stress hormone which, while it suppresses inflammation, may potentiate both diabetes and aging. Melatonin may be able, therefore, to retard the development of some of these conditions.

Although light striking the retina has been thought to control melatonin production, a rather astonishing study published in *Science* in January 1998 showed that a blue light shined on the back of the knee influences melatonin production just as effectively as daylight striking the retina. In both these areas (the retina and behind the knee), blood vessels are very close to the surface. The blue light apparently influences chemical molecules in the blood, whether via the retina or at the back of the knee. The scientists who made the discovery suggested that blue-light therapy may be useful in treating jet lag, insomnia, and other melatonin-regulated body functions.

Light has an impact on our emotional as well as our physical well-being by regulating seasonal (as well as daily) rhythms. The absence of sunlight in winter creates a syndrome known as *seasonal affective disorder* (SAD) in susceptible individuals. SAD's symptoms include insomnia, depression, weight gain, moodiness, and loss of sex drive. George Brainard, a neurophysiologist at Thomas Jefferson University (in Philadelphia), has demonstrated the positive effects of ultraviolet light on the brain chemistry of laboratory animals. The body's entire supply of blood circulates through the retina every twenty minutes, where it is exposed to light. Therefore, chemicals in the blood that influence brain chemistry are also exposed to light every twenty minutes.

As little as thirty minutes of moderate light (even artificial light from a light box) can change people's outlooks and alleviate the SAD syndrome, without damaging the eyes, according to research published in the *American Journal of Ophthalmology* in February 1995. Pamela Gallin, M.D., of the Columbia-Presbyterian Medical Center in New York, and an international team of colleagues found a 75 percent clinical remission from SAD after treating patients with bright-light therapy. Gallin and her colleagues also found that long-term bright-light treatment (three to six years) produced no eye damage in seventeen patients studied. Although concluding that bright-light therapy is effective for SAD and apparently does not damage the eyes, they urged extreme care in providing this treatment to patients with preexisting eye conditions or those who are taking photosensitizing drugs.

Refraction

The lens is positioned approximately one-quarter of the length of the eye behind the cornea. If the eye is longer, the lens is positioned differently, influencing where light focuses. In nearsighted (myopic) people, the eye is longer than normal ("normal" being around 23–24 mm, or about 1 inch), and light comes to its focus too soon, falling short of the retina. Therefore, what the retina experiences is a blur. Individuals with long eyes (i.e., those who suffer from nearsightedness) must walk closer to an object or hold it in their hand to bring it into focus.

The contrary is true for farsighted people—those with short eyes (less than 22.5 mm long). In this case, the image focuses *behind* the retina, which also produces a blurry image. The farther away an object, the more likely its image is to focus on the retina. Farsighted people's *best vision* is at distance.

A *diopter* is the unit of focus power (i.e., the unit in which focus power is measured) of a lens that can focus light coming from a great distance (twenty feet or more) to a point 1 meter away from that lens. The eye has about 60 diopters of focus power, the amount necessary to focus light on a 1-inch-long eye. Two-thirds, or forty diopters, of focusing light is done by the cornea; only one-third is performed by the lens.

Since twenty feet was agreed upon by all eye doctors as "light coming from a distance," eye doctors' examining lanes used to be twenty feet long. Today, lenses placed in a device called a *phoropter* are arranged in front of the patient to measure *refraction*—the amount of glasses' correction required. The methods of measuring refraction are (1) subjective, in which the patient helps make the decision, or (2) objective, in which the optometrist or ophthalmologist makes the decision. There are also machines that give an objective refraction, which may require fine-tuning by the doctor. In the subjective variety, trial and error can be used, or the patient's previous spectacle correction can be used as a starting point. In objective examinations for young children, and in difficult situations, a special light is flashed across the eye and the image is neutralized. Three variables are then measured: (1) the spherical correction (nearsighted/farsighted, i.e., more or less lens power); (2) the amount of astigmatism; and (3) the axis of the astigmatism. If someone with a significant amount of astigmatism is not corrected on the right axis, he will not see well. Each of these three components, therefore, must be judged correctly by the eye doctor.

What Medicare Pays for in Your Eye Examination

- Test of visual acuity (does not include determination of refractive error)
- Test of gross visual field by confrontation
- Test of ocular motility including primary gaze alignment
- Inspection of bulbar and palpebral conjunctiva
- Examination of ocular adnexa, including lids (e.g., ptosis or lagophthalmos), lacrimal glands, lacrimal drainage, orbits, and preauricular nodes
- Examination of pupils, irises (including shape), direct and consensual reaction (afferent pupil), size (e.g., anisocoria), and morphology

- Slit lamp examination of the corneas, including epithelium, stroma, endothelium, and tear film
- Slit lamp examination of anterior chambers, including depth, cells, and flare
- Slit lamp examination of the lenses, including clarity, anterior and posterior capsule, cortex, and nucleus
- Measurement of intraocular pressures (except in children and patients with trauma or infectious disease)
- Ophthalmic examination through dilated pupils (unless contraindicated) of: Optic discs, including size, C/D ratio, appearance (e.g., atrophy, cupping, tumor elevation), and nerve fiber layer; posterior segments including retina and vessels (e.g., exudates and hemorrhages)

Appendix B: The Cataract Epidemic (Chapter 6)

Incidence of Cataracts

Four out of ten patients between 52 and 64 years of age have some precataract changes; about 50 percent of individuals between the ages of 65 and 74 begin to develop cataracts; and 70 percent of people over 75 years of age have some degree of cataract development. Women have a higher rate of cataract formation than men. Because most women who develop cataracts are postmenopausal, it's thought that estrogen may have a protective effect against cataracts.

Numerous studies now support the correlation between exposure to UV light in sunlight and the development of cataracts. One of the best known of these studies is the Chesapeake Bay study of watermen, which quantified exposure to UV light, taking into account the type of work done, leisure activities pursued, and type of headgear and eye protection used while in the sun, and correlated UV light exposure with the development of cataract. It was found that the relative risk of developing cataracts increased with the annual amount of UV exposure. The men who developed cataracts were found to have a 21 percent higher average annual UV exposure than men who did not develop cataracts. Like many other studies, the Chesapeake Bay study found that the effects of exposure to UV light accumulate over a lifetime.

Other research supports the Chesapeake Bay study. The Beaver Dam study in Wisconsin found an association between UV exposure and cataract formation. In Australia, a study of aborigines found that cataract development correlated with the number of hours a person was exposed to sunlight daily. In Nepal (in the Himalayan study), investigators also found a positive association between exposure to UV rays in sunlight and the development of cataracts. And the Salisbury (Maryland) Eye Evaluation Project showed a positive correlation between UVB exposure and the development of cortical cataracts.

The United States is experiencing a cataract surgery epidemic. Nearly two million cataract surgeries are performed every year in the United States, at a cost of $3.5 billion. Cataract surgery is the number-one item on the Medicare budget.

Much can be done to stop the cataract surgery epidemic, including protecting our eyes from UV light and consuming enough antioxidants (through diet and supplementation) to fight the free-radical damage created, not only by UV light but also by smoking, stress, environmental pollutants, alcohol, and prescription drugs.

Anatomy and Physiology of Cataracts

The lens of the eye, which focuses light on the retina, develops from the same kinds of cells as skin. It has no blood supply and no nerves (and, therefore, no feeling). The lens has a thickened capsule on the outside, unlike skin, where the thickened capsule lies beneath the surface layers. Unlike the skin, which can shed externally, the lens compacts internally, contributing to its opacification with age.

Just as the eye is controlled by the muscles that encircle it, the lens is controlled by fine ligaments called *zonules*. In younger people, when the *ciliary body* (the circular muscle of the eye) contracts during focusing, the lens can change shape so that near objects remain in focus. As we grow older, the ciliary body's flexibility diminishes, which means that the lens's *accommodation* (its ability to focus light) diminishes, too. At the same time, the lens begins to yellow and cloud over a certain amount from lifetime exposure to UV light.

Even though cataract formation is not inevitable, the aging of the eye contributes to cataracts. We know, for instance, that the curvature of the lens changes as we age (which is why many older people require reading glasses). Dr. Richard P. Hemenger and colleagues at the University of Auckland in New Zealand examined how changes in the curvature and opacity of the lens affect vision with age, and they discovered that changes in the lens's curvature and opacity parallel each other over the years.

When the lens is damaged (by sunlight, smoking, diabetes, drugs, or injury), it becomes cloudy or opaque, and is no longer able to focus light properly. As a cataract develops, the lens becomes denser, which also interferes with the focusing of light. Cataracts impair distance vision more than near vision, which means that people with cataracts generally become more nearsighted. As cataracts worsen, vision gradually becomes dim, distorted, or is lost entirely.

Cataract Surgery

In my practice, patients undergo presurgery tests and counseling. If the surgery is going to be done in the outpatient surgical center, fewer tests are required. If the surgery is to be done in the hospital, patients need to have an electrocardiogram and blood tests. Patients on multiple medications need to have their electrolytes checked (to make sure there's no imbalance of minerals, especially potassium, in the blood), and most patients should have a blood count taken to make sure they aren't anemic, don't have a bacterial infection, and have the proper amount of bloodclotting cells (platelets). Of course, patients need to have their eyes measured (the length of the eye and the curvature of the cornea) to determine the type of lens implant needed. Every patient is unique, and there are many options for the vision produced by intraocular lens implants, including reproducing the patient's previous nearsightedness, if this is what is requested. There is even a bifocal lens that can be implanted. While this sounds as if the patient will not have to wear glasses, the reality is that they may.

The morning of surgery, I always greet my patient ahead of time to make sure he or she is as relaxed as possible and that the pupil is adequately dilated. I talk with the nurses and the patient's family. The eye is not only dilated (with eyedrops), but is already anesthetized with a single drop of anesthetic (nonpreserved 4 percent xylocaine or lidocaine). People who may have had previous reactions to local anesthetic have usually had a reaction to the adrenaline in the solution. Our drops, however, contain no adrenaline.

I then push the stretcher down the hall to the hospital operating room or our outpatient surgery center where the nurse anesthetist and circulating nurse introduce themselves. In our surgery centers, the patient may be walked in. I make sure the patient is in the most comfortable position possible under the microscope in the operating room. I place another drop of 4 percent xylocaine on the outside of the eye. I then explain our regular routine to the patient. A sticky drape is used to keep the eyes open. Most people feel relieved to hear this because they've wondered how they're going to avoid blinking. I tell them that we'll numb the eye several more times, using a couple of different techniques, and that they will feel no pain. The difficult part is looking at the bright light of the microscope. In order to minimize the brightness of the light, I cover the eye while preparing for the surgery. At the beginning of the operation, I take the little cover off the eye and place another drop of anesthetic in the eye. I take a small Q-tip and rub anesthetic on the side of the eye adjacent to where I will be working.

I make an initial incision on the edge of the cornea, while the eye is still covered. I then remove the cover and explain to the patient that it's necessary to look at the light for five quick steps. At the end of this time, a small wound (three-sixteenths of an inch) has been made in the eye, and the anesthetic (1 percent nonpreserved xylocaine) has been injected in the eye to numb it completely for the operation.

The front of the cataract capsule is removed. Saline (salt water) is injected into the lens. This reduces the glare, also making the patient much more comfortable during the surgery. Patients often say to me during surgery, "It's really amazing to see those beautiful lights without having them be too bright!" High-speed sound, or *phacoemulsification*, is used to break up the center part of the lens, called the *nucleus*. After the nucleus is fragmented and absorbed, the soft cortical portion of the cataract is removed. The back of the lens capsule is polished, if there is residual debris. At this point, a visco-elastic material is placed in the chamber so the anterior chamber does not collapse and the pupil does not get smaller. The remains of the cataract, which is now an empty bag filled with the visco-elastic material I inserted, is ready to receive the implant, a plastic lens.

The commonest plastic lens materials are silicone, acrylic, and collagin because they are foldable. Some surgeons still use old-fashioned hard plastic lenses, but they require a larger incision in the eye. After the implant is put into the eye, the visco-elastic material inserted to keep the eye from collapsing is removed. The edges of the wound are usually injected with a small amount of saline so that the wound will be self-secure, without needing stitches. If the wound does not look as if it will hold together by itself, it is sutured. At the end of the procedure, a contact lens that has been soaked in antibiotics and anti-inflammatory steroid drops is placed on the eye. An additional antibiotic drop is placed in the eye before the patient leaves the operating room. Glasses or a plastic shield may be placed over the patient's eye.

Most patients are rather amazed that the procedure is over so fast and that it was painless. In the holding area, I show the patient and family how to place eyedrops in the eye, by lying on the floor and doing it myself, into a closed eye. (Even a patient who has had a small amount of sedative will remember this rather vivid demonstration.) I recommend using antibiotic eyedrops hourly that day to prevent infection.

I always call my surgical patients later in the day to see how they are doing. If the patient is having any difficulty at all, I evaluate it immediately, instead of allowing them to spend the night in any kind of discomfort. Ninety percent of patients have no discomfort, but may have a small amount of tearing. Some, who have more discomfort, can take the analgesic pill or use the ointment in the bag of medication I give them after surgery. Patients are given the medications that they will require for the first week.

The day after the surgery, I see the patient in my office and remove the contact lens, which is no longer necessary. The patient usually has good vision by the first day (although it can vary for a number of reasons), and should be able to lift, bend, and perform most activities. I personally prefer that the patient wear an eye shield at bedtime and in the shower for the first three days. The wound is self-sealing and strong enough to resist pressure, even force.

Cataract surgery, which can improve quality of life enormously in such a short period of time, is probably one of the most worthwhile operative procedures in modern medicine. People's vision is often better than it has been for twenty to forty years because the amount of light entering the eye after surgery (and implantation of the artificial lens) is greater than the normal adult lens allows. People may even be able to see gradations of colors (that is, different parts of the visual spectrum) that they have not been able to see in recent years. My patients often tell me they are amazed at the brightness of the world and their friends' wrinkles.

Appendix C: Thief of Sight: Glaucoma (Chapter 7)
Models of Glaucoma Causality

Glaucoma is a group of diseases that damage the optic nerve and cause vision loss. We still do not understand exactly how that vision loss is caused, but two different models attempt to explain it.

The first applies to high-pressure glaucoma (in which eye pressure is elevated). The *mechanical model* postulates that, when pressure inside the eye increases, its fluid presses on the tiny, vulnerable blood vessels (capillaries) that nourish the optic nerve. This causes a loss of blood supply to nerve fibers, which damages them, resulting in isolated blind spots that might not be immediately obvious to the patient. Gradually, however, this area of sight will be more affected so that, for instance, the patient might miss an overhead traffic light in that area of visual loss. The patient's other, healthy eye usually masks the defect, which can delay diagnosis. Glaucoma is usually a nonsymmetrical disease, so the progressive loss in one eye may be masked by the good vision in the healthy eye.

In contrast to high-pressure glaucoma is low-pressure glaucoma, in which the internal eye pressure is not only elevated, but may actually be a little low (13 mm of pressure or lower). The second model, the *circulatory model*, could explain how both low-pressure and high-pressure glaucoma develop. The circulatory model suggests that deficient blood flow to the optic nerve damages it and is the direct cause of vision loss. Whereas the mechanical model suggests that increased pressure indirectly damages the nerves in the eye, the circulatory model suggests that inadequate blood flow to the retina is primarily responsible for nerve damage. That is, lack of adequate blood supply leads to the death of optic nerve cells, and therefore to loss of vision.

In the mid-1990s, investigators suggested that the lack of adequate blood supply observed in low-pressure glaucoma might be due to *vasospasm* (constriction and release of blood vessels). Alon Harris, a researcher at Indiana University, has found that as many as 50 to 60 percent of patients with low-pressure glaucoma exhibit some type of vascular abnormality or vasospasm. Vasospasm is a mechanism that also occurs to different degrees in migraine headache, chronically cold hands and feet (Raynaud's disease), heart disease, and stroke. Harris diagnoses these conditions using a combination of laser ophthalmoscopy and new techniques that actually quantify the blood flow to the back of the eye. He found that using drugs like beta-blockers, that reverse vasospasm, also reverse glaucoma. Magnesium, an important intracellular mineral, often counteracts vasospasm.

Another possible cause of glaucoma is *glutamate toxicity*. Glutamate is an amino acid that is required for nerves to work properly. Some studies, however, have found elevated amounts of glutamate in the eyes of glaucoma patients, suggesting it may be toxic in high levels. In one study, researchers found twice as much glutamate in the vitreous humor of glaucoma patients than they found in control patients who had cataracts. In monkeys with glaucoma, even higher amounts of glutamate were found in the vitreous. While we need this excitatory amino acid in small amounts in the retina, it's possible that excessive amounts damage this delicate nervous tissue.

Glutamate has also been found to be significantly elevated in the blood of people suffering from *amyotrophic lateral sclerosis*, or Lou Gehrig's disease. Many central nervous system diseases—including Alzheimer's disease, Parkinson's disease, and multiple sclerosis—are now thought to be caused in part by the accumulation of toxic chemicals that damage nerves. This is one reason I urge glaucoma patients—and all my patients, for that matter—to avoid substances that are known to be toxic to nerves (including the retina), like MSG (which contains glutamate) and artificial sweeteners.

Classification and Characteristics of Glaucoma

Many doctors and patients believe that elevated eye pressure defines glaucoma, but it does not. As many as 50 percent of people who experience elevated eye pressure at some time in their lives never develop optic nerve damage and its accompanying vision loss. And at least 25 percent of elderly people with damaged optic nerves never have elevated eye pressure.

There are six major types of glaucoma:

1. The usual type of glaucoma in the United States is chronic *open-angle glaucoma* (also called chronic simple or primary open-angle glaucoma). In open-angle glaucoma, there is plenty of room in the angle between the iris and the cornea for the eye's fluid to exit. It is thought that open-angle glaucoma develops because the trabecular meshwork doesn't filter the circulating aqueous fluid very well. When the doctor puts on a special contact lens called a *goniolens* (*gonio* means angle), he or she will see an open angle that has some pigment accumulation, resembling a clogged drain. In other words, the spigot is running, but the drain is partially blocked, and so the fluid cannot drain from inside the eye. In Africa and the Caribbean, the prevalence is four to six times higher than it is in Caucasian populations.

2. A less frequent type of glaucoma in the U.S. (although it makes up almost 50 percent of this disease in Asia and other areas of the world) is *angle-closure glaucoma*, in which the base of the iris is too close to the cornea. Angle-closure glaucoma usually occurs in farsighted people. Because their eyes are short, the inner parts of the eye are very close together. Many of these patients have the chronic form (not the acute attack form) of glaucoma, so they are asymptomatic and don't realize they have it. However, early cataract changes in people with short eyes may force the lens to swell and shift forward, pushing the iris forward and nearly closing the angle. In this situation, elevated eye pressure or even a dilated pupil can close the angle completely, preventing any fluid from exiting the eye. Angle-closure glaucoma arises most often as a sudden attack with severe pain and visual halos, accompanied by a precipitous increase in eye pressure. The pain can be so intense that the entire head aches and the patient feels nauseous and actually vomits. *This is a true emergency.*

3. The third type is called *secondary glaucoma*, because it develops secondary to other conditions such as inflammation, injury, or blood in the eye. Secondary glaucoma may also be seen after the patient takes steroid medications. Steroid eyedrops, which are useful for red eyes, can cause increased eye pressure in up to 30 percent of people (this reaction generally occurs only after numerous weeks of treatment), and can lead to secondary glaucoma. Whether this increased pressure is marked or mild, it creates a complicated situation that must be evaluated by an opthalmologist as soon as possible. Fortunately, secondary glaucoma is easily diagnosed and monitored by most eye doctors; visits to a glaucoma specialist are necessary when the eye pressure cannot be controlled.

4. The fourth type is *low-tension glaucoma*, which has been thought to develop most often in elderly patients with other diseases like high blood pressure. As many as 40 percent of patients with open-angle glaucoma have normal or low eye pressure, and develop the usual optic nerve changes and progressive visual loss without ever having elevated pressure. The fundamental defect in low-tension glaucoma is *ischemia*, or poor blood supply to the back of the eye. Most doctors try to lower the pressure as much as possible without starving the entire eye of its source of nutrition. These individuals often have pressure changes in their eyes at night when their blood pressure is low and not supplying the optic nerve sufficiently. Some medications to lower eye pressure or enhance circulation, therefore, should be given at bedtime. In treating this condition, we need to improve circulation to the eye to nourish the optic nerve.

Since doctors are just beginning to realize how often glaucoma occurs in the absence of elevated eye pressure, it's important to know which other conditions can mimic low-tension or normal-tension glaucoma. Foremost is blockage of the carotid artery, which may produce no other symptoms unless the patient has a stroke. There can be optic nerve lesions, caused by brain tumors, carotid artery aneurysm, Leber's hereditary optic nerve disease, or toxic drugs or chemicals (especially methanol). *An eye exam may be the key to diagnosing this life-threatening condition.*

5. Congenital glaucoma is unusual, but can occur in the first few months of life. Its occurs in one out of every 5000 to 10,000 babies. Since the child's eye is still growing, the cornea can enlarge, become extremely swollen, and develop the bluish haze first noted by the ancient Greeks. Congenital glaucoma is extremely serious, and only aggressive surgery can blunt progression of the disease. There may or may not be

a family history of this type of disorder (in other words, it may or may not be genetic), and there may not be any other eye problems.

6. The sixth form of glaucoma is *ocular hypertenson,* or *glaucoma suspect.* In this condition, the patient has elevated internal eye pressure, but no optic nerve damage. Patients with glaucoma suspect need to be followed carefully, because it is impossible to predict who will go on to develop the vision loss indicative of glaucoma.

Appendix D: Starvation of the Retina: Macular Degeneration (Chapter 8)

Incidence

The incidence of macular degeneration increases with age, as several studies have demonstrated. The Beaver Dam Eye Study found that macular degeneration occurs in 14.4 percent of people aged 55 to 64, in 19.4 percent of people aged 65 to 74, and in 36.8 percent of those 75 and older.

The amount of degeneration reported varies both according to the patient and to the doctor-observer involved. At least 14 million Americans over the age of 65 have macular degeneration listed on their Medicare fee slip. The number of patients with macular degeneration in both the United Kingdom and Japan is growing as rapidly as the number in the United States, as the total number of people 65 and older increases throughout the world.

Macular degeneration develops in one eye at a time, and may or may not develop in the other eye. A five-year study found that macular degeneration developed in the other eye at a rate of 8.8 percent per year, indicating that the risk of the condition developing in the second eye increases with time.

Research on Nutritional Treatment and Prevention

Although most ophthalmologists will tell you that nothing can be done to stop or reverse macular degeneration, there is ample evidence in the scientific literature showing that nutrition and supplementation can indeed halt this blinding disease's progression.

The Age-Related Eye Disease Study (AREDS), the first major study to track the natural history of macular degeneration followed over 3,600 participants for eight years. This major study has produced evidence that antioxidant nutrients, along with zinc, may help reduce the risk of developing AMD or even retard its progression if the condition is already present. (See page 384.)

In addition, a three-year pilot study conducted at Veterans Administration hospitals across the country concluded for the first time in 1996 that macular degeneration is associated with decreased B vitamin and magnesium intake, and confirmed the known association with lack of vitamin E and zinc.

There is also evidence that maintaining high antioxidant levels—keeping the antioxidant bank account at healthy levels—will not only protect against macular degeneration but also help prevent cataract formation. A study published in the *Journal of the American Medical Association* in 1995 found that people in the highest twentieth percentile of dietary intake of carotenoids had a 43 percent lower risk of developing AMD.

A very important study of nutrition's impact on the risk of developing AMD was performed by Max Snodderly, M.D., of the Schepens Eye Research Institute in Boston, using monkeys. The dietary antioxidants that Snodderly found to be protective against AMD (because they protect against light-induced damage, he hypothesized) are the carotenes (particularly lutein and zeaxanthin) and the vitamins E and C. Snodderly determined that lutein and zeaxanthin are highly concentrated in the macula, and that these particular carotenoids (as opposed to the more widely known alpha- and beta-carotene) serve very specific structural purposes in the macula, facilitating the flow of nutrients. Furthermore, the areas of the retina in which lutein, zeaxanthin, and vitamin E are at lowest concentration were the areas where macular disease developed first in Snodderly's monkeys when they were fed diets extremely deficient in these nutrients, and correspond to areas where AMD develops in humans. Vitamin C deficiency has also been shown to lead to retinal degeneration according to Snodderly, apparently because this vitamin protects against the damaging effects of UV light.

In high-risk groups, Snodderly found a 50 percent or greater reduction of lutein and zeaxanthin in the macular area, a finding that has also been shown at autopsy. And in a study of identical twins, during which one twin was fed a diet deficient in lutein and the other a high-lutein diet, the twin with the high-lutein diet had greater carotene levels in the macula than the twin eating the lutein-deficient diet—a result which effectively removed heredity from the equation.

In a 1995 study, Snodderly also found that UV and blue-light damage leads to the breakdown of cell membranes, producing substances that are highly toxic to the retina. Blue light is particularly injurious to the retina, but its damage can be limited by zeaxanthin and lutein. Therefore, it's important to protect our eyes against blue light as well as UV light.

A study directed by Lawrence Yannuzzi, M.D., at the Manhattan Eye and Ear and Throat Hospital in New York City found that moderate intake of carotenoids (including lutein and zeaxanthin) resulted in halving the amount of macular degeneration.

Appendix E: Diabetes: Is Blindness Inevitable? (Chapter 9)

Systemic Complications of Diabetes

Cardiovascular-renal (heart-kidney) disease is the leading cause of death among diabetics, who appear to be more at risk for developing heart disease and hardening of the arteries (atherosclerosis) than the general public. Kidney disease (renal disease or nephropathy) also can develop subsequent to hardening of the arteries. Therefore, conditions that contribute to heart and kidney disease, such as high blood pressure, must be tightly controlled in diabetics.

Native Americans have higher rates of diabetic retinopathy and kidney disease than do other Americans. Kidney disease (nephropathy) is linked to the development of diabetic eye disease, particularly in people who have Type I (childhood) diabetes. Nephropathy leading to diabetic retinopathy appears to occur at much higher rates at earlier ages in Native Americans (at age 26, as compared to age 33 in the general population). Poverty is one of the reasons suggested for this discrepancy. The incidence of diabetic retinopathy (with or without kidney disease) is much higher in some Southwestern tribes than even in other Native Americans.

Hypoglycemia (low blood sugar) occurs when the blood sugar level falls too far. This may be a warning symptom of diabetes. Before insulin failure, the pancreas becomes extremely sensitive to the presence of sugar and produces too much insulin, resulting in hypoglycemia. It is commonly referred to as *insulin shock*, because the blood sugar level drops quickly and the brain is deprived of its essential energy source. The first sign of insulin shock is hunger, followed by dizziness, sweating, palpitations, confusion, and eventual loss of consciousness. Usually there's enough time (ten minutes) to get the patient some orange juice or a candy bar to rectify the condition. In some cases, the only effective measure is an intravenous injection of glucose, but that is quite unusual.

Appendix F: Eye Aerobics

Few cases of eyestrain have been developed by looking on the bright side of things.

—Anonymous

This particular area has been difficult for me to address in the past because, as an ophthalmologist, I've always been taught by ophthalmology professors that eye exercises and vision therapy more closely resemble voodoo than modern medicine. Of course, that's also what physicians used to be taught about such alternative therapies as chiropractic, massage, and acupuncture which now are accepted by many traditional physicians as being very effective in certain circumstances. There is always a time lag between the introduction of new therapies or medical concepts and their widespread acceptance within the medical establishment. Now, however, many medical schools even offer courses in alternative therapies like mind/body healing, Chinese herbs and acupuncture, and similar subjects, which would have been unthinkable even just a decade ago. This doesn't mean that every doctor should immediately adopt every alternative therapy he or she studies. Responsible physicians should combine curiosity and open-mindedness about new therapies with concern about their safety and effectiveness, and investigate fully before recommending them to patients.

Despite its lack of acceptance by most mainstream ophthalmologists, I've long been fascinated by articles in the lay press about eye exercises that help tired eyes and reduce the need for glasses. Traveling in India and Nepal, I learned that eye exercises have been used for generations in these areas of the world to help improve vision. Vision therapy, which is primarily utilized by optometric specialists in the United States, corrects vision problems associated with learning disabilities in some individuals, according to my behavioral optometrist colleagues in Delaware who specialize in vision therapy.

One problem that vision therapy and eye exercises attempt to treat is eyestrain. Like fatigue, we currently have no way to measure eyestrain. Our standard methods of evaluating vision, like the eye chart, are unable to measure a number of subtle eye and vision problems, including several that can lead to eyestrain.

Eyestrain can be caused by physical/environmental conditions (like insufficient or too-bright lighting, exposure to smoke, staring at a computer screen for too long without blinking, or doing close work for long periods without stopping) or emotional stress (which can lead to eye muscle strain and poor attention). Many cases of eyestrain are caused by not having the correct glasses prescription. Eyestrain occurs in all kinds of situations, but it is almost epidemic in offices. Sitting at a desk doing one task for twenty minutes without stopping constricts the mind as well as the eyes. When the eyes are irritated, so is the brain.

In 1996, H. S. Seung, M.D., published a report in the *Proceedings of the National Academy of Sciences USA* demonstrating that the brain is able to hold the eye still in one position because it stores a memory of that position in the visual cortex. This research demonstrated that, just as the brain controls the position of the eye, the eye's position influences the brain.

The whole head and neck are involved in keeping the eye focused on a specific spot. Try, for instance, following a bouncing tennis ball without moving your head and neck. It's very difficult. The eyes, head, and neck work as a team. Head and neck movements are naturally integrated with eye movements, and keeping the eyes, head, and neck still (while working at a computer, for example) tenses the head and neck muscles and can cause headache.

Relaxing the body relaxes the eye, and anything that relaxes the eye causes the mind to be more relaxed as well. The goal of most eye exercises is to improve vision by relaxing the eye.

In Japan, Tibet, India and many other places, there are written records of eye exercises that date back thousands of years. There's no question that these exercises, still commonly practiced in these countries, must have some value in promoting eye health and quality of vision, even though their value has not been proved in the Western scientific press. One reason they haven't been proved to be of value, of course, is that they haven't been tested by Western doctors. There is no question, however, that some people can feel more comfortable, suffer less eyestrain, and possibly reduce the need for glasses for short periods of time by performing eye exercises.

Numerous studies of the effects of vision therapy exercises have been published in the medical literature. Harold A. Solan, O.D., summarized the evidence supporting vision therapy in the March 1998 *Review of Ophthalmology*, describing several studies showing that more than 50 percent of children with various types of focusing disorders (convergence insufficiency, accommodation insufficiency, and convergence excess) experienced improvement after undergoing vision therapy. He also suggested that vision therapy exercises might help some children with learning difficulties or disabilities.

Crossed eyes and other focusing problems can be helped by specific eye exercises like "pencil push-ups" or "edging," which I will explain and teach you about later in this chapter. I've found that, despite the lack of controlled studies—which should definitely be performed—a growing number of people are being helped by vision therapy techniques.

It can be difficult to remember to do eye exercises regularly unless you have eyestrain or a headache. People who do a lot of indoor, close work have a greater tendency to become nearsighted, and people who often look into the distance—like farmers—remain farsighted. I believe it's important to maintain a balance between close and distance vision. If you do a lot of close work, like accounting, computer, law, editing, or studying of any sort, you need to take occasional breaks and, "shake the eyes out," so to speak.

I recommend a number of exercises for people who are suffering from eyestrain or eye fatigue from their work, reading, or even from wearing strong glasses. The first task is to relax the eyes, a method of relieving eyestrain and promoting better vision first suggested by William H. Bates, M.D., in his 1920 book *Better Eyesight Without Glasses*. Dr. Bates argued that mental tension is the root of eye problems, and that bad habits contribute to bad eyesight. His recommendation to correct this tension was to rest the eyes properly. Although his methodology was not accepted by traditional ophthalmologists, optometrists quickly adopted it.

To relax your eyes, first bathe them, using cool water to energize them. The eye is used to seeing fire—bright light—and it needs periodic cooling. Then just look around the outskirts of the room you're in in a panoramic circle. Close your eyes gently and concentrate on breathing, while you warm your hands by rubbing them together for about twenty seconds. Place a hand over each eye with a cupped palm so that the fingertips are on the forehead and the base of the palms is on your cheekbones, not actually touching the eye. Look into the darkness with your eyes closed; you may even see some shimmering light. Continue to look at the darkness, concentrating on taking deep breaths, relax your mind and, along with it, your eyes.

Eye Exercises

A number of eye exercises relax the eyes—as well as improving outlook and vision function—by relaxing the eye muscles, both those on the outside of the eyelids and those around the eye (the *extraocular muscles* inside the skull).

1. *Pencil Push-Ups.* This exercise is the standard way of developing focusing power (accommodation and convergence). Take a pencil, hold it at arm's length (12 to 14 inches from your eye), and look at the tip

of the pencil facing the ceiling (eraser or point). Focus on the tip of the pencil, and bring it in toward your nose until you can no longer keep it in focus and the image becomes blurry. At this point, relax and stop trying to focus your eyes. Perform the exercise three more times. My recommendation is to do this exercise twice a day, once when you first get up and once before you go to sleep, even if you're doing other exercises. Continue on this schedule until you feel that you no longer need this exercise.

2. *Accommodation jump.* This exercise is sometimes called *thumbing.* Extend your arm with your thumb pointed upward, and look beyond it at a distant target. After fifteen to twenty seconds of looking at the distant target, look at your thumb. An alternative is to watch a ball bounce, or attend a ball game or other sports event with a constantly moving target—like tennis, basketball, Ping Pong, or hockey. This is an opportunity for the eye muscles, and even the neck muscles, to move freely. Repeat either one of these exercises (choose the one that works best for you, or alternate them) any number of times until your eyes and neck feel more relaxed.

3. *Edging.* Cover one eye with your hand, and look around the room with the other eye. This helps extend the extraocular muscles toward all four quadrants. Another method of using those muscles is to look at the four quadrants individually (looking straight up for a few seconds until it hurts, straight down, to the right, and to the left, in the same manner), which accomplishes the same objective. Another technique used by Tibetans is to place a butterfly-like picture on the wall. Get as close to the picture as possible, and trace the pattern of the butterfly's wings with your eyes until fatigue sets in. "Edging," or outlining the work space, is also good for the neck and eye muscles. Use either technique, and repeat the exercise as many times as you feel are necessary, until your eyes feel tired and it is relaxing to stop.

4. *Whole-body relaxation.* Stand up, stretch, and move at the waist, shake the hands, and standing on one foot, shake the other foot gently. You can even make circles with your shoulders. Swing the neck around slowly in four directions without creating any discomfort. This will help relax the body as well as the eyes—there's nothing like the seventh-inning stretch! This is especially helpful for computer users.

5. *Distant vision practice.* If you wear glasses, take them off and try to look at a distant point, even if it's blurry, for about half a minute to a full minute several times a day. Remember to breathe evenly and deeply at the same time. This will help relax the eye muscles. Studies have shown that nearsightedness (myopia) is most prevalent in areas

of the world in which the most close work is done on a regular basis. If we examine rates of myopia around the world, the highest rate occurs in Taiwan, which has a prevalence of 80 percent. In the United States, 20 to 25 percent of people are myopic. In rural Rwanda, 3.6 percent of people are nearsighted, but in the cities (urban areas of Rwanda), 19.7 percent have myopia. The lesson to be gained from this information is not, of course, that we should stop engaging in intellectual pursuits or avoid professions that require close work, but that we should take care to use our distance vision as often as possible so that the muscles that control accommodation (focusing) can relax by performing a different task.

6. *Imaging.* If you are in a small space and cannot look at something far away, close your eyes and imagine a scene in front of you. This is the beginning of visual imagery technique, in which you control your mental scenery to accomplish an inner physical or psychological purpose.

Choose from among these exercises the ones that are good for you. (There are also a number of books on eye exercises that you can consult to find more exercises.) Create your own personal group of exercises that is effective and fits into the time you have available. Remember, if you feel comfortable and your eyes feel more relaxed after doing eye exercises, add them to your own self-help manual.

Massaging the Eyes

To improve eye comfort and release fatigue, blurred vision, and stress, you can perform a number of ocular massaging techniques. Millions of Chinese schoolchildren perform acupressure eye exercises regularly. They are applied to the face and head, and take advantage of the acupressure points that are believed to influence the eyes.

1. Place your index or middle finger on the center of each orbit above the eye but under the brow, and massage gently for approximately ten seconds, and then press gently in the same spot for about three seconds and release. If you feel any discomfort, stop. Repeat the pressure and release, trying to feel the release. Massage gently in the same way under the orbit, at the position where 6:00 would be if your eye were a clock face.

2. Take the index and middle fingers and place them on the sides of the nose and the upper orbit. Massage the area gently for a few

seconds, then press gently for three seconds and finally, release. This can even be done while massaging skin creams in and around the eyes. Next, place the thumbs at the temple areas on the face, slightly in front of and at the top of your ears. There will be a slight discomfort, but press for five to ten seconds, and you will notice that the discomfort disappears; there is no need to press harder. Relax and feel the comfort. Repeat this for ten seconds on both temples simultaneously, and relax. This can actually be done while looking at the computer screen.

3. I've begun recommending an acupuncture exercise to reduce bags under the eyes. The fluid that accumulates under the lids, other than pockets of actual fat, is due to water retention, toxins, allergies, and sleeping face- or side-down. Sleeping on your back with your head slightly elevated is helpful in minimizing fluid-filled bags under the eyes. There are also two acupressure points that can be gently massaged. The first is at the lateral side (the outside) of the eye's orbit, just outside the bony rim and level with the eye. The second point is under the center of the eye, in the notch of the lower orbital rim. Before pressing on these trigger points, rub your hands together enough to warm and energize them. Then apply gentle pressure in the spots I've described with the index (first) or middle finger to the first point for seven seconds. Release the pressure without moving your finger, and repeat two more times for seven-second counts. Then find the notch under the eye socket (the second point I described), and repeat the same process. When finished, tap gently around the eye with one or two fingers, several times. This is an easy way to unload unnecessary "baggage." If it doesn't work for you, you haven't found the right points, so if you want to proceed to investigate acupressure, find an instructor.

4. Proceed to the jaw's joint, called the TMJ point, which is another site of stress, headaches, and even grinding the teeth at night. Feel underneath the bony arch of the cheek, approximately one inch in front of the ear's opening on each side. Use your thumb to find a slightly uncomfortable spot, which indicates the joint, and with your mouth slightly open, massage, press for ten seconds and release. Repeat this procedure once or twice, suddenly releasing the pressure. Then move your jaw gently and feel the reduced tension in the jaw and eyes. If this doesn't feel good, either you've missed the spot or are pressing on it too hard.

Vision Therapy

Vision therapy is taught at optometry schools; ophthalmologists know very little about it. If you asked an optometrist about vision therapy, he or she would probably say it works quite well. Behavioral optometrists feel that vision can be actively influenced and that seeing well is a malleable process that can be learned. Most ophthalmologists view vision as a passive optical event which cannot be influenced by a behavioral approach. My opinion is somewhere in between. We know very little about the brain, learning, and reading, and how the eyes interact with the brain. I believe that people can learn to improve their sense of comfort and may even be able to improve their eyesight, but not everyone is open to it or willing to commit the required time. Vision therapy has been used by some practitioners to improve concentration in children with learning disabilities, ADD, and ADHD.

Dyslexia, for instance, is often an inherited condition, and scientists have even discovered the location of the genes that contribute to or cause dyslexia. Other research has shown that dyslexic eyes have trouble focusing and refocusing from near to far. This means a child's eyes may skip lines of type while reading, or the eyes don't travel smoothly from one printed line to the next, or even from one paragraph to the next. Research performed by Dr. Sally Shaywitz's group at Yale University School of Medicine provides more proof that this particular vision/learning disorder originates in the brain. Shaywitz used a brain scan called *functional magnetic resonance imaging* (functional MRI) to monitor the mental activity of 61 children, and mapped which areas of the brain are active at different times. The MRI scans showed that dyslexic children have very little activity in the areas of the brain that translate letters on a page into words that can be recognized and spoken. (See Chapter 12.)

Vision therapy attempts to correct several types of vision problems, including:

- Eyes that don't track together (inefficiency in using eyes together)
- Eyes that don't focus on the same point (accommodation disorders)
- One eye that may shut off during reading (lazy eye or amblyopia)
- Misalignment of the eyes (strabismus or crossed eyes)
- Visual information processing disorders (learning disabilities like dyslexia)
- Visual rehabilitation after stroke or other brain injury

Vision therapy exercises are designed to keep the eyes working together. To read quickly and understand what is being read, the eyes must see clearly and move together. If your child is having trouble in school, a first step toward identifying possible problems is for him (or her) to have complete physical and eye examinations. It's also important to realize that some children, particularly boys, are not ready to read at age four or five. As I already pointed out, the problems these children experience may be genetic. If your child is having trouble learning because of vision and/or learning disabilities (dyslexia and others), please realize that your child is not dumb or incapable of learning. He or she may just need a little extra help learning, as well as his parents' patience and understanding.

If vision therapy can improve one's ability to track, read, learn, and ultimately function well in school and other learning situations, it will transform self-image. It can change people's life, as it has for President Lyndon Baines Johnson's daughter Lucy, whose dyslexia was helped greatly by vision therapy. She is now an active campaigner for vision therapy techniques. If you are interested in pursuing vision therapy, find an expert in your area to guide you. Vision therapy is not for everyone.

Eye Movement Desensitization Reprocessing

California psychologist Francine Shapiro made a startling accidental discovery in 1987: a technique combining rapid eye movements and hearing distracting sounds sometimes helps to process and release disturbing thoughts and memories. She suggests that the technique she originated, called *eye movement desensitization reprocessing* (EMDR), acts on the unconscious mind to resolve traumatic memories as they are sometimes worked out during rapid eye movement (REM) sleep. During EMDR, according to Shapiro, memories are moved from the portion of the brain where they are perceived as threatening events that are currently happening to another portion of the brain, where they can be processed without a sense of imminent disaster or panic.

EMDR has been adopted by perhaps 2000 psychiatrists, psychologists, and social workers in the mental health field. This innovative therapeutic technique is used to treat posttraumatic stress disorder (PTSD) patients (a condition often diagnosed in veterans who've seen combat), to alleviate anxiety related to disturbing memories (as can occur in rape victims), and to help people deal with the stress of daily life. It appears to help people with eating disorders, depression, low self-esteem, and perhaps even chronic fatigue, for reasons that are not yet understood. The rapid eye movements seem to stimulate the patient's innate information processing system to transform dysfunctional, disturbing thoughts into less threatening, more palatable information that is easier to endure.

In performing EMDR, the therapist has the patient recount the traumatic event while following a rapidly moving object (often the therapist's hand) and hearing certain sounds for short periods of time. As details of the disturbing experience emerge from the patient's memory, the patient is asked to describe them. As the therapy proceeds over time, even events that previously produced a state of panic can be remembered without stress and experienced as a memory of the past, not as a currently threatening situation, according to EMDR practitioners.

Bessel van der Kolk, M.D., professor of psychiatry at Boston University, is an expert on trauma who was extremely skeptical of EMDR until he performed brain scans of trauma patients before and after EMDR. He found that EMDR stimulates both the left and right sides of the brain. Before EMDR, the part of the brain that controls the fear response was constantly activated. After EMDR, Dr. van der Kolk found that the fear-response area of the brain was no longer activated, and the frontal lobe, which processes present-day information (as opposed to memories), became activated. EMDR appears to help degrade the stress level of the image and make it less threatening by processing it out of the brain's fear center along normal brain pathways. Isn't it amazing how the mind works?

Another visionary technique comes from the Technion Institute in Israel. Doctors there are helping to improve vision by having patients use short-term memory while watching an object on a computer screen. These investigators found that this technique could improve vision in healthy individuals with good vision. They are now planning to examine patients with vision problems to see if they can enhance their eyesight. This exciting research, which is still in the experimental state, may have some application for many people in the future.

In Germany, Bernhard Sabel, Ph.D., and his research team used vision therapy via computers to enlarge the visual fields in brain-injured patients. Ninety-five percent of their patients showed improvement after six months.

Robert-Michael Kaplan, M.D., author of *Seeing Without Glasses* and *The Power Behind Your Eyes*, advocates doing eye exercises as a way to take responsibility for your vision. I agree that performing eye exercises can relax not only the eyes, but also the body and the mind, making not only our vision but all our efforts more effective in the long run. We may not be able to change our refractive error, but we can certainly make our eyes feel better.

Appendix G: Vitamins: Historical Comparison of RDIs, RDAs, and DRIs, 1968 to Present

VITAMIN	RDI[1]	1968 RDA[2]	1974 RDA[2]	1980 RDA[2]	1989 RDA[2]	DRIs[3]
Vitamin A	5000 IU	5000 IU	1000 RE (5000 IU)	1000 RE	1000 RE	900 mcg (3000 IU)
Vitamin C	60 mg	60 mg	45 mg	60 mg	60 mg	90 mg
Vitamin D	400 IU (10 mcg)	400 IU (10 mcg)	400 IU (10 mcg)	10 mcg (400 IU)	10 mcg (400 IU)	15 mcg (600 IU)
Vitamin E	30 IU (20 mg)	30 IU (20 mg)	15 IU (10 mg)	10 mg (15 IU)	10 mg (15 IU)	15 mg[4]
Vitamin K	80 mcg	—	—	70–140 mcg	80 mcg	120 mcg
Thiamin	1.5 mg	1.5 mg	1.5 mg	1.5 mg	1.5 mg	1.2 mg
Riboflavin	1.7 mg	1.7 mg	1.8 mg	1.7 mg	1.8 mg	1.3 mg
Niacin	20 mg	20 mg	20 mg	19 mg	20 mg	16 mg
Vitamin B_6	2 mg	2 mg	2 mg	2.2 mg	2 mg	1.7 mg
Folate	0.4 mg (400 mcg)	400 mcg	400 mcg	400 mcg	200 mcg	400 mcg food, 200 mcg synthetic[5]
Vitamin B_{12}	6 mcg	6 mcg	3 mcg	3 mcg	2 mcg	2.4 mcg[6]
Biotin	(300 mcg)	150–300 mcg	100–300 mcg	100–200 mcg	30–100 mcg	30 mcg
Pantothenic acid	10 mg	5–10 mg	5–10 mg	4–7 mg	4–7 mg	5 mg
Choline	—	—	—	—	—	550 mg

1. The Reference Daily Intake (RDI) is the value established by the Food and Drug Administration (FDA) for use in nutrition labeling. It was based initially on the highest 1968 Recommended Dietary Allowance (RDA) for each nutrient, to assure that needs were met for all age groups.

2. The RDAs were established and periodically revised by the Food and Nutrition Board. Value shown is the highest RDA for each nutrient, in the year indicated for each revision.

3. The Dietary Reference Intakes (DRIs) are the most recent set of dietary recommendations established by the Food and Nutrition Board of the Institute of Medicine, 1997–2001. They replace previous RDAs, and may be the basis for eventually updating the RDIs. The value shown here is the highest DRI for each nutrient.

4. Historical vitamin E conversion factors were amended in the DRI report, so that 15 mg is defined as the equivalent of 22 IU of natural vitamin E or 33 IU of synthetic vitamin E.

5. It is recommended that women of childbearing age obtain 400 mcg of synthetic folic acid from fortified breakfast cereals or dietary supplements, in addition to dietary folate.

6. It is recommended that people over 50 meet the B_{12} recommendation through fortified foods or supplements, to improve bioavailability.

Appendix H: Minerals: Historical Comparison of RDIs, RDAs, and DRIs, 1968 to Present

MINERAL	RDI[1]	1968 RDA[4]	1974 RDA[2]	1980 RDA[2]	1989 RDA[2]	DRIs[3]
Calcium	1000 mg	1300 mg	1200 mg	1200 mg	1200 mg	1300 mg
Phosphorus	1000 mg	1300 mg	1200 mg	1200 mg	1200 mg	1250 mg (700 mg adult)
Iron	18 mg	18 mg	18 mg	18 mg	15 mg	18 mg
Iodine	150 mcg	150 mcg	150 mcg	150 mcg	150 mcg	150 mcg
Magnesium	400 mg	400 mg	400 mg	400 mg	400 mg	420 mg
Zinc	15 mg	10–15 mg	15 mg	15 mg	15 mg	11 mg
Selenium	70 mcg	—	—		70 mcg	55 mcg
Copper	2 mg	—	—	2–3 mg	1.5–3 mg	0.9 mg
Manganese	2 mg	—	2.5–7 mg	2.5–5 mg	2–5 mg	2.3 mg
Chromium	120 mcg	—	—	50–200 mcg	50–200 mcg	35 mcg
Molybdenum	75 mcg	—	45–500 mg	150–500 mcg	75–250 mcg	45 mcg

1. The Reference Daily Intake (RDI) is the value established by the Food and Drug Administration (FDA) for use in nutrition labeling. It was based initially on the highest 1968 Recommended Dietary Allowance (RDA) for each nutrient, to assure that needs were met for all age groups.

2. The RDAs were established and periodically revised by the Food and Nutrition Board. Value shown is the highest RDA for each nutrient, in the year indicated for each revision.

3. The Dietary Reference Intakes (DRIs) are the most recent set of dietary recommendations established by the Food and Nutrition Board of the Institute of Medicine, 1997–2001. They replace previous RDAs, and may be the basis for eventually updating the RDIs. The value shown here is the highest DRI for each nutrient.

Bibliography

Chapter 4

Bacotti, Joseph; "Progressive Lenses: The First Choice for Presbyopes"; *Refractive Eyecare for Ophthalmologists* 2(2):1, March/April 1998.

Berson, Frank G. ed., *Basic Ophthalmology for Medical Students and Primary Care Residents*, 7th Ed.; American Academy of Ophthalmology (San Francisco), 1999.

Blakeslee, Sandra; "Study Offers Surprise on Working of Body's Clock"; *New York Times*, January 16, 1998.

Brody, Jane E.; "Personal Health: When Eyes Betray Color Vision"; *New York Times*, October 21, 1997.

———. "Personal Health: Safety Rules for Contact Lenses"; *New York Times*, February 17, 1998.

———. "Personal Health: New Tack Promising on Winter Depression"; *New York Times*, March 31, 1998.

Bruneni, Joseph L.; *The Polycarbonate Handbook*; Polycarbonate Lens Council (Torrance, CA), 1998.

Campbell, Scott S., and Patricia J. Murphy; "Extraocular Circadian Phototransduction in Humans"; *Science* 279(5349):396, January 16, 1998.

Cohen, Stuart; "Shedding New Light on Sun Lenses"; *Eyewear*, January 1998.

Durrie, Daniel S.; "Touching-Up Over- and Undercorrections in Refractive Surgery"; *Refractive Eyecare for Ophthalmologists*, March/April 1998.

Edelson, Edward R.; "Rose-Colored Glasses, Sort Of"; *Newsday*, January 27, 1998.

Gallin, Pamela F., et al.; "Ophthalmologic Examination of Patients with Seasonal Affective Disorder, Before and After Bright-Light Therapy"; *American Journal of Ophthalmology* 119:202–210, February 1995.

Gilbert, Susan; "Polycarbonate Eyeglass Lenses Found Significantly Safer in Study"; *New York Times*, January 8, 1997.

Jaffe, Glenn J., and Irmgard S. Wood; "Retinal Phototoxicity from the Operating Microscope: A Protective Effect by the Fovea"; *Archives of Ophthalmology* 106:445, April 1988.

Lerman, Sidney; *Radiant Energy and the Eye*, Macmillan (New York), 1980.

Marcus, Mary Brophy; "The Next Miracles"; *U.S. News & World Report*, March 30, 1998.

Pierpaoli, Walter, and William Regelson with Carol Colman; *The Melatonin Miracle*; Simon & Schuster (New York), 1995.

Raloff, J.; "Eyes Possess Their Own Biological Clocks"; *Science News* 149:245, April 20, 1996.

Rosenthal, Norman E.; *Winter Blues: Seasonal Affective Disorder*, Guilford (New York), 1993.

Sardi, Bill; "Benefits of Light"; *Townsend Letter for Doctors*, p. 950, November 1992.

Schmid, Randolph E.; "Solar Warning Index Sounds Cancer Alarm"; *Wilmington News Journal*, June 29, 1994.

Schrier, Michael; "Shrewdest Eye Safety"; *Bottom Line Health,*, November 1, 1996.

Singer, Henry W.; "Experiment Suggests that Post-PRK Haze Can Be Linked to UV Exposure"; *Ocular Surgery News*, December 15, 1997.

Slon, Steven; "See 20/20 at 40-Plus"; *Prevention*, September 1997.

Smyth, Angela; *Seasonal Affective Disorder*, HarperCollins (Glasgow), 1991.

Strickland, Carol; "Low Vision Experts Debate Bioptic Driving Controversy"; *Ophthalmology World News*, June 1996.

Wu, Corinna; "Supernormal Vision"; *Science News* 152:312, November 15, 1997.

Young, R.W.; "Solar Radiation and Age-Related Macular Degeneration"; *Survey of Ophthalmology* 32:252–69, 1988.

Rosenthal, N.E.; "Diagnosis and Treatment of Seasonal Affective Disorder"; *JAMA* 270:2717–20, 1993.

Lenses & Technology: Annual Resource Guide, Jobson (St. Paul, MN), December 1997.

Men's Health; "Armor for Your Eyeballs"; November 1997.

Refractive Errors; American Academy of Ophthalmology (San Francisco), 1997.

Review of Ophthalmology, Supplement A:12A; "Understanding PRK Techniques and Technology," May 1996.

SunNet News, Autumn 1996; "Research Updates."

Chapter 5

Berson, Frank G.; *Basic Ophthalmology for Medical Students and Primary Care Residents*, 6th Ed.; American Academy of Ophthalmology (San Francisco), 1993.

Das, G. K., R. M. Pandey, and N. R. Biswas; "Comparative Double-Masked Randomized Placebo-Controlled Clinical Trial of a Herbal Eye Drop Preparation in Trachoma and Conjunctivitis"; *Journal of the Indian Medical Association* 93(10):383–84, October 1995.

Donnenfeld, E. D., et al.; "Controlled Evaluation of a Bandage Contact Lens and a Topical Nonsteroidal Anti-Inflammatory Drug in Treating Traumatic Corneal Abrasions"; *Ophthalmology* 102(6):979–84, June 1995.

Ehlers, William H.; "Maintaining Contact Lens Wear During Allergy Season"; *Refractive Eyecare for Ophthalmologists*, March/April 1998.

Eisenberg, Anne; "Focusing on Computer Users' Eyestrain"; *New York Times*, June 11, 1998.

Friedlaender, Mitchell H.; "Update on Allergic Conjunctivitis"; *Review of Ophthalmology*, March 1997.

Frucht-Pery, J., and E. Sagi; "The Use of Doxycycline and Tetracycline in Ocular Rosacea"; *Ocular Immunology and Inflammation* 1:99–103, 1993.

Hoang-Xuan, Thanh, Oliver Prisant, Daniele Hannouche, and Hervé Robin; "Systemic Cyclosporine A in Severe Atopic Keratoconjunctivitis"; *Ophthalmology* 104:1300–1305, 1997.

Jenkins, M. S., S. I. Brown, Lempert, S. L., and R. J. Weinberg; "Ocular Rosacea"; *Metabolic, Pediatric, and Systemic Ophthalmology* 6:189–96, 1982.

Kagi, M. K., B. Wuthrich, and S. G. Johansson; "Compari-Orange Anaphylaxis due to Carmine Allergy"; *Lancet* 344: 60–1, 1994.

Lazarus, S. M.; "The Use of Yoked Base-Up and Based-In Prism for Reducing Eyestrain at the Computer"; *Journal of the American Optometric Association* 57(4):204–8, April 1996.

Lowe, N., et al.; "Topical Metronidazole for Severe and Recalcitrant Rosacea: A Prospective Open Trial"; *Cutis* 43:283–86, 1989.

Metsahonkala, L., et al.; "Outcome of Early School Age Migraine"; *Cephalgia* 17:662–65, 1997.

Moles, Virginia Leoni; "9 Ways to Look Better"; *Men's Health*, January/February 1998.

Murata, K., et al.; "Accumulation of VDT Work-Related Visual Fatigue Assessed by Visual Evoked Potential, Near Point Distance and Critical Flicker Fusion"; *Industrial Health* 34(2):61–69, 1996.

Rechichi, C., C. A. De Moja, and L. Scullica; "Psychology of Computer Use: XXXVI. Visual Discomfort and Different Types of Work at Videodisplay Terminals"; *Perceptual & Motor Skills* 82:935–38, June 1996.

Rehm, Donald; "The Truth About Nearsightedness"; *Here's to Your Health*, September 1998

Roberts, Major Sanford; "Healthy Home"; *Bottom Line Health*, January 1998.

Schwartz, Brian S., et al.; "Epidemiology of Tension-Type Headache"; *Journal of the American Medical Association* 279(5):381–388, February 4, 1998.

Tanne, J. H.; "Viewing With Alarm"; *New York Times*, February, 1988.

Tervo, K., T. Latvala, V. P. Suomalamen, T. Tervo, and I. Immonen; "Cellular

Fibronectin and Tenascin in Experimental Perforating Scleral Wounds with Incarceration of the Vitreous"; *Grafes Archive for Clinical and Experimental Ophthalmology* 233(3):168–72, March 1995.

Ukai, K., K. Tsuchiva, and S. Ishikawa; "Induced Papillary Hippus Following Near Vision: Increased Occurrence in Visual Display Unit Workers"; *Ergonomics* 40:120–11, 1997.

Welch, K. M. A.; "A 27-year-old Woman with Migraine Headaches"; *Journal of the American Medical Association* 278(4):322–28, 1997.

Bottom Line Health; "Halogen Danger"; January 1998.

Harvard Men's Health Watch; "New Treatments for Migraines"; June 1997.

Morbidity and Mortality Weekly Report; "Alcohol-Related Traffic Fatalities Involving Children—United States, 1985–1996, 46:1130–33, 1997.

Chapter 6

Abel, Robert, Jr., and Ari D. Abel; "Perioperative Antibiotic, Steroid, and Nonsteroidal Anti-Inflammatory Agents in Cataract Intraocular Lens Surgery"; *Current Opinion in Ophthalmology* 8;I:29–32, 1997.

Abel, Robert, Jr., Stuart P. Richer, and Bill Sardi; "The Case for Nutrition as Preventive Eye Care"; Patient Care, *Review of Optometry*, August 1996.

Aesoph, Lauri M.; "Eat Right for Sharp Eyesight"; *Delicious!*, June 1997, p. 22.

Awashthi, Sanjay, Sanjay K. Srivatava, John T. Piper, Sharad S. Singhal, Meena Chaubey, and Yogesh C. Awasthi; "Curcumin Protects Against 4-hydroxyl-2-trans-nonenal-induced Cataract Formation in Rat Lenses"; *American Journal of Clinical Nutrition* 64:761–66, 1996.

Bando, Masayasu, and Hajime Obazawa; "Soluble Ascorbate Free Radical Reductase in the Human Lens"; *Japanese Journal of Ophthalmology* 38:1–9, 1994.

Beswick, H.T., and J.J. Harding; "Conformational Changes Induced in Bovine Lens Alpha-Crystallin by Carbamylation. Relevance to Cataract"; *Biochem. J.* 223:221–27, 1984.

Bland, Jeffrey S.; "Eye on Nutrition"; *Delicious!*, September 1996, p. 26.

Borchman, Douglas, W. Craig Byrdwell, and M. Cecilia Yappert; "Regional and Age-Dependent Differences in the Phospholipid Composition of Human Lens Membranes"; *Investigative Ophthalmology & Visual Science* 35(11):3938–42, October 1994.

Braidi, Susan M.; "Ancient Medical Practice in the Twentieth Century"; *Enquiry*, Summer 1989, p. 7.

Bravetti, G.; "Preventive Medical Treatment of Senile Cataract with Vitamin E and Anthocyanosides: Clinical Evaluation"; *Ann. Ottamol. Clin. Ocul.* 115:109, 1989.

Brown, Harriet; "The *AH* Guide to the Female Eye"; *American Health*, May 1997.

Charman, W. N.; "Ultraviolet Radiation and Cataract"; Correspondence, *British Journal of Ophthalmology* 79:196, 1994.

Christen, W. G., H. Manson, J. E., Seddon, J. M., et al.; "A Prospective Study of Cigarette Smoking and Risk of Cataract in Men"; *Journal of the American Medical Association* 268:989–93, 1992.

Christen, W. G., Jr.; "Antioxidants and Eye Disease"; *American Journal of Medicine* 97(3A):14S–17S, September 26, 1994.

Dolin, Paul J.; "Ultraviolet Radiation and Cataract: A Review of the Epidemiological Evidence"; *British Journal of Ophthalmology* 78:478–82, 1994.

———. "Ultraviolet Radiation and Cataract"; Correspondence, *British Journal of Ophthalmology* 79:196, 1994.

Drews, Robert C.; "Alcohol and Cataract"; *Archives of Ophthalmology* 111:1312, 1993.

Enstrom, J. E., et al.; "Vitamin C Intake and Mortality Among a Sample of the United States Population"; *Epidemiology* 3(3):194–202, May 1992.

Firshein, Richard N.; *Reversing Asthma: Reduce Your Medications with This Revolutionary New Program*, Warner Books (New York), 1998.

Ganea, E., Rixon, K. C., and J. J. Harding; "Binding of Glucose, Galactose, and Pyridoxal Phosphate to Lens Crystallins"; *Biochem. Biophys. Acta* 1226:286–90, 1994.

Garbe, Edeltraut, et al. "Corticosteroids Increase the Risk of Cataract"; *Journal of the American Medical Association* 280:539–43, 1998.

Gross, Neil; "Innovations"; *Business Week*, October 27, 1997, p. 156.

Gupta, S. K., Sujata Joshi, T. Velpandian, and S. D. Varma; "Protection Against Cataract by Pyruvate and Its Ocular Kinetics"; *Annals of Ophthalmology* 29(4):243–48, 1997.

Harding, John J.; "Cigarette Smoking and Risk of Cataracts"; Correspondence, *Journal of the American Medical Association* 269(6):747, February 10, 1993.

———. "Cigarettes and Cataract: Cadmium or a Lack of Vitamin C?"; Editorial, *British Journal of Ophthalmology* 79(3):199, March 1995.

Harkinson, S. E., M. J. Stampfer, J. M. Seddon, G. A. Colditz, B. Rosner, F. E. Speizer, and W. C. Willett; "Nutrient Intake and Cataract Extraction in Women: A Prospective Study"; *British Medical Journal* 305(6849):335–39, August 8, 1992.

Harkinson, S. E., et al.; "A Prospective Study of Cigarette Smoking and Risk of Cataracts in Women"; *Journal of the American Medical Association* 268(8):994–98, 1992.

Hemenger, Richard P., Leon F. Garner, and Chuan S. Ooi; "Change with Age of the Refractive Index Gradient of the Human Ocular Lens"; *Investigative Ophthalmology & Visual Science* 36(3):703, March 1995.

Jacques, P. F., and L. T. Chylack, Jr.; "Epidemiologic Evidence of a Role for the Antioxidant Vitamins and Carotenoids in Cataract Prevention"; *American Journal of Clinical Nutrition* 53(1 Suppl):352S–55S, January 1991.

Klein, Barbara E. K., Ronald Klein, and Linda L. Ritter; "Is There Evidence of an Estrogen Effect on Age-Related Lens Opacities?"; *Archives of Ophthalmology* 112:85–91, January 1994.

Langer, Stephen,; "New Insights Into Better Vision"; *Better Nutrition*, July 1997.

Leske, M. C., L. T. Chylack, Jr., and S. Y. Wu; "The Lens Opacities Case-Control Study: Risk Factors for Cataract"; *Archives of Ophthalmology* 109(2):244–51, February 1991.

Mares-Perlman, Julie A., William E. Brady, Barbara E. K. Klein, Ronald Klein, Mari Palta, Phyllis Bowen, and Maria Stacewicz-Sapuntzakis; "Serum Carotenoids and Tocopherols and Severity of Nuclear and Cortical Opacities"; *Investigative Ophthalmology & Visual Science* 36(2):276–88, February 1995.

Newsome, D. A., et al.; "Oral Zinc in Macular Degeneration"; *Archives of Ophthalmology* 106:192–98, 1988.

Olson, R. J.; "Supplementary Dietary Antioxidant Vitamins and Minerals in Patients with Macular Degeneration"; Abstract; *Journal of the American College of Nutritionists* 10(5):550, 1991.

Ravenholt, R. T.; "Cigarette Smoking and Risk of Cataracts"; Correspondence, *Journal of the American Medical Association* 269(6):747, February 10, 1993.

Robertson, J. M., A. P. Donner, and J. R. Trevithick; "A Possible Role for Vitamins C and E in Cataract Prevention"; *American Journal of Clinical Nutrition* 53(1 Suppl.):346S–51S, January 1991.

Roy, Hampton; "Cigarette Smoking and Risk of Cataracts"; Correspondence, *Journal of the American Medical Association* 269(6):747, February 10, 1993.

Salchert, John J.; "Cigarette Smoking and Risk of Cataracts"; Correspondence, *Journal of the American Medical Association* 269(6):747, February 10, 1993.

Sardi, Bill; "Eradicating Cataracts"; *Townsend Letter for Doctors*, June 1995.

————. "How Eight Eye Signs Can Reveal Your Nutritional Health"; *Alternative Medicine Digest*, Issue 19. Health Spectrum Publishers.

————. "Artificial Sweeteners and the Eyes"; *Nutrition and the Eyes*, Vol. II, 1994, pp. 89–93. Health Spectrum Publishers.

Schoenfeld, Elinor Randi, M. Cristina Leske, and Suh-Yuh Wu; "Recent Epidemiologic Studies on Nutrition and Cataract in India, Italy, and the United States"; *Journal of the American College of Nutrition* 12(5):521–26, 1993.

Seddon, J. M., W. G. Christen, J. E. Manson, F. S. LaMotte, R. J. Glynn, J. E. Buring, and C. H. Hennekens; "The Use of Vitamin Supplements and the Risk of Cataract Among U.S. Male Physicians"; *American Journal of Public Health* 84(5):788–92, May 1994.

Spector, Abraham, Guo-Ming Wang, Ren-Rong Wang, William H. Garner, and Hans Moll; "The Prevention of Cataract Caused by Oxidative Stress in Cultured Rat Lenses. I: H_2O_2 and Photochemically Induced Cataract"; *Current Eye Research* 12(2):163–79, 1993.

————. "The Prevention of Cataract Caused by Oxidative Stress in Cultured Rat Lenses. II: Early Effects of Photochemical Stress and Recovery"; *Experimental Eye Research* 57:659–67, 1993.

Sperduto, R. D., T. S. Hu, R. C. Milton, et al.; "The Linxian Cataract Studies: Two Nutrition Intervention Trials"; *Archives of Ophthalmology* 111(9):1246–53, September 1993.

Sperduto, R. D., F. L. Ferris III, and N. Kurinij; "Do We Have a Nutritional Treatment for Age-Related Cataract or Macular Degeneration?"; *Archives of Ophthalmology* 108:1403–5, 1990.

Taylor, A.; "Effect of Photooxidation on the Eye Lens and Role of Nutrients in Delaying Cataract"; *EXS* 62:266–79, 1992.

Taylor, Allen, Paul F. Jacques, and Esther M. Epstein; "Relations Among Aging, Antioxidant Status, and Cataract"; *American Journal of Clinical Nutrition* 62(supppl):1439S–47S, 1995.

Varma, Schambhu D.; "Scientific Basis for Medical Therapy of Cataracts by Antioxidants"; *Journal of Clinical Nutrition* 53:335S–45S, 1991.

Varma, S. D., P. S. Devamanoharan, and S. M. Morris; "Prevention of Cataracts by Nutritional and Metabolic Antioxidants"; *Critical Reviews in Food Science and Nutrition* 35(1&2):111–29, 1995.

Ward, J.; "Free Radicals, Antioxidants, and Preventive Geriatrics"; *Australian Family Physician* 23(7):1297–301, July 1994.

Weil, Andrew; "Protect Your Vision Naturally"; *Self-Healing*, June 1997, p. 2.

West, Sheila, et al.; "Sunlight Exposure and Risk of Lens Opacity in a Population-Based Study"; *Journal of the American Medical Association* 280:714–18, 1998.

West, Sheila; "Cataract: Can We Prevent It?" Research to Prevent Blindness Science Writers Seminar, April 25–28, 1993.

Yeum, Kyung-Jim, Allen Taylor, Guangwen Tang, and Robert M. Russell; "Measurement of Carotenoids, Retinoids, and Tocopherols in Human Lenses"; *Investigative Ophthalmology & Visual Science* 36(13):2756–61, December 1995.

EyeWorld Week, Vol. 3, No. 6, February 9, 1998.

Harper's Biochemistry 22nd Ed.; Murray, R. K., et al.; Appleton & Lange (Norwalk, CT), 1990.

Health News; "Excess Weight Linked to Cataracts"; October 31, 1995.

Health News; "Asthma Inhalers Linked to Cataracts"; August 4, 1997.

Nutritional Influences on Illness, 2nd Ed.; Werbach, M. R.; Third Line Press (Tarzana, CA), 1993.

Review of Optometry; "Research Report: New Drug Prevents Cataracts"; July 1992.

Chapter 7

Abel R., Jr., and A. D. Abel; "Ocular Diseases" in *Drug Therapy*, 4th Ed. (ed. Spraight); Adis Press, New Zealand, pp. 592–99, 1997.

Akyol, N., et al.; "Aqueous Humour and Serum Zinc and Copper Concentrations of Patients with Glaucoma and Cataract"; *British Journal of Ophthalmology* 74(11):661–62, 1990.

Asregadoo, E. R.; "Blood Levels of Thiamine and Ascorbic Acid in Chronic Open-Angle Glaucoma"; *Annals of Ophthalmology* 11(7):1095–1100, 1979.

Bajracharya, Vaidya Mana, with Robert Abel, Jr., and Allan Tillotson; *Ayurvedic Ophthalmology: Treatment Strategies and Formulas for 76 Eye Diseases*; published by Nature's Herbs, 1992.

Berens, C., et al.; "Allergy in Glaucoma. Manifestations of Allergy in Three Glaucoma Patients as Determined by the Pulse-Diet Method of Coca"; *Annals of Allergy* 5:526–35, 1947.

Brody, Jane E.; "For Glaucoma Risk Group, Ignorance Is Blindness"; *New York Times*, January 20, 1998.

Carels, Robert A., Andrew Sherwood, and James A. Blumenthal; "High Anxiety and White-Coat Hypertension"; Letter to the Editor; *Journal of the American Medical Association* 279(3):197, January 21, 1998.

Charters, Lynda; "Studies Shed Light on Glutamate Toxicity"; *Ophthalmology Times*, December 1, 1997, p. 23.

Christen, William Gerard, Jr.; "Antioxidants and Eye Disease"; *American Journal of Medicine* 97(suppl. 3A): September, 1994, 14S–17S.

Davis, R. H.; "Does Caffeine Ingestion Affect IOP?" (Letter); *Ophthalmology* 96(11): 1680–81, 1989.

Dreyer, Evan B.; "Glutamate Antagonists Find a New Role in the Eye"; *Glaucoma*, January 1, 1998.

Edelson, Ed; "Genetic Advances May Answer Glaucoma Questions"; *Ophthalmology Times*, December 1, 1997, p. 21.

Evans, S. C.; "Ophthalmic Nutrition and Prevention of Eye Disorder and Blindness"; *Nutr. Metab.* 21(Suppl. 1):268–72, 1977.

Fishbein, S. L., and S. Goldstein; "The Pressure-Lower Effect of Ascorbic Acid"; *Annals of Ophthalmology* 4:498–91, 1972.

Garbe, E., J. Lelorier, J. Boivin, et al.; "Inhaled and Nasal Glucocorticoids and the Risks of Ocular Hypertension or Open-Angle Glaucoma"; *JAMA* 277:722–27, 1997.

Harris, Alon, and Hak Sung Chung; "Ocular Blood Flow in Glaucoma"; *Mediguide to Ophthalmology*, Vol. 7, Issue 4, published by Merck & Co., Inc. (West Point, PA).

Heijl, Anders, Ellen Strahman, Thordur Sverrisson, Olaf Brinchman-Hansen, Tuomo Puustjarvi, and Robert Tipping; "A Comparison of Dorzolamide and Timolol in Patients with Pseudoexfoliation and Glaucoma or Ocular Hypertension"; *Ophthalmology* 104:137–142, 1997.

Higginbotham, E. J., et al.; "The Effect of Caffeine on IOP in Glaucoma Patients"; *Ophthalmology* 96(5):624–26, 1989.

Jou, Diana, and David A. Lee; "Glaucoma Medications: First, Do No Harm"; *Review of Ophthalmology*, June 1998.

Lane, B. C.; "Diet and the Glaucomas" (abstract); *J. Am. Coll. Nutr.* 10(5):536, 1991.

———. "Evaluation of IOP with Daily, Sustained Closework Stimulus to Accommodation, Lowered Tissue Chromium, and Dietary Deficiency of Ascorbic Acid"; 3rd International Conference on Myopia, Cophenhagen & The Hague, *Doc. Ophthalmol.* 28:149–55, 1981.

Lee, P., et al.; "Aqueous Humor Ascorbate Concentration and Open-Angle Glaucoma"; *Archives of Ophthalmology* 95(2):308–10, 1977.

Linner, E.; "The Pressure-Lowering Effect of Ascorbic Acid in Ocular Hypertension"; *Acta Ophthalmol.* (Copenhagen) 47:685–89, 1969.

———. "Eye Pressure Regulation and Ascorbic Acid"; *Acta Soc. Med. Upsala.* 69:225–32, 1964.

Liu, K. M., et al.; "Inhibition of Oxidative Degradation of Hyaluronic Acid by Uric Acid"; *Current Eye Research* 3(8):1049–53, 1984.

Martin, Wayne; "Prevention and Treatment of Glaucoma" (Letter); *Townsend Letter for Doctors & Patients*, February/March 1997, p. 107.

McGuire, Rich; "Fish Oil Cuts Lower Ocular Pressure"; *Medical Tribune*, August 19, 1991, p. 25.

Mehra, K. S.; "Relationship of pH of Blood and Aqueous with Vitamin C"; *Annals of Ophthalmology* 10(1):83–92, 1978.

Netland, Peter A.; "Low-Tension Glaucoma"; *Mediguide to Ophthalmology*, Vol. 7, Issue 1, published by Merck & Co., Inc. (West Point, PA).

Passo, M. S., L. Goldberg, D. L. Elliott, et al.; "Exercise Training Reduces Intraocular Pressure Among Subjects Suspected of Having Glaucoma"; *Archives of Ophthalmology* 109:1096–98, 1991.

Raymond, L. F.; "Allergy and Chronic Simple Glaucoma"; *Annals of Allergy* 22:146–50, 1964.

Robin, Alan L.; "Glaucoma Management: Beyond Intraocular Pressure"; *Ophthalmology Times*, Supplement 2, December 1997, p. S2.

Shen, T-M., and M-C. Yu; "Clinical Evaluation of Glycerin-Sodium Ascorbate Solution in Lowering IOP"; *Chinese Medical Sciences Journal* 1:64–68, 1975.

Sommer, Alfred, et al.; "Relationship between Intraocular Pressure and Primary Open Angle Glaucoma among White and Black Americans"; *Archives of Ophthalmology* 109:1090–95, 1991.

Tielsch, James M., J. Katz, A. Sommer, H. A. Quigley, and J. C. Javitt; "Family History and Risk of Primary Open Angle Glaucoma: The Baltimore Eye Study"; *Archives of Ophthalmology* 112:69–73, 1994.

Todd, G. P.; *Nutrition, Health and Disease*, The Donning Company (Norfolk, VA), 1985.

Eye Net (a publication of the American Academy of Ophthalmology), March 1998.

EyeWorld Week, Vol. 3, No. 6, February 9, 1998 (published by ASCRS Ophthalmic Services Corp., Fairfax, VA).

Chapter 8

Atkins, Robert; "Macular Medicine"; *Dr. Robert Atkins' Health Revelations*, Vol. 5, No. 3, March 1997.

Allikmets, Rando, et al.; "Mutation of the Stargardt Disease Gene (ABCR) in Age-Related Macular Degeneration"; *Science* 277:1805, September 19, 1997.

Bishop, Jerry E.; "Team of Researchers May Have Found Treatment for Major Cause of Blindness"; *Wall Street Journal*, May 8, 1992.

Brody, Jane E.; "The Aging Eye: Researcher Aims to Stop the Clock"; *New York Times*, October 14, 1997.

Carlisle, Tamsin; "Mother's Blindness Spurs New Therapy"; *Wall Street Journal*, October 21, 1997.

Chandra, R. K.; "Effect of Vitamin and Trace Element Supplementation on Immune Responses and Infection in Elderly Subjects"; *The Lancet* 340:1124–27, 1992.

Eastman, Peggy; "When the Light Fades: Macular Degeneration in the Spotlight"; *AARP Bulletin*, Vol. 37, No. 7, July-August 1996.

Hammond, B. R., Jr., K. Fuld, and J. Curran-Calentano; "Macular Pigment Density in Monozygotic Twins"; *Investigative Ophthalmology* 36:2531–41, 1995.

Hankinson, Susan, and Meir J. Stampfer; "Editorial: All That Glitters Is Not Beta-Carotene"; *Journal of the American Medical Association* 272(18):1455, November 9, 1994.

Hartstein, Jack, Umberto Pace, Morris E. Hartstein, Rudolph E. Tanzi, and Ashley I. Bush; "Editorial: Zinc and Macular Degeneration"; *Annals of Ophthalmology-Glaucoma*, 27(4):194, July/August 1995.

Klein, Ronald, Barbara E. K. Klein, Susan C. Jensen, and Stacy M. Meuer; "The Five-year Incidence and Progression of Age-Related Maculopathy: The Beaver Dam Eye Study"; *Ophthalmology* 104:7–21, 1997.

————. "The Relation of Cardiovascular Disease and Its Risk Factors to the 5-year Incidence of Age-Related Maculopathy: The Beaver Dam Eye Study"; *Ophthalmology* 104:1804–12, 1997.

Krall, Charles; "Nutritional Treatment Program and Age-Related Macular Degeneration: Improved Vision One Year Later"; *Townsend Letter for Doctors & Patients*, January 1997.

Kugler, Hans; "Ask Your Doctor"; *Journal of Longevity* 3(11):45, 1997.

Levin, Leonard A.; "Ophthalmology"; *Journal of the American Medical Association* 273(21):1703, June 7, 1995.

Maguire, Maureen G.; "More Pieces for the Age-Related Macular Degeneration Puzzle"; *Ophthalmology* 104(1):5, January 1997.

Mares-Perlman, Julie A., et al.; "Serum Antioxidants and Age-Related Macular Degeneration in a Population-Based Case-Control Study"; *Archives of Ophthalmology* 113:1518–23, December 1995.

Morris, Dexter L., Stephen B. Kritchevsky, and C. E. Davis; "Serum Carotenoids and Coronary Heart Disease"; *Journal of the American Medical Association* 272(18):1439, November 9, 1994.

Nataloni, Rochelle; "Nutrition and the Eye: Supplements' Role Studied"; *Ocular Surgery News* 12(14):1, July 15, 1994.

Newsome, David; "Vitamin-Mineral Supplements and Retinal Health"; *Ocular Surgery News*, December 15, 1995, p. 32.

———. "Straight Talk on Nutrition and the Eye"; *Review of Ophthalmology*, July 1994, p. 49.

Pratt, Steven G.; "What We Now Know About AMD and Nutrition"; *Review of Ophthalmology*, August 1998.

Richer, S.; "Is There a Prevention and Treatment Strategy for Macular Degeneration?"; *Journal of the American Optometric Association* 64(12), 1993.

———. "Atrophic ARMD—A Nutrition-Responsive Chronic Disease"; *Journal of the American Optometric Association* 67:50–57, 1996.

Sardi, Bill; "Nutrients to Help Reverse Macular Degeneration"; *Alternative Medicine Digest*, No. 16, p. 63.

Schwab, Ivan; "The Avian Eye"; *EyeNet*, May 1998, p. 29.

Seddon, Johanna M., et al.; "Dietary Carotenoids, Vitamins A, C, and E, and Advanced Age-Related Macular Degeneration"; *Journal of the American Medical Association* 272(18):1413, November 9, 1994.

Snodderly, D. Max; "Evidence for Protection Against Age-Related Macular Degeneration by Carotenoids and Antioxidant Vitamins"; *American Journal of Clinical Nutrition* 62(suppl.): 1448S–61S, 1995.

Stuen, Cynthia; "Measuring the Impact of Macular Degeneration"; *Aging & Vision News*, Vol. 9, No. 2, Fall 1997.

The Mindell Letter; "Macular Degeneration"; April 1997.

Ophthalmology Times; "Support Grows for Vitamin/Mineral Supplements for ARMD"; February 15, 1993.

Retina/Vitreous; "To Battle Macular Degeneration, Researchers Offer Time-Tested Advice: Eat Right and Exercise"; January 15, 1998.

Review of Ophthalmology, "News & Trends," June 1995.

Science News 152:198; "New Treatments for Macular Degeneration"; September 27, 1997.

Chapter 9

Breecher, Maury M.; "Two New Drugs Show Promise in Treating Obesity"; *Diabetes Wellness Letter*, December 1997.

————. "Managed Care Message: Patients Receive Better Diabetes Care from Specialists"; *Diabetes Wellness Letter*, December 1997.

Choate, Clinton; "Diabetes Mellitus from Western and TCM Perspectives"; *East/West Perspectives*, December 8, 1997.

Crane, M. G., et al.; "Regression of Diabetic Neuropathy and Total Vegetarian (Vegan) Diets"; *Journal of Nutritional Medicine* 4:431–36, 1994.

DCCT Research Group (Box NDIC/DCCT, Bethesda, MD 20892); "Clustering of Long-Term Complications in Families with Diabetes in the Diabetes Control and Complications Trial"; *Diabetes* 46:1829–39, 1997.

Flynn, Harry W., Emily Y. Chew, Brad D. Simons, et al.; "Pars Plana Vitrectomy in the Early Treatment Diabetic Retinopathy Study"; *Ophthalmology* 99:1351–57, 1992.

Gijsman, H., et al.; "Double-Blind, Placebo-Controlled, Dose-Finding Study of Rizatriptan (MK-462) in the Acute Treatment of Migraine"; *Cephalalgia* 17:647–51, 1997.

Hoffman, Joseph; "Who Is at Greatest Risk for Diabetic Retinopathy?"; *Ocular Surgery News*, December 1, 1997.

Sardi, Bill; "Diabetic Retinopathy, Insulin and Laser vs. Diet and Nutritional Supplements, Part I: The Disappointment of Modern Therapy"; *Townsend Letter for Doctors & Patients*, April 1996.

————. "Diabetic Retinopathy, Insulin and Laser vs. Diet and Nutritional Supplements, Part II: The Real Way to Save Sight"; *Townsend Letter for Doctors & Patients*, May 1996.

Scharrer, A., and M. Ober; "Anthocyanosides in the Treatment of Retinopathies"; *Klin. Monatsbl. Augenheilkd* 178:386–9, 1981 (in German).

Sharma, K. R, R. P. Bhatia, and V. Kumar; "Role of the Indigenous Drug Saptamrita Lauha in Hemorrhagic Retinopathies"; *Annals of Ophthalmology* 24(1):5–8, January 1992.

Shaw, Donna; "Antitumor Test Starts for a Compound from Shark"; *Philadelphia Inquirer*, p. 1, December 16, 1997.

Sotaniemi, Eero Al, Eila Haapakoski, and Arja Rautio; "Ginseng Therapy in Non-Insulin-Dependent Diabetic Patients"; *Diabetes Care* 18(10):1373, October 1995.

Stametz, Paul, and C. Dusty Wu Yao; "Mycomedicinals: Information on Medicinal Mushrooms"; *Townsend Newsletter for Doctors*, issue 179, pp. 152–67.

Chapter 10

Abel, Robert Jr.; "Gift of Sight Helps People Become Self-Sufficient"; *The Dialog* (Wilmington, DE), March 20, 1997.

Alster, Yair, et al.; "Delay of Corneal Wound Healing in Patients Treated with Colchicine"; *Ophthalmology* 104:118–19, 1997.

Brody, Jane E.; "Beyond Ragweed, Allergenic Combinations"; *New York Times*, September 6, 1995.

Ehlers, William H.; "Treating GPC"; *Refractive Eyecare for Ophthalmologists*; March/April 1998.

Sandler, Gregory; "The State-of-the Art Corneal Transplant"; *EyeWorld*, November 1997.

Wilson, Steven E.; "Keratocyte Apoptosis: Response to Corneal Epithelial Injury"; *EyeWorld*, January 1998.

Wright, Jonathan V.; "Buffered Vitamin C and Eye Problems"; *Let's Live*, February 1991.

Eye Donation: Giving the "Gift of Sight"; Lions Eye Bank of Delaware Valley; 2000 Hamilton Street, Rodin Place, Suite 202, Philadelphia, PA 19130–722.

Chapter 11

Abel R., Jr., and A. D. Abel; "Ocular Diseases" in *Drug Therapy*, 4th Ed. (ed. Spraight), Adis Press, New Zealand, pp. 592–99, 1997.

Brody, Jane E.; "Beyond Ragweed, Allergenic Combinations"; *New York Times*, September 6, 1995.

―――. "When Eyes Have That Sandpaper Grit Feeling"; *New York Times*, October 28, 1997.

Childers, Norman Franklin; *A Diet to Stop Arthritis*; Somerset Press, 1981.

Das, G. K., R. M. Pandey, and N.R. Biswas; "Comparative Double-Masked Randomized Placebo-Controlled Clinical Trial of a Herbal Eye Drop Preparation in Trachoma and Conjunctivitis"; *Journal of the Indian Medical Association* 93(10):383–84, October 1995.

Donnenfeld, E. D., B. A. Selkin, H. D. Perry, K. Moadel, G. T. Selkin, A. J. Cohen, and L. T. Sperber; "Controlled Evaluation of a Bandage Contact Lens and a Topical Nonsteroidal Anti-Inflammatory Drug in Treating Traumatic Corneal Abrasions"; *Ophthalmology* 102(6):979–84, June 1995.

Hoang-Xuan, Thanh, Oliver Prisant, Daniele Hannouche, and Hervé Robin; "Systemic Cyclosporine A in Severe Atopic Keratoconjunctivitis"; *Ophthalmology* 104:1300–1305, 1997.

Kobayashi, T. K., et al.; "Effect of Retinol Palmitate as a Treatment for Dry Eye: A Cytological Evaluation"; *Ophthalmologica* 211:358–361, 1997.

Pullman-Mooar, S., et al.; "Alteration of the Cellular Fatty Acid Profile and the Production of Eicosanoids in Human Monocytes by Gamma-Linolenic Acid"; *Arthritis and Rheumatism* 33(10):1526–33, 1990.

Scerra, Chet; "Researchers Work to Unravel Cortisol Link to Disease"; *Ophthalmology Times*, March 15, 1998.

Tervo, K., T. Larvala, V. P. Suomalainen, T. Tervo, and I. Immonen; "Cellular Fibronectin and Tenascin in Experimental Perforating Scleral Wounds with Incarceration of the Vitreous"; *Graefes Archive for Clinical & Experimental Ophthalmology* 223(3):168–72, March 1995.

"Research Finds Genital Herpes Soaring Among Young Whites"; Associated Press, *New York Times*, October 21, 1997.

American Journal of Ophthalmology, vol. 118, p. 81.
The PDR for Ophthalmology, 25th Ed., Medical Economics Company (New Jersey), 1997.

Chapter 12

American Academy of Pediatrics, Committee on Nutrition; "The Practical Significance of Lactose Intolerance in Children"; *Pediatrics* 62:240–50, 1978.

Associated Press; "Girls' Body Fat Isn't Related to Cholesterol Levels, Study Finds"; *New York Times*, June 17, 1997.

Barr, Ronald G., Melvin D. Levine, and John B. Watkins; "Recurrent Abdominal Pain of Childhood Due to Lactose Intolerance"; *New England Journal of Medicine*, pp. 1449–52, June 28, 1979.

Begley, Sharon, with Mary Hager; "Pesticides and Kids' Risks"; *Newsweek*, June 1, 1998.

Flatz, Gebhard and Hans Werner Rotthauwe; "Lactose Nutrition and Natural Selection"; *The Lancet*, pp. 76–77, July 14, 1973.

Liebman, William M.; "Recurrent Abdominal Pain in Children: Lactose and Sucrose Intolerance: A Prospective Study"; *Pediatrics* 641:43–45, 1979.

Matsumura, T., T. Kuroume, and K. Amanda; "Close Relationship Between Lactose Intolerance and Allergy to Milk Protein"; *Journal of Asthma Research*, pp. 13–29, Septemper 1971.

Owens, Jennifer; "Study: Baby Food Has Unsafe Pesticide Levels"; SN, February 9, 1998.

Shapiro, Laura; "Is Organic Better?"; *Newsweek*, June 1, 1998.

Talan, Jamie; "Study Ties Attention Disorders, Fatty Acid"; *Newsday*, April 24, 1998.

Walker, W. A.; "Antigen Absorption from the Small Intestine and Gastrointestinal Disease"; *Pediatr. Clinc., North Am.* 22:731–46, 1975.

Chapter 13

Adour, K. K.; "Medical Management of Idiopathic Bell's Palsy"; *Otolaryngologic Clinics of North America* 24:663–73, 1991.

Berson, E.L., et al.; "Evaluation of Patients with Retinitic Pigmentosa Receiving Electric Stimulation, Ozonated Blood, and Ocular Surgery in Cuba"; *Archives of Ophthalmology* 114(5):560–63, May 1996.

Buo, Yin, and Lu Shao Ping; "Two Case Histories: Optic Neuritis"; *Journal of Chinese Medicine*, 1992.

Hughes, G. B.; "Practical Managmeent of Bell's Palsy"; *Otolaryngology, Head and Neck Surgery* 102:658–63, 1990.

Keeney, A. H., et al.; "Carcinogenesis and Nicotine in Malignant Melanoma of the Choroid"; *American Ophthalmologic Society* 80:131–42, 1982.

Kodish, Eric, Georgia L. Wiesner, Maxwell Mehlman, and Thomas Murray;

"Genetic Testing for Cancer Risk: How to Reconcile the Conflicts"; *Journal of the American Medical Association* 279(3):179, January 21, 1998.

Morgan, M., and D. Nathwani; "Facial Palsy and Infection: The Unfolding Story"; *Clinical Infectious Diseases* 14:263–71, 1992.

Ritch, Robert, series ed.; "Rounds: What Is Diagnosis?"; *Ophthalmology Times,* January 15, 1998.

Sabbagh, Leslie B; "Managing the Great Masquerader"; *EyeWorld,* November 1997.

Schena, Lori Baker; "Retina/Vitreous: Face-Down Positioning, the Debate Continues"; *EyeNet,* April 1998.

New England Journal of Medicine 338:73–78; "Radiotherapy Followed by Prednisone Best Treatment for Graves' Hyperthyroidism"; 1998.

Nutrition & Healing; "Nutritionally-Oriented Physical Exam"; May 1998.

Chapter 14

Abel, Robert, Jr., Stuart P. Richer, and Bill Sardi; "The Case for Nutrition as Preventive Eye Care"; *Review of Optometry,* August 15, 1995.

Absher, Kenneth,; "Why Eye Problems Are Increasing"; *Journal of Longevity* 4(6):7, 1998.

Albert, Christine M., et al.; "Fish Consumption and Risk of Sudden Cardiac Death"; *Journal of the American Medical Association* 279(1):23, January 7, 1998.

Anderson, Curt; "U.S. Tries to Define What is 'Organic' "; Associated Press, December 16, 1997.

Aronne, Louis; "High-Protein Diets: Why They're Dangerous"; *Bottom Line/ Health,* January 1998.

Atkins, Robert C.; *Dr. Atkins' New Diet Revolution;* M. Evans (New York), 1998.

Bao, Weihand, et al.; "Longitudinal Changes in Cardiovascular Risk from Childhood to Young Adulthood in Offspring of Parents with Coronary Artery Disease: The Bogalusa Heart Study"; *Journal of the American Medical Association* 278(21):1749, December 3, 1997.

Breneman, J. C.; "Allergy Elimination Diet as the Most Effective Gallbladder Diet"; *Annals of Allergy* 26:83–87, 1968.

Brody, Jane E.; "New Guide Puts Most Americans on the Fat Side"; *New York Times,* June 9, 1998.

———. "A Recipe for Woe: High-Fat, High-Protein Diets Are Back"; *New York Times,* December 25, 1996.

Burros, Marian; "Fat Substitute May Cause Disease, a Top Researcher Says"; *New York Times,* June 11, 1998.

Carper, Jean; *Food, Your Miracle Medicine;* Harper Perennial (New York), 1993.

Christen, W. G., Jr.; "Antioxidants and Eye Disease"; *American Journal of Medicine* 97 (Suppl 3A):14S–17S, 1994.

Clifford, A. J., et al.; "Delayed Tumor Onset in Transgenic Mice Fed an Amino

Acid-Based Diet Supplemented with Red Wine Solids"; *American Journal of Clinical Nutrition* 64(5):748–56, November 1996.

Collins, Richard; "The Cooking Cardiologist"; *GreatLife*, January 1998.

Constant, J.; "Alcohol, Ischemic Heart Disease, and the French Paradox"; *Coronary Artery Disease* 8(10):645–49, October 1997.

Coughlin, Carol; "A Feast for the Eyes"; *Vegetarian Times*, August 1997.

Crayhon, Robert; *Nutrition Made Simple*; M. Evans (New York), 1994.

Duke, James; *The Green Pharmacy*; Rodale Press (Emmaus, PA), 1997.

Erasmus, Udo; *Fats that Heal Fats That Kill*; Alive Books (Burnaby, BC, Canada), 1993.

Fenech, M., C. Stockley, and C. Aitken; "Moderate Wine Consumption Protects Against Hydrogen Peroxide-induced DNA Damage"; *Mutagenesis* 12(4)289–96, July 1997.

Fox, Arnold; "Why the French Have Healthier Hearts"; *Journal of Longevity* 3(11):7, 1997.

Gelatt, Kirk N.; ed.; *Veterinary Ophthalmology*, 2nd Ed., Lea & Febiger (Philadelphia) 1991.

Gin, H., P. Morlat, J. M. Ragnaud, and J. Aubertin; "Short-Term Effect of Red Wine (Consumed During Meals) on Insulin Requirement and Glucose Tolerance in Diabetic Patients"; *Diabetes Care* 15(4):546–8, April 1992.

Haas, Elson M.; *The Detox Diet*, Celestial Arts (Berkeley, CA), 1996.

———. *Staying Healthy with Nutrition*; Celestial Arts (Berkeley, CA), 1992.

Hendler, Sheldon Saul; *The Doctors' Vitamin and Mineral Encyclopedia*, Simon & Schuster (New York), 1990.

Hibbeln, Joseph R.; "Fish Consumption and Major Depression"; *The Lancet* 351:1213, April 18, 1998.

Hodis, Howard N., et al.; "Serial Coronary Angiographic Evidence That Antioxidant Vitamin Intake Reduces Progression of Coronary Artery Atherosclerosis"; *Journal of the American Medical Association* 273(23):1849, June 21, 1995.

Jang, Pezzuto, et al.; "Cancer Chemopreventive Activity of Resveratrol, and Natural Product Derived from Grapes"; *Science* 275:218–20, 1997.

Kennedy, Ron; "How Poor Digestion Leads to Illness"; *Journal of Longevity* 3(11):33, 1997.

Keuneke, Robin; *Total Breast Health*, Kensington (New York), 1998.

Klein, Ronald, Barbara E. K. Klein, and Susan C. Jensen; "The Relation of Cardiovascular Disease and Its Risk Factors to the 5-year Incidence of Age-Related Maculopathy: The Beaver Dam Eye Study"; *Ophthalmology* 104:1804–12, 1997.

Kolata, Gina; "New Clue to Heart Disease: A Vitamin Lack"; *New York Times*, July 4, 1995.

Krinsky, N. J., M. D. Russert, G. J. Handelman, and D. M. Snodderly; "Structural and Geometrical Isomers of Carotenoids in Human Plasma"; *Journal of Nutrition* 120(12):1654–63, December 1990.

Kromhout, Daan; "Editorial: Fish Consumption and Sudden Cardiac Death"; *Journal of the American Medical Association* 279(1):65, January 7, 1998.

Lahnborg, G., K.-G. Hedstrom, and C.-E. Nord; "The Effect of Glucan—A Host Resistance Activator—and Ampicillin on Experimental Intra-Abdominal Sepsis"; *Journal of the Reticuloendothelial Society* 32:347-52 (1982).

Lane, Ben C.; "What Patients Eat May Affect What They See"; *Review of Optometry*, July 15, 1995.

Leibovitz, Brian; "Nutritional Treatment of Heart Disease: CCME"; *Journal of Optical Nutrition*, Vol. 3(3), 1994.

Linde, K., et al.; "St. John's Wort for Depression: An Overview and Meta-Analysis of Randomised Clinical Trials"; *British Medical Journal* 313:253–58, 1996.

Littlewood, J. T., et al.; "Red Wine as a Cause of Migraine"; *Lancet* 1 (8585):558–59, 1988.

Miyagi, Y., K. Miwa, and H. Inoue; "Inhibition of Human Low-Density Lipoprotein Oxidation by Flavonoids in Red Wine and Grape Juice"; *American Journal of Cardiology* 80(12):1627-31, December 15, 1997.

Morgan, Brian L. G.; *Nutrition Prescription*, Crown (New York), 1987.

Murray, Michael T.; *Encyclopedia of Nutritional Supplements*; Prima (Rocklin, CA), 1996.

Pi-Sunyer, F. Xavier; "Editorial: The Fattening of America"; *Journal of the American Medical Association* 272(3):238, July 20, 1994.

Plotnick, G. D., M. C. Corrett, and R.A. Voge; "The Effect of Antioxidant Vitamins in the Transient Impairment of Endothelium-Dependent Brachial Artery Vasoactivity Following a Single High-Fat Meal"; *JAMA* 278:1682–86, 1997.

Privitera, James; "Studies Reveal Surprising Diet/Hearing Connection"; *Journal of Longevity*, July 1998.

Pullman-Mooar, S., et al.; "Alteration of the Cellular Fatty Acid Profile and the Production of Eicosanoids in Human Monocytes by Gamma-Linolenic Acid"; *Arthritis and Rheumatism* 33(10):1526–33, 1990.

Raloff, Janet; "Soya-nara, Heart Disease"; *Science News* 153:348, May 30, 1998.

Recer, Paul; "U.S. Weight Problem Takes on New Proportions"; Associated Press, May 29, 1998.

Rimm, Eric B., et al.; "Vegetable, Fruit, and Cereal Fiber Intake and Risk for Coronary Heart Disease Among Men"; *Journal of the American Medical Association* 275(6):447, February 14, 1996.

Robinson, E. E., S. R. Maxwell, and G. H. Thorpe; "An Investigation of the Antioxidant Activity of Black Tea Using Enhanced Chemiluminescence"; *Free Radical Research* 26(3):291–302, March 1997.

Salaman, Maureen Kennedy; "The Prevention of Cancer Through Diet"; *Total Health*, October 1996.

Sardi, Bill; "Soy for Sight"; *Brandywine Valley Weekly*, November 28, 1997.

Sears, Barry; *Mastering the Zone*; HarperCollins (New York), 1997.

Sherwin, Robert, and Thomas R. Price; "Fat Chance: Diet and Ischemic Stroke";

editorial, *Journal of the American Medical Association* 278(24):2185, December 24/31, 1997.

Simopoulos, Artemis P.; "Preventing Illness with Fish or Fish Oil"; *Bottom Line/ Health*, April 1998.

Simopoulos, Artemis P., and Jo Robinson; *The Omega Plan*, HarperCollins (New York), 1998.

Somer, Elizabeth; *The Essential Guide to Vitamins and Minerals*, Harper Perennial (New York), 1992.

Sun, Y.; "Free Radicals, Antioxidant Enzymes, and Carcinogenesis"; *Free Radic. Biol. Med.* 8(6):583–599, 1990.

Tabbara, Khalid F.; "Nutritional Blindness: Vitamin A Deficiency." In *Prevention of Eye Disease* (ed. M. H. Friedlaender), Mary Ann Liebert, Publishers (New York), 1988.

Talorico, Patricia; "Fruit for All Seasons"; *The News Journal* (Wilmington, DE), January 28, 1998.

Taylor, Allen, Paul F. Jacques, and Esther M. Epstein; "Relations Among Aging, Antioxidant Status, and Cataract"; *American Journal of Clinical Nutrition* 62(supppl):1439S–47S, 1995.

Wald, George; *Science*, 101:653; 1945.

Walzer, Matthew et al.; "The Allergic Reaction in the Gallbladder"; *Gastroenterology* 1:565-72, 1943.

Wantke, F., M. Gotz, and R. Jarisch; "The Red Wine Provocation Test: Intolerance to Histamine as a Model for Food Intolerance"; *Allergy Proceedings* 15(1):27–32, 1994.

Waterhouse, A., et al.; "Inhibition of Human LDL Oxidation by Resveratrol"; *The Lancet* 341:1103–4, 1993.

Wright, Jonathan V., "Your Nutritionally Oriented Physical Examination"; *Nutrition & Healing*, April 1998.

60 Minutes; "The French Paradox"; November 5, 1995.

American Institute for Cancer Research Newsletter; "More Than a Hill of Beans: Soy Research Takes Off"; Issue 49, Fall 1995.

Mayo Clinic Health Letter 10(7):1; "Fruits and Vegetables"; July 1992.

Medical Tribune; "Glutathione May Hold Key to HIV Survival"; March 20, 1997.

New England Journal of Medicine, November 20, 1997.

The Nutrition Reporter; "Alpha-Lipoic Acid May Be of Particular Benefit in Stroke, Other Brain Disorders"; February 1997.

Science News 149:20; "Myrrh: An Ancient Salve Dampens Pain."

Chapter 15

Associated Press; "Experts: Drug May Replace Estrogen"; May 13, 1998.

———. "As a Medicine, Garlic Gets a Big "Phew"; June 17, 1998.

Atkins, Robert C.; *Dr. Atkins' New Diet Revolution*; M. Evans (New York), 1998.

Awasthi, S., et al.; "Curcumin Protects Against 4-Hydroxy-2-trans-Nonenal-

Induced Cataract Formation in Rat Lenses"; *American Journal of Clinical Nutrition* 64(5):761–66, 1996.

Black, M. R., et al.; "Zinc Supplements and Serum Lipids in Young Adult White Males"; *American Journal of Clinical Nutrition* 47(6):970–75, 1988.

Blumenthal, Mark; "Focus on Rainforest Remedies"; *Journal of Well-Being*, March-April 1995.

Brody, Jane E.; "Adding Cumin to the Curry: A Matter of Life and Death"; *New York Times*, March 5, 1998.

———. "Behind the Hoopla Over a Hormone: DHEA"; *New York Times*, February 3, 1998.

———. "Experimental Evidence Is Lacking for Melatonin as Cure-All"; *New York Times*, September 27, 1995.

———. "Reasons for Garlic's Benefits are Uncovered"; *New York Times*, July 27, 1994.

Chandra, R. K.; "Effect of Vitamin and Trace Element Supplementation on Immune Responses and Infection in Elderly Subjects"; *Lancet* 340:1124–27, 1992.

Cheng, Vicki; "328 Useful Drugs Are Said to Lie Hidden in Tropical Forests"; *New York Times*, June 27, 1995.

Coleman, A. L., et al.; "Topical Timolol Decreases Plasma High-Density Lipoprotein Cholesterol Level"; *Archives of Ophthalmology* 108:1260–63, 1990.

Collins, Richard; "The Cooking Cardiologist"; *GreatLife*, January 1998.

Croom, Edward M., and Larry Walker; "Botanicals in the Pharmacy: New Life for Old Remedies"; *Drug Topics*, November 6, 1995.

Cruickshanks, K. J., R. Klein, and B. E. Klein; "Sunlight and Age-Related Macular Degeneration: The Beaver Dam Eye Study"; *Archives of Ophthalmology* 111:514–18, 1993.

Day, Kathleen; "Rain Forest Remedies"; *Washington Post*, September 19, 1995.

Duke, James; "The Botanical Alternative"; *HerbalGram* 28:48, 1993.

———. *The Green Pharmacy*; Rodale Press (Emmaus, PA), 1997.

Erasmus, Udo; *Fats That Heal Fats That Kill*; Alive Books (Vancouver, Canada), 1993. Available by mail order from Flora (1-800-498-3610).

Farnsworth, Norman R.; "Relative Safety of Herbal Medicines"; *HerbalGram* 29, 1993.

Fraley, Ellingwood; *American Materia Medica, Therapeutics and Pharmacognosy*; Eclectic Medical Publication (Sandy, OR), 1919 (reissued 1998).

Goldberg, J., et al.; "Factors Associated with Age-Related Macular Degeneration: An Analysis of Data from the First National Health and Nutrition Examination Survey"; *American Journal of Epidemiology* 128(4):700–710, 1988.

Gordon, Dafna W., et al.; "Chaparral Ingestion: The Broadening Spectrum of Liver Injury Caused by Herbal Medications"; *Journal of the American Medical Association* 273(6):489, 1995.

Gregor, Alison; "Ethnobotanist Preserves Healing Tradition"; *Jackson Hole News*, February 22, 1995.

Haas, Elson M.; *The Detox Diet*; Celestial Arts (Berkeley, CA), 1996.

————. *Staying Healthy With Nutrition*; Celestial Arts (Berkeley, CA), 1992.

Harkinson, S. E., et al.; "Nutrient Intake and Cataract Extraction in Women: A Prospective Study"; *British Medical Journal* 305:335–39, 1992.

Hendler, Sheldon Saul; *The Doctors' Vitamin and Mineral Encyclopedia*; Simon & Schuster (New York), 1990.

Heusel, Catherine; "Herb-Drug Risks Cited"; *Newsday*, May 5, 1998.

Keuneke, Robin; *Total Breast Health*, Kensington (New York), 1998.

Khalsa, Karta Purkh Singh; "Heart-Warming Herbs"; *Let's Live*, December 1997.

Kilham, Chris; "Kava, the Tranquil Plant"; *Total Health* 20(2):22.

Klein, Ronald, Barbara E. K. Klein, and Susan C. Jensen; "The Relation of Cardiovascular Disease and Its Risk Factors to the 5-year Incidence of Age-Related Maculopathy: The Beaver Dam Eye Study"; *Ophthalmology* 104:1804–12, 1997.

Kuczynski, Alex; "DHEA: Anti-Aging Potion or Poison?"; *New York Times*, April 12, 1998.

Langer, Stephen; "Garlic: The New Cancer-Fighting Candidate"; *Better Nutrition*, June 1991.

Liles, M. R., D. A. Newson, and P. D. Oliver; "Antioxidant Enzymes in the Aging Human Retinal Pigment Epithelium"; *Archives of Ophthalmology* 109:1285–88, 1991.

Morales, A. J., J. J. Nolan, J. C. Nelson, and S. S. Yen; "Effects of Replacement Dose of Dehydroepiandrosterone in Men and Women of Advancing Age"; *Journal of Clinical Endocrinological Metabolism* 78:1360–67, 1994.

Morgan, Brian L. G.; *Nutrition Prescription*, Crown (New York), 1987.

Murray, Michael T.; *Encyclopedia of Nutritional Supplements*; Prima (Rocklin, CA), 1996.

Newsome, D. A., et al.; "Oral Zinc in Macular Degeneraation"; *Archives of Ophthalmology* 106:192–98, 1988.

Packer, Mark, and James D. Brandt; "Ophthalmology's Botanical Heritage"; *Survey of Ophthalmology* 36(5), March/April 1992.

Reader, August L. III; "What to Tell Patients About Nutritional Supplements"; *Review of Ophthalmology*, August 1998.

Robertson, J. M.; "A Possible Role for Vitamins C and E in Cataract Prevention"; *American Journal of Clinical Nutrition* 53:346, 1991.

Roeback, J. R., et al.; "Effects of Chromium Supplementation on Serum High-Density Lipoprotein Cholesterol Levels in Men Taking Beta-B Blockers"; *Annals of Internal Medicine* 115(12):917–24, 1991.

dos Santos, Father Joao; "Ethiopia Oriental"; in *Records of South-Eastern Africa*, printed in the Dominican convent at Evora in 1609. Also in *General Collection of the Best and Most Interesting Voyages and Travels in All Parts of the World*, 1808, London.

Simopoulos, Artemis P., and Jo Robinson; *The Omega Plan*, HarperCollins (New York), 1998.

Somer, Elizabeth; *The Essential Guide to Vitamins and Minerals*, Harper Perennial (New York), 1992.

Schulick, Paul; *Ginger, Common Spice and Wonder Drug*, Herbal Free Press Ltd., 1994.

Tabbara, Khalid F.; "Nutritional Blindness: Vitamin A Deficiency." In *Prevention of Eye Disease* (ed., M. H. Friedlaender), Mary Ann Liebert, Publishers (New York), 1988.

Tribelli, Angela; "St. John's Wort, the Downtown Herb du Jour"; *New York Times*, December 14, 1997.

West, S. K.; "Exposure to Sunlight and Other Risk Factors for Age-Related Macular Degeneration"; *Archives of Ophthalmology* 107:875–79, 1989.

Wolf, Robert V.; "A Cut Above: Kinder Surgery"; *Vegetarian Times*, September 1997.

Wright, Jonathan V.; *Nutrition and Healing*, Publisher's Management Corp. (Phoenix, AZ), June 1998.

Consumer Reports; "Herbal Roulette"; November 1995.

GreatLife; "Nutrition News: Nut News is Good News"; January 1998.

Harvard Men's Health Watch; "The DHEA Express"; July 1997.

Chapter 16

Brody, Jane E.; "Aches and Pains of a Joyous Season"; *New York Times*, December 23, 1997.

Cohen, Kenneth; *The Way of Qi Gong*; Ballantine Books (New York), 1997.

de Lateur, Barbara de Lateur;"Application of Exercise to Fat Reduction"; *Physical Medicine and Rehabilitation Clinics of North America*, Vol. 5, No. 2, May 1994.

Hakim, Amy A., Helen Petrovitch, Cecil M. Burchfield, et al.; "Effects of Walking on Mortality Among Nonsmoking Retired Men"; *New England Journal of Medicine* 338:94–99, 1998.

Lee, Martin, Emily Lee, and Jo Ann Johnstone; *Ride the Tiger to the Mountain: Tai Chi for Health*; Stanford University Press (Stanford, CA).

Liang, Master T. T.; *T'ai Chi Chu'an for Health and Self-Defense*; Vintage (New York), 1977.

Silva Mehta, Mira Mehta, and Shayam Mehta; *Yoga The Iyengar Way*; Alfred Knopf (New York), 1996.

Soulsman, Gary; "Middle Age Mixes Its Blessings"; *The News Journal* (Wilmington, DE), November 1997.

Health & Wellness Report; "Yoga: Stretching Your Mind and Body"; ed., Catherine Tishkoff; published by Oxford Medicare Advantage (New York), July/August 1997.

Chapter 17

Cho, Z. H., et al.; "New Findings of the Correlation Between Acupoints and Corresponding Brain Cortices Using Functional MRI"; *Proceedings of the National Academy of Sciences USA* 95(5):2670–73, March 3, 1998.

Ketham, Katherine, and Jason Elias; *The Five Elements of Self-Healing*; Harmony Books (New York), 1998.

Kolata, Gina; "A Child's Paper Poses a Medical Challenge"; *New York Times*, April 1, 1998.

Lubec, Walter; *The Complete Reiki Handbook*; Lotus Life Publications (Twin-lakes, WI), 1994.

Stein, Diane; *Essential Reiki: A Complete Guide to an Ancient Healing Art*; Crossing Press (Freedom, CA), 1995.

Underwood, Anne; "The Magic of Touch"; *Newsweek*, April 6, 1998.

Chapter 18

Altman, Lawrence K.; "More Orgasms, More Years of Life?"; *New York Times*, December 23, 1997.

Associated Press; "Doctors Lead in Hormone Therapy"; *New York Times*, December 23, 1997.

———. "NIH Scientific Panel Weighs Cancer Risk Posed by Power Lines"; *Wall Street Journal*, June 25, 1998.

———. "Misuse of Prescription Drugs Harming Older Americans"; *Wall Street Journal*, June 25, 1998.

Bjorneboe, G. E., et al.; "Diminished Serum Concentration of Vitamin E in Alcoholics"; *Ann. Nutr. Metab.* 32(2):56–61, 1988.

Brody, Jane E.; "A Cold Fact: High Stress Can Make You Sick"; *New York Times*, May 12, 1998.

Christen, W. G., et al.; "A Prospective Study of Cigarette Smoking and Risk of Cataract in Men"; *Journal of the American Medical Association* 268(8):989–93, 1992.

Dossey, Larry; *Healing Words: The Power of Prayer and the Practice of Medicine*; HarperCollins (New York), 1997.

Fiering, Alice; "Waters of Life"; *New Age*, March/April 1998.

Hampton, Aubrey; *Natural Organic Hair and Skin Care*; Organic Press (Tampa, FL), 1987.

Harkinson, S. E., et al.; "A Prospective Study of Cigarette Smoking and Risk of Cataract in Women"; *Journal of the American Medical Association* 268(8):994–98, 1992.

Harman, D.; "Nutritional Implications of the Free-Radical Theory of Aging"; *Journal of the American College of Nutrition* 1(1):27–34, 1982.

Harris, Kathryn; "Don't Just Accept Depression"; *The News Journal* (Wilmington, DE), July 6, 1998.

Howard, George, et al.; "Cigarette Smoking and Progression of Atherosclerosis"; *Journal of the American Medical Association* 279(2):157, January 14,1998.

Keenan, J.; "The Japanese Tea Ceremony and Stress Management"; *Holistic Nursing Practice* 10(2):30–37, January 1996.

Ketham, Katherine, and Jason Elias; *The Five Elements of Self-Healing*; Harmony Books (New York), 1998.

Kolata, Gina; "Study of Brains Alters the View on Path of Multiple Sclerosis"; *New York Times*, January 29, 1998.

Lamberg, Lynne; "New Manual Tells A to ZZZs of Sleep Diagnosis"; *Journal of the American Medical Association* 279(3):187, January 21, 1998.

Martin, Dale; "UCSF/Mount Zion Researchers Find Correlation Between Stress and Disease Activity in Multiple Sclerosis"; *BW HealthWire*, March 26, 1998.

Matthews, Dale; *The Faith Factor: Proof of the Healing Power of Prayer*; Viking (New York), 1998.

Mills, Dixie; "Since Columbus, Smokers Knew Tobacco's Risk, Witness Testifies"; *The News Journal* (Wilmington, DE), March 25, 1998.

Nowell, Peter D., et al.; "Benzodiazepines and Zolpidem for Chronic Insomnia"; *Journal of the American Medical Association* 278(24):2170–77, December 24/31, 1997.

Ornish, Dean; *Love and Survival: The Scientific Basis for the Healing Power of Intimacy*; HarperCollins (New York), 1998.

Robinson, Mike; "Illinois Deli's Potato Salad May Have Sickened 4,500"; *The News Journal* (Wilmington, DE), June 24, 1998.

Ruhl, R. A., C. Chang, G. M. Halpern, and M. E. Gershwin; "The Sick Building Syndrome: Assessment and Regulation of Indoor Air Quality"; *Journal of Asthma* 30(4):297–308, 1993.

Russell, R. M.; "New Views on the RDAs for Older Adults"; *J. Am. Diat. Assoc.* (97):515–518, 1997.

Scerral, Chet; "Researchers Work to Unravel Cortisol Link to Disease"; *Ophthalmology Times*, March 15, 1998.

Solberg, Y., et al., "The Association Between Cigarette Smoking and Ocular Diseases"; *Survey of Ophthalmology* 42(6):535–47, 1998.

Talen, Jamie; "Study: Smoking Worsens Seniors' Mental Functions"; *Newsday*, April 30, 1998.

Weil, Andrew, M.D.; *Spontaneous Healing*; Fawcett Columbine (New York), 1995.

Werner, Rachel M., and Thomas A. Pearson; "Editorial: What's So Passive About Passive Smoking?"; *Journal of the American Medical Association* 279(2):157, January 14, 1998.

Wolverton, William; *How to Grow Clean Air: 50 Houseplants That Purify Your Home or Office*, Penguin Books (New York), 1998.

Zommers, Ingrid; "Is Your Home Making You Sick?"; *Natural Living Today*, September/October 1997.

Energy Times; "Environmental Estrogens"; January 1998.
New York Times, February 11, 1994.
The Sciences; "Fried Couch Potatoes"; March/April 1998.

Chapter 19

Johnson, J. F.; "Considerations in Prescribing for the Older Patient"; *Clinical Pharmacy Review* Vol. 8, No. 1, 1998 (published by PCS Health Systems Inc., a subsidiary of Eli Lilly and Co.).

Fraunfelder, F. T.; *Drug-Induced Ocular Side Effects*, 4th Ed., Williams & Wilkins (Baltimore), 1996.

Heusel, Catherine; "Herb-Drug Risks Cited"; *Newsday*, May 5, 1998.

Magnan, June; "Some Drugs That Can Interact with Foods"; *MMC Bulletin*, January 1998.

Mark, S. D., W. Wang, and J. S. Fraumeni Jr.; "Do Nutritional Supplements Lower the Risk of Stroke or Hypertension?"; *Epidemiology* 9:9–15, 1998.

Moore, Thomas J.; *Prescription for Disaster: The Hidden Dangers in Your Medicine Cabinet*; Simon & Schuster (New York), 1998.

Pelton, R. O.; *Drug Induced Nutrient Depletion Handbook*, 2nd Ed.; Lexi-Comp Inc., 2001.

Safran, A.B., et al.; "Topical Timolol Maleate Might Adversely Affect Serum Lipoproteins"; *International Ophthalmology* 17:109–110, 1993.

Vargas, E., et al.; "Effect of Adverse Drug Reactions on Length of Stay in Intensive Care Units"; *Clinical Drug Invest.* 15(4):353–60, 1998.

Clinical Drug Investigations 14(3):243, September 1997.

New York Times; "Doctors Lead in Hormone Therapy"; Associated Press, December 23, 1997.

Chapter 20

Abelson, Reed; "A Medical Resistance Movement"; *New York Times*, March 24, 1998.

Gerber, Suzanne; "New Medicine Man"; *Vegetarian Times*, February 1998.

Gilbert, Susan; "Forget About Bedside Manners, Some Doctors Have No Manners"; *New York Times*, December 23, 1997.

Goodman, Ellen; "Patients' Rights and Wrongs: HMO Anxiety Is Worse Than Anti-Regulation Fever"; *The News Journal* (Wilmington, DE), December 16, 1997.

Kilbourn, Peter T.; "Looking Back at Jackson Hole"; *New York Times*, March 22, 1998.

Marion, Matt; "Full Body Tune-Up"; *Men's Health*, May 1, 1998.

NIH Office of Alternative Medicine Clearinghouse; "Frequently Asked Questions"; March 1997.

Chapter 23

Abel, R., Jr.; *The DHA Story: How Life's Supernutrient Can Save Your Life,* Basic Health Publications (North Bergen, NJ), 2002.

AREDS Investigators; "A Randomized Placebo-Controlled Clinical Trial of High Dose Supplementation with Vitamins C and E, Beta-Carotene and Zinc for Age-Related Macular Degeneration and Vision Loss"; *Archives of Ophthalmology* 119:1417–36, 2001.

AREDS Research Group; "Risk Factors Associated with Age-Related Macular Degeneration"; *Ophthalmology* 107:2224–32, 2000.

Babizhayer, M. A., et al.; *Peptides* N-acetyl carnosine, a natural histadine-containing dipeptide, as a potent ophthalmic drug in treatment of human cataract 22:979–94, 2001.

Bechmann, M., M. J. Thiel, B. Roesen, et al.; "Central Corneal Thickness Determined with Optical Coherence Tomography in Various Types of Glaucoma"; *British Journal of Ophthamology* 84: 1233–37, 2000.

Begley, S.; "Science Journal: Marketplace"; *Wall Street Journal,* August 23, 2002.

Bendich, A., and L. Langseth; "Safety of Vitamin A"; *American Journal of Clinical Nutrition* 49:358–71, 1989.

Bernstein, P. S., N. A. Balashov, E. D. Tsong, R. K. Rando, et al.; "Retinal Tubulin Binds Macular Carotenoids"; *Invest Ophthalmology Visual Science* 38:167–75.

Boer, D., M. Maiello, and M. Lorenzo; "Increased Presence of Microthrombosis in Retinal Capillaries of Diabetic Individuals"; *Diabetes* 50:1432–39, 2001.

Bohmer, H. A., B. Selhaus, and N. F. Schroge; "Effects of Ascorbic Acid on Retinal Pigment Epithelial Cells"; *Current Eye Research* 23:206–14, 2001.

Bone, R. A., J. T. Landrum, S. T. Mayne, et al.; "Macular Pigment in Donor Eyes With and Without AMD"; *Investigative Ophthalmology and Visual Science* 42:235–40, 2001.

Brody, J. E.; "Diabetes Candidates Can Reduce the Risk"; *New York Times,* Health Section, January 15, 2002.

Christian, P., S. K. Khatry, S. Yamini, et al.; "Zinc Supplementation Might Potentiate the Vitamin A in Restoring Night Vision in Pregnant Nepalese Women"; *American Journal of Clinical Nutrition* 73:1045–51, 2001.

Chung, H. S., J. Harris, J. K. Christiansson, et al.; "Ginkgo Biloba Extract Increases Ocular Blood Flow Velocity"; *Ocular Pharmacologic Therapy* 15:233–40, 1999.

Coleman, M. D., et al.; *Environmental Toxicology Pharmacology* 10:167–72, 2001.

Cruickshank, K. J., R. Klein, B. E. Klein, et al.; "Sunlight and the 5-Year Incidence of Early Age-Related Maculopathy"; *Archives of Ophthalmology* 119:246–50, 2001.

Frank, R. N.; "Potential New Therapies for Diabetic Retinopathy: Protein Kinase C Inhibitors"; *American Journal of Ophthalmology* 133:693–98, 2002.

Freeman, E. E., B. Munoz, O. Schein, et al.; "Hormone Replacement Therapy and Lens Opacities"; Salisbury Eye Evaluation Project; *Archives of Ophthalmology* 119:1687–92, 2001.

Gale, C. R., N. F. Hall, D. I. Phillips, et al.; "Plasma Antioxidant Vitamins and Carotenoids and Age-Related Cataract"; *Ophthamology* 108:1992–98, 2001.

Goldberg, D., A. Gitomer, and R. Abel, Jr.; *The Best Supplements for Your Helath*, Kensington (New York), 2002.

Gottfredsdottir, M. S., R. R. Allingham, M. B. Shields, et al.; "Physician Guide to Interaction Between Glaucoma and Systemic Medication"; *Journal of Glaucoma* 6:377–83, 1997.

Heuberger, R. A., J. A. Mares-Perlman, R. Klein, et al.; "The Relationship of Dietary Fat to Age-Related Maculopathy in the Third National Health and Nutritional Examination Survey"; *Archives of Ophthalmology* 119:1833–38, 2001.

Iezzi, R.; "New Advances in Artificial Vision"; *Review of Ophthalmology*, August 2002, pp. 64–66.

Jacobs, L. D., et al.; "Intramuscular Interferon Beta-1A Therapy Initiated During the First Demyelinating Event in Multiple Sclerosis"; *New England Journal of Medicine* 343:898, 2000.

Jacques, P. F., L. T. Chylack, Jr., S. E. Hankinson, et al.; "Long-Term Nutrient Intake and Early Age-Related Nuclear Lens Opacities"; *Archives of Ophthalmology* 119:1009–19, 2001.

Kaufman, D. W., J. P. Kelly, L. Rosenberg, et al.; "Recent Patterns of Medication Use in the Ambulatory Adult Population of the United States"; *Journal of the American Medical Association* 287:337–44, 2002.

Khaw, K. T., S. Bingham, E. Welch, et al.; "Relation Between Plasma Ascorbic Acid and Mortality in Men and Women in EPIC-Norfolk Perspective Study"; *Lancet* 357:657–63, 2001.

Knight, J. A.; "The Biochemistry of Aging"; *Advances in Clinical Chemistry* 35:1–62, 2000.

Kountouras, J., N. Mylopoulos, D. Chatzopoulos, et al.; "Eradication of Heliobacter Pylori May Be Beneficial in the Management of Chronic Open-Angle Glaucoma"; *Archives of Internal Medicine* 162:1237–44, 2002.

Kuzniarz, M., P. Mitchell, R. G. Cumming, et al.; "Use of Vitamin Supplements and Cataract: The Blue Mountains Eye Study"; *American Journal of Ophthalmology* 132:19–26, 2001.

Lal, B., A. K. Kapoor, O. P. Asthana, et al.; "Efficacy of Curcumin in the Management of Chronic Anterior Uveitis"; *Phytotherapy Research* 13:318–22, 1999.

Lee, J. B., C. H. Ryu, J. Kim, et al.; "Comparison of Tear Secretion and Tear Film Instability After Photorefractive Keratectomy and LASIK"; *Journal of Cataract and Refractive Surgery* 26:1326–31, 2000.

Levy, J., E. Bosin, E. Feldman, et al.; "Lycopene Is a More Potent Inhibitor of Human Cancer Cell Proliferation Than Either Alpha or Beta Carotene"; *Nutrition and Cancer* 24:257–66, 1995.

Linkenhuker, B., and E. Knudson; "Incremental Training Increases the Plasticity of the Auditory Space Map in Adult Barn Owls"; *Nature* 419:293–96, 2002.

Mares-Perlman, J. A., B. J. Lyle, R. Klein, et al.; "Vitamin Supplement Use and Incident Cataracts in a Population-Based Study"; *Archives of Ophthalmology* 118:1556–63, 2000.

McCarthy, C. A., B. N. Mukesh, C. L. Fu, et al.; "Risk Factors for Age-Related Maculopathy"; *Archives of Ophthalmology* 119:1455–62, 2001.

Owsley, C., G. McGwin, Jr., M. Sloane, et al.; "Impact of Cataract Surgery on Motor Vehicle Crash Involvement by Older Adults"; *Journal of the American Medical Association* 288:841–49, 2002.

Parthsarathy, H.; "Neurobiology, Plasticity and the Older Owl"; *Nature* 419:258–59, 2002.

Pavlidis, I., N. L. Eberhardt, and J. A. Levine; "Seeing Through the Face of Deception"; *Nature* 415:38, 2002.

Pediatric Eye Disease Investigative Group; "A Randomized Trial of Atrophine Versus Patching for Treatment of Moderate Amblyopia in Children"; *Archives of Ophthalmology* 120:268–78, 2002.

Rezaie, T., A. Child, R. Hitchings, et al.; "Adult Onset Primary Open-Angle Glaucoma Caused by Mutation in Optineurin"; *Science* 295:1077–79, 2002.

Schaumberg, D. A., J. E. Buring, D. A. Sullivan, et al.; "Hormone Replacement Therapy and Dry Eye Syndrome"; *Journal of the American Medical Association* 286:2114–19, 2001.

Schaumberg, D. A., R. J. Glynn, W. G. Christen, et al.; "Relations of Body Fat Distribution and Height with Cataract in Men"; *American Journal of Clinical Nutrition* 72:1495–502, 2000.

Seddon, J. M., et al.; "Dietary Carotenoids, Vitamins A, C, and E, and Advanced Age-Related Macular Degeneration"; *Journal of the American Medical Association* 272:1413, 1994.

Seddon, J. M., B. Rosner, and R. D. Sperduto; "Dietary Fat and Risk for Advanced Age-Related Macular Degeneration"; *Archives of Ophthalmology* 119:1191–99, 2001.

Smith, W., P. Mitchell, and S. R. Leeder; "Dietary Fat and Fish Intake and Age-Related Maculopathy"; *Archives of Ophthalmology* 118:401–4, 2000.

Solomon, P. R., F. Adams, A. Silver, et al.; "Ginkgo for Memory Enhancement"; *Journal of the American Medical Association* 288:835–40, 2002.

Sweeney, A. D., and J. Bennet; "Cracking the Code of Retinal Disease"; *Review of Ophthalmology*, 9:58–64, 2002.

TAP Study Group; "Photodynamic Therapy of Subfoveal Choroidal Neovascularization in Age-Related Macular Degeneration with Verteporfin"; *Archives of Ophthalmology* 119:198–207, 2001.

Taylor, A., P. F. Jacques, I. T. Chylack, Jr., et al.; "Long-Term Intake of Vitamins and Carotenoids and Odds of Early Age-Related Cortical and Posterior Subcapsular Lens Opacities"; *American Journal of Ophthalmology* 75:540–49, 2002.

Tillotson, A. K.; Trifola and glaucoma; personal comunication.

Trubo, R.; "Guidelines Clarify Migraine Treatment"; *Eyenet*, April 2001, pp. 29–30.

Wang, J. S., P. Mitchell, J. M. Simpson, et al.; "Visual Impairments, Age-Related Cataract, and Mortality"; *Archives of Ophthalmology* 119:1186–90, 2001.

Wax, M. B.; "Emergency Perspectives in Glaucoma: Optimizing 24-Hour Control of Intraocular Pressure"; *American Journal of Ophthalmology* 133:S1–S10, 2002.

About the Author

Dr. Robert Abel, Jr., is a graduate of Wesleyan University and Jefferson Medical College. He performed his ophthalmology training at Mount Sinai Hospital in New York City and a cornea transplant fellowship at the University of Florida. Dr. Abel cofounded the alternative medicine curriculum at Thomas Jefferson University, where he was a clinical professor of ophthalmology. He has helped found eye banks, holds patents on artificial corneas, and has developed a nutritional supplement for the eyes. Dr. Abel has long been a nationally renowned teacher of conventional eye therapy and is the recipient of the senior honor award from the American Academy of Ophthalmology. He assisted with the translations of ancient Ayurvedic eye therapies and coauthored *The One Earth Herbal Sourcebook* and *The Best Supplements for Your Health*. He has also written *The DHA Story*. His mission is to bring mind-body medicine to twenty-first-century eye care. Dr. Abel is also a practitioner of Tai Chi Ch'uan and lives in Wilmington, Delaware, with his wife.

Index